Challe
in Pediatric
Diagnosis

FROM "INDEX OF SUSPICION"
A Section of *Pediatrics in Review*

Edited by Lawrence F. Nazarian, MD, FAAP

American Academy of Pediatrics
141 Northwest Point Boulevard, PO Box 927
Elk Grove Village, Illinois 60009-0927

Library of Congress Catalog No.: 99-76725
ISBN: 1-58110-049-3
MA0151

Quantity prices on request. Address all inquiries to:
American Academy of Pediatrics
141 Northwest Point Boulevard, PO Box 927
Elk Grove Village, Illinois 60009-0927

The recommendations in this publication do not indicate an exclusive course of treatment or serve as a standard of medical care. Variations, taking into account individual circumstances, may be appropriate.

Introduction

Clinicians learn best by caring for patients. The practitioner who is asked about rheumatic fever will recall those patients he or she has known who had rheumatic fever. Knowledge of medicine is linked with clinical experience. This principle forms the rationale for creating "Index of Suspicion."

The first issue of *Pediatrics in Review* was published in 1979. A new phase of the journal began in 1992, when a number of modifications were made. Among other changes was the addition of several special features that present clinically relevant material in formats different from the traditional review article. "Index of Suspicion" was the first of those new formats and has enjoyed continuing popularity with readers. By the end of the year 2000, we plan to have published 257 cases, including those presented in the annual CD-ROM issues.

Case presentations represent a time-honored element of the practice of medicine, and this teaching tool is employed by many journals in a variety of formats. "Index of Suspicion" incorporates two characteristics that contribute to its particular flavor. Most clinical experiences add small chunks of knowledge to the slowly expanding database that all practitioners acquire. We wanted "Index" cases to make a few important points, but did not design them to present an exhaustive discourse on specific disorders. When the feature was young, a reader expressed his disappointment that the presentations seemed superficial and did not offer the comprehensive immersion in a clinical situation that was provided by the case presentations of a particular prestigious journal. Our response to that reader was that our intention differed from that of the other journal. We felt that a briefer format, concentrating primarily on the diagnostic aspects of a condition and making a few selected points, would be effective for the clinician in a way that more ponderous presentations would not.

Another aspect of "Index of Suspicion" that is not found in most other journals is the standing invitation for readers to submit interesting cases they have encountered. We are able in this way to tap into the vast experience of more than 60,000 subscribers around the world and to give clinicians who might not otherwise do so the opportunity to add to the medical literature. At first, the cases were written by editorial board members, starting with particular content specifications of the American Board of Pediatrics on which both recertification examinations and the content of *Pediatrics in Review* are based. These initial cases often were composites of patients whom the authors had encountered in the past.

After those first few years, though, virtually all of the cases published have been submitted by individual readers and are based on specific patients. In fact, submissions by readers have grown to the point where we now have our "Index" slots filled 1 year in advance and still have a backup pool of fine cases. Each new case of publishable quality that is submitted goes into the pool; three are chosen each month for the journal issue scheduled 1 year from that month. We have received cases from all over the United States as well as from Canada, Guam, India, Israel, Norway, Saudi Arabia, Spain, and Sri Lanka. Authors have included practitioners, junior and senior faculty, residents, and medical students.

One characteristic of material submitted by readers is the inevitable variability in quality, both in terms of writing and of science. All cases receive some stylistic revision to make them clearer and more readable; then they are sent to specialist reviewers, primarily members of our editorial board. The comments of the reviewers are incorporated into a final revision, which is sent to the author for approval.

To compile this book, we examined the 216 cases published or scheduled for publication in the years 1992 through 1999. From these, 100 were selected for the book. The selection process admittedly was arbitrary; I will assume total responsibility for the choices. Several principles, however, were used in making the selections. When there was more than one case dealing with the same disorder, only one was picked, except in a few instances where two cases of the same condition offered significantly different perspectives. There was a bias against very unusual syndromes and toward unusual presentations of common conditions. Some cases stood out by virtue of the way they were written or because of a specific twist they offered. To all authors whose cases are not included, I can say only that their material was worth sharing, as evidenced by previous publication of their contributions in the journal, but this particular selection process favored others.

Because some of these cases were published as long ago as 1992, all were examined from the vantage point of whether they might need revision. Whenever it seemed that a diagnostic procedure or therapy mentioned in the case might be outdated, expert input was sought and, if indicated, an update note was appended to the case discussion. We did not rewrite the cases in any way; they appear as they did in the journal, except for new headings. Despite this screening process, the reader is urged to consider the possibility that all of this material—as with any element of medical education—is subject to the need for revision because new approaches constantly appear in both diagnostic and therapeutic realms.

It has taken many people with diverse talents to bring "Index of Suspicion" to life in the journal and in this book, and I would like to mention those to whom I owe deep gratitude. The American Academy of Pediatrics, especially through Drs Errol Alden and Robert Perelman, has nurtured *Pediatrics in Review* and its parent program, PREP, and has provided constant support to all of us involved in the production of these teaching tools. Equally supportive has been the superb staff of the Academy, with Kent Anderson, Angela Brooks Green, Theresa Tracy, and Michelle Adams providing much of the insight and hard work that brought this volume to publication.

Dr Robert Haggerty has guided *Pediatrics in Review* from the very beginning and is its heart and soul. He was my department chief when I was an intern and has been my mentor, role model, cheerleader, and friend ever since. Cindy Sutherland, our editorial assistant, has served as right arm for both of us.

The many authors who have shared their experiences with their colleagues deserve special praise, as do the reviewers who allow us to publish clear, accurate, useful teaching examples. Deb Kuhlman, our copy editor, has worked her special magic, in the journal and in this book, to make sure that what is printed is of the highest quality. A special measure of appreciation is due to my wife, Sharon, who has offered constant encouragement and shows infinite patience when I retreat to my home office for hours at a time to edit.

Most of all, each of must offer deep and sincere thanks to those people whose welfare and happiness are the goals of our work and who gratify and teach us constantly—our patients.

Lawrence F. Nazarian, MD
Editor

Table of Contents

Persistent Throat Infection, Despite Antibiotics

PRESENTATION

A 9-year-old girl is brought to the office having a 1-week history of bilateral neck swelling. She does not have fever, malaise, or other specific complaints. She has been diagnosed in the past as having beta thalassemia minor. Her immunizations are complete. On physical examination, she does not appear ill, and her temperature is 37.2°C (99°F) orally. Several tender lymph nodes that are approximately 1.5 cm in size are palpable on both sides of the submandibular area. There is a white-yellow exudate on her tonsils. You obtain a throat culture and initiate therapy with amoxicillin because she has refused to take penicillin V in the past due to the taste. As suspected, the culture grows group A beta-hemolytic Streptococcus.

The child returns 5 days later. Despite taking the antibiotic faithfully, she now has a sore throat and feels more tired. A red, maculapapular rash is noted on her trunk and extremities. She is still afebrile and does not look very ill.

What is your differential diagnosis at this point?
Are there any elements of history or physical examination that would help you?
What additional diagnostic studies would you like performed?

DISCUSSION

Although infectious mononucleosis (IM) is a common infection that in its typical presentation is not difficult to diagnose, this case illustrates several important points. The presence of a streptococcal throat infection does not rule out IM; it is not unusual for streptococci to cause superinfection in a throat already inflamed by a viral infection. Ampicillin and its congeners commonly induce a rash in patients who have IM, although about 5% of patients who have IM will have a maculapapular rash as part of the infection. In addition, many patients, especially younger ones, will not present in typical fashion.

Clinical Findings

IM is a viral infection caused by the Epstein-Barr virus (EBV), one of the herpesvirus group. In its complete manifestation, IM is characterized by malaise, fatigue, fever, pharyngitis with exudate, enlarged lymph nodes, splenomegaly, and hepatomegaly. Two other helpful physical findings are petechiae on the soft palate and bilateral edema of the eyelids. The infection can be mild or even asymptomatic, especially among preschool children, and the clinician may encounter a great variety of clinical manifestations.

This disease is present throughout the world. In developing countries or underprivileged communities, almost all children are EBV-seropositive by age 6 years; primary infection occurs later in developed countries. Eventually, almost all adults will evidence EBV infection, although they may not recall symptoms. The virus is transmitted through the saliva from person to person, and it can be detected in saliva as long as 6 months beyond the acute period. The incubation period is estimated to be 30 to 50 days. Other conditions that should be included in the differential diagnosis of IM are cytomegalovirus infection, toxoplasmosis, infectious hepatitis A, streptococcal pharyngitis, adenoviral infection, and rubella. It is worth emphasizing that the classic signs and symptoms do not appear in every patient, and sometimes, as in this case, we must suspect IM on the basis of selected clinical findings.

Diagnosis
Results of laboratory testing are of great help in diagnosing this disorder. Lymphocytosis is usual, with atypical lymphocytes often constituting more than 10% of the total leukocytes. Liver enzymes often are elevated to a mild or moderate degree. In this patient, the aspartate aminotransferase (AST; SGOT) was 208 IU/L and the alanine aminotransferase (ALT; SGPT) was 334 IU/L.

A complete discussion of the serology of IM is beyond the scope of this discussion, but the reader should know that the "instant" slide tests for IM employ treated horse erythrocytes and detect the presence of Paul-Bunnell heterophil antibodies, which are present in 90% of cases of EBV IM in older children and adults (but often missing in preschool-age children). Some of the tests have additional reagents for absorption of the serum, making the procedure even more specific. Paul-Bunnell heterophil antibodies, however, are in themselves considered nonspecific for IM; the most accurate diagnosis requires demonstration of specific antibodies (immunoglobulins M and G) against EBV in the serum. In most cases, testing for Paul-Bunnell antibodies is sufficient for clinical purposes. Be aware that results of rapid tests involving horse erythrocytes may remain positive for more than 1 year.

Treatment
Treatment of IM is symptomatic, and recovery may take weeks or months. Short courses of corticosteroids can be used for patients who have upper airway obstruction or severe hematologic or hepatic complications. The prognosis is excellent if there are no complications, which are infrequent but numerous. They include splenic rupture, encephalitis, Guillain-Barré syndrome, myocarditis, hemolytic anemia, aplastic anemia, and upper airway obstruction due to tonsillar hypertrophy, and mucosal edema. Syndromes of chronic fatigue have been ascribed to EBV; the relationship of such illness to the virus is still unclear. It should be noted that EBV is involved in the etiology of Burkitt lymphoma, lymphoproliferative disorders, and nasopharyngeal carcinoma.

Lesson for the Clinician
The clinician is well advised to keep in mind the broad clinical spectrum associated with infectious mononucleosis.

Juan J. Jiménez Garcia, MD, Madrid, Spain

A Sudden, Painless Inability to Walk

PRESENTATION

A 5-year-old girl is brought to the office because she has been unable to walk since awakening this morning. Last night her family returned from a 4-day summer camping trip during which she was active and healthy. Her past medical history is unremarkable, and she is fully immunized. There is no evidence of infectious, drug, or toxic exposures.

On physical examination, the child is alert and cooperative but unable to stand or walk, although she denies pain. Deep tendon reflexes cannot be elicited in her lower extremities. Her cranial nerve function is normal, as are her vital signs and the remainder of her physical examination.

What is your differential diagnosis at this point?
Are there any elements of history or physical examination that would help you?
What additional diagnostic studies would you like performed?

DISCUSSION

An engorged tick was found cloistered in the hair in the child's occipital area. Within hours of its removal, strength returned to her lower extremities, and she recovered fully by 24 hours.

Etiology

Tick paralysis is a neurologic disorder characterized by an ascending paralysis in association with the attachment of certain ticks. In North America, *Dermacentor andersoni* (the wood tick, a Rocky Mountain resident) and *Dermacentor variabilis* (the dog tick, an inhabitant of the midwest) are the primary arachnids involved in this disorder. Female ticks are implicated most often because they remain firmly attached for a longer time than male ticks, which usually drop off.

Coincident with maximal tick activity, tick paralysis is a spring and summer malady that most commonly affects infants and children. Girls are affected twice as often as boys, perhaps because the ticks find wider sanctuary in their scalps and, thus, escape notice. Other concealed areas of attachment include the ear canal, axilla, popliteal fossa, and perianal area. Dark-haired persons are said to be more susceptible, but this observation may be due to dark hair camouflaging the tick, thereby hindering detection.

Presentation

Symptoms appear after a latent period of 4 to 10 days following tick attachment and often begin with irritability, anorexia, and lethargy for 12 to 24 hours. Thereafter, ataxia and weakness occur in the lower extremities and progress rapidly until the patient no longer is able to walk. The ascending paralysis progresses so rapidly that some involvement of the upper extremities may be seen within hours of paralysis in the lower extremities.

Bulbar signs follow, with lower cranial nerves being involved initially, usually in the form of dysphagia and dysarthria. Besides weakness, the patient may experience numbness and tingling of the extremities or face. Delay in treatment after the appearance of bulbar signs may result in death from respiratory paralysis or aspiration.

Abnormal physical findings usually are confined to the obvious weakness and absent deep tendon reflexes in the lower extremities. Sensory changes rarely are noted. The engorged tick usually does not cause pain and may be mistaken for a pedunculated mole or wart.

Treatment

Removal of the tick results in reversal of paralysis and return to normal function, usually within hours; in rare cases, recovery may take weeks. The tick is extracted by strong constant traction on its body with forceps. If the patient does not recover after tick removal, further search for another tick is indicated because there may be more than one culprit. Analysis of the tick is unnecessary, so it should be discarded appropriately. However, because ticks are associated with other clinical disorders, it may be prudent in some clinical situations to save an extracted tick in a glass jar for possible examination in the future.

In contrast to other tick-borne diseases, no infectious agent has been identified in tick paralysis. Toxins present in the salivary glands of female ticks of certain species are believed to be the paralytic agents. A toxin from the Australian *Ioxedes* tick has been partially purified; parenteral injection of this agent produces paralysis in dogs within 48 hours. The action of the toxin, although poorly understood, is postulated to be production of a conduction block in the peripheral branches of motor fibers that results in acetylcholine not being liberated at the neuromuscular junction.

Laboratory tests are not helpful in establishing the diagnosis of tick paralysis.

Differential Diagnosis

The differential diagnosis of tick paralysis includes Guillain-Barré syndrome, myasthenia gravis, poliomyelitis, diphtheria, acute transverse myelitis, botulism, heavy metal poisons, and spinal cord tumors. The most common of these conditions to consider is Guillain-Barré syndrome. Elevated cerebrospinal fluid protein in the absence of pleocytosis should help to identify this neuropathy, although these abnormalities may be absent in the first several days of Guillain-Barré syndrome.

A travel history and diligent search for the tick should result in cure of this uncommon but potentially lethal condition.

Dennis J. McCarthy, MD, Butte, MT

Gross Hematuria and Bleeding Gums

PRESENTATION

An 8-year-old autistic boy is brought to the office for evaluation of gross hematuria. Four days ago he was seen for abdominal pain, had normal findings on physical examination, and was treated symptomatically. The pain persisted and he went to an emergency department, where he was found to have microscopic hematuria without pyuria; a sulfonamide was prescribed for a presumed urinary tract infection. That evening he developed gross hematuria.

His history includes multiple episodes of otitis media, hearing loss, and speech delay. He now communicates in short sentences. The only medication he is receiving is methylphenidate. There is no history of recent travel or known ingestion or any family history of coagulopathy.

On physical examination, the boy appears alert but frightened. His blood pressure is 100/58 mm Hg (110/90 mm Hg when agitated), pulse is 110 beats/min, and temperature is 37.9°C (101°F). There is dried blood in his nares and oozing of blood at his gum lines. His mother recalls a nosebleed last evening. There are healing impetiginous lesions on his legs, and he has mild periumbilical tenderness. His urine is grossly bloody. His hemoglobin is 1.83 mmol/L (11.8 g/dL), white blood cell count is 12.8 x 10^9/L (12.8 x 10^3/mcL), and platelet count is 488 x 10^9/L (488 x 10^3/mcL). No clot forms during plasma prothrombin time testing, and his partial thromboplastin time is greater than 100 sec. The fibrinogen and D-dimer (DIC) levels are normal.

His father arrives and supplies the history that leads to the diagnosis.

What is your differential diagnosis at this point?
Are there any elements of history or physical examination that would help you?
What additional diagnostic studies would you like performed?

DISCUSSION

The boy's father recalled placing a readily available brand of rat poison under the furniture several months earlier. Although the family had seen no evidence that the bait had been disturbed, ingestion of the poison was the cause of this child's illness.

Presentation

There was no history to suggest a congenital coagulopathy in this patient or his family. The prolongation of both his prothrombin time (PT) and partial thromboplastin time (PTT) suggested a more global factor deficiency rather than the most common isolated congenital deficiencies (factor VIII hemophilia and von Willebrand disease). He did not have any underlying illness that would produce disseminated intravascular coagulation; indeed, the fibrinogen and fibrinogen split products levels were normal.

The initial signs of hematuria, hypertension (albeit temporary and with some agitation), and impetigo indicated the possibility of acute streptococcal glomerulonephritis. That condition was no longer a concern once the signs of a coagulopathy became evident. An antistreptolysin O titer was negative.

Treatment

The child was treated presumptively for ingestion of a superwarfarin-like substance, specifically brodifacoum, the active ingredient in the poison. He was given 25 mg of vitamin K subcutaneously and a unit of fresh frozen plasma (FFP). His PT became 17 sec (control, 11 to 13.9 sec) and his PTT became 42.8 sec (control, 0 to 37.6 sec).

However, he subsequently developed a shock-like state, with pallor, decreased strength of his radial pulse, and lethargy. His hemoglobin concentration diminished from 1.83 mmol/L (11.8 g/dL) to 1.27 mmol/L (8.2 g/dL) and his hematocrit from 0.36 (36%) to 0.264 (26.4%), presumably due to the gross hematuria. Two units of packed red blood cells and two additional units of FFP were administered in response to the blood loss and shock, and he improved. His gross hematuria and abdominal pain resolved rapidly, and his peripheral perfusion and activity level normalized. At this point, the PT and PTT were prolonged only mildly, and he was begun on oral vitamin K at 25 mg twice a day. His PTT normalized after a fourth unit of FFP and an increase of the vitamin K to 25 mg three times a day.

Laboratory studies confirmed the ingestion. There was suppression of clotting factors II, VII, IX, and X, all of which were less than 20% of normal, and the brodifacoum level was 120 ng/mL. The child was weaned gradually from the vitamin K over the next 8 months. His PT and PTT have remained normal, and he has had no more episodes of unusual bleeding.

Etiology

The coumarin anticoagulants (warfarin and dicumarol) impair carboxylation of the vitamin K-dependent factors, which are prothrombin (factor II) and factors VII, IX, and X. The coumarin nucleus is chemically similar to vitamin K, and both interact at a common receptor site. It is the carboxylated factor residues that bind calcium and orient the clotting factors, thus permitting the generation of thrombin. The drugs known as superwarfarins are used in many commercial rat baits and are more potent and persistent anticoagulants than warfarin. Brodifacoum, a 4-hydroxy-coumarin derivative, was the active ingredient in the rat poison ingested by this child.

Because these compounds are so potent, the amount of poison that a child must ingest to cause a coagulopathy is not substantial. It is estimated that a child weighing 10 kg must eat a mouthful (about one third of a box of the bait) to affect coagulation. This patient weighed 36 kg, but might have eaten a larger amount because of his size and developmental status.

Clinical Manifestations

The clinical manifestations of hemorrhage include epistaxis, bleeding gums, hematuria, and abdominal pain, as in this patient, as well as hemoptysis, gastrointestinal bleeding, and bruising. Intracranial hemorrhage is the most common complication that has long-term consequences. It is of interest that this child was referred initially to a urologist because of his hematuria before it was determined that his bleeding was due to a bleeding disorder. As an additional complication, his renal bleeding caused clots in his urinary collecting system, leading to intermittent hydronephrosis.

Management

Management of warfarin ingestion depends on the seriousness of the bleeding. The superwarfarins can be expected to have more profound and prolonged effects. In the absence of significant bleeding, the child is removed from the source of the anticoagulant and coagulation times are monitored. PT and PTT should be obtained immediately. The PT will be prolonged within 24 hours of ingestion and maximally prolonged in 36 to 72 hours. Factor assays II, VII, IX, and X may be abnormal in patients who have normal PT and PTT, and those circumstances warrant treatment with vitamin K.

Plasma is given to patients who have massive hemorrhage and prolonged PT. (Although whole blood will supply both erythrocytes and vitamin K-dependent factors, it rarely is available.) FFP can be used to raise the levels of vitamin K-dependent factors to hemostatic levels (above 30% to 40% of normal), and 15 mL/kg is a reasonable initial pediatric dose. Vitamin K should be administered as well; in warfarin ingestions, it will correct factor VII levels in several hours and normalize hemostasis within 1 to 2 days. When administered intravenously, vitamin K has resulted in rare severe anaphylactic-like reactions. Subcutaneous administration lessens the risks while still producing a rapid response.

Oral vitamin K treatment may need to be tapered over several months to 1 year in superwarfarin ingestions because of the prolonged effect of these agents. Early discontinuation of vitamin K can result in recurrence of the coagulopathy and the risk of serious bleeding complications, such as intracranial bleeding. Inadequate dosing, noncompliance with therapy, or reingestion will be detected by careful monitoring of the PT.

Fatalities and irreversible neurologic deficits can follow ingestion of household rodent poison. Specific questions about rat bait should be asked when managing a child who has a coagulopathy consistent with warfarin overdose.

M. Joyce Neal, MD, John T. Duelge, MD, Albany, GA

Waxing and Waning Rash With Exposure to Cold Water

PRESENTATION

A 13-year-old boy who had been in good health previously comes to the pediatric clinic with a history of a pruritic red rash that waxes and wanes for several hours after he has been swimming. This rash has been a problem for the past 5 days.

Two days ago, after swimming, he developed a diffuse rash, periorbital edema, and a burning sensation on his back. He suddenly became lightheaded and collapsed into his mother's arms, losing consciousness briefly. By the time he arrived at the emergency department, the rash was gone and results of his physical examination was normal. No treatment was prescribed.

Yesterday, while washing the family car with cold soapy water, his right arm and hand swelled and turned solidly red in a "glove" distribution. These changes resolved within 1 hour. Results of his physical examination today are normal.

What is your differential diagnosis at this point?
Are there any elements of history or physical examination that would help you?
What additional diagnostic studies would you like performed?

DISCUSSION

Diagnosis

A 5-minute cold stimulation time test was performed, resulting in localized erythema, edema, and urticaria. Results of the following laboratory tests were normal: complete blood count, erythrocyte sedimentation rate, antinuclear antibody, infectious mononucleosis spot test, serum complement (C3, C4), blood glucose, blood urea nitrogen, serum creatinine, electrolyte levels, aspartate aminotransferase (AST, SGOT), and creatine phosphokinase (CPK). Serum lactate dehydrogenase (LDH) was 776 U/L (normal, 313 to 618 U/L). Cryoglobulin and cryofibrinogen were absent from the serum.

Cold urticaria syndromes are characterized by the development of urticaria or angioedema after exposure to cold. The diagnosis is confirmed by performing a cold stimulation test, in which ice is applied to the skin, directly or in a glass beaker, for 3 to 5 minutes. A positive test consists of the development of a wheal or angioedema after rewarming of the skin, usually within 10 minutes after the ice is removed.

Primary acquired cold urticaria is diagnosed in the patient who acquires wheals or angioedema when exposed to cold and demonstrates no evidence of underlying disease. Secondary cold urticaria syndromes have been associated with underlying diseases such as leukemia, infectious mononucleosis, syphilis, bee stings, and cryoglobulinemia, among others.

Potential Sequelae

Although these syndromes are considered benign and self-limiting (symptoms may persist for a few months to years), patients who have cold urticaria syndromes are susceptible to shock-like reactions during aquatic activities. It is imperative that all affected patients be informed fully of these risks to prevent potential drownings. It is recommended that those who have these syndromes avoid aquatic activities until the symptomatology has resolved. Some authorities recommend that patients have ANA Kits® available.

Treatment

Histamine$_1$ (H$_1$) antihistamines, such as diphenhydramine, hydroxyzine, and cyproheptadine, have suppressed cold urticarial reactions successfully. Some clinicians prefer cyproheptadine because they believe it is a more specific antihistamine for cold urticaria than are other H$_1$ blockers. Treatment with a combination of H$_1$ and H$_2$ receptor antagonists, such as hydroxyzine and cimetidine, also has been effective. Corticosteroids have been shown to be ineffective in the treatment of cold urticaria. Hydroxyzine, 25 mg at bedtime, dramatically prevented further urticaria in this patient; he is being followed off medication.

John C. Leopold, MD, Ehrling Bergquist Hospital, Offutt Air Force Base, NE

Metabolic Imbalance in the Presence of Cardiac Disease

PRESENTATION

A 2-year-old girl presents with a 1-day history of diarrhea, vomiting, and lethargy. She underwent surgical correction of atrial and ventricular septal defects in the first year of life and later developed cardiomyopathy, for which she is receiving digitalis and an angiotensin-converting enzyme inhibitor. She also has a history of tethered spinal cord and chronic constipation.

On physical examination, the child appears drowsy and severely dehydrated. Her temperature is 36.5°C (97.7°F), pulse is 140 beats/min, blood pressure is 58/33 mm Hg, and respiratory rate is 40 breaths/min with a Kussmaul breathing pattern. Her abdomen is markedly distended and tympanitic on percussion. Bowel sounds are diminished, and there is evidence of fecal impaction on rectal examination. She also has tetany, demonstrating carpopedal spasms and a positive Chvostek sign.

Her blood levels are: sodium, 141 mmol/L (141 mEq/L); potassium, 6 mmol/L (6 mEq/L); chloride, 110 mmol/L (110 mEq/L); bicarbonate, 14 mmol/L (14 mEq/L); blood urea nitrogen, 8.57 mmol urea/L (24 mg/dL); creatinine, 88.57 mcmol/L (1.0 mg/dL); calcium, 1.3 mmol/L (5.2 mg/dL); phosphate, 3.01 mmol/L (9.4 mg/dL); and magnesium, 0.95 mmol/L (1.9 mg/dL). Capillary blood gases are: pH, 7.21; Pco_2, 54 torr; total bicarbonate, 12 mmol/L (12 mEq/L); and base deficit, 15 mmol/L (15 mEq/L). Electrocardiography shows prolongation of the QT interval (corrected QTc, 0.53 sec).

A detailed history reveals the cause of her metabolic imbalance.

What is your differential diagnosis at this point?
Are there any elements of history or physical examination that would help you?
What additional diagnostic studies would you like performed?

DISCUSSION

Diagnosis

The child's symptoms appeared a few hours after the administration of one adult Fleet® enema. She had been receiving weekly pediatric Fleet® enemas over the previous 6 months. Intravenous correction of her fluid deficit and several doses of intravenous calcium gluconate led to rapid correction of the hypocalcemic manifestations and to normalization of the serum calcium and phosphate levels. The vomiting and dehydration were not caused by the enema and may have been related to a viral illness or the chronic constipation, but the dehydration accentuated the adverse effects of the enema. Rectal biopsy performed later excluded an underlying congenital megacolon. Surgery for her tethered cord is being planned.

Etiology

The relationship between serum phosphate and calcium levels is well known, with the body's homeostatic mechanisms attempting to maintain the product of the two serum levels as close to 30 as possible. Consequently, hyperphosphatemia is associated with hypocalcemia and hypophosphatemia with hypercalcemia. Individuals who have chronic renal failure can have hyperphosphatemia with hypocalcemia, and the same pattern is seen in patients who are undergoing chemotherapy in which there is massive lysis of tumor cells that have high intracellular phosphate concentrations.

Pediatric Fleet® enema contains 9.5 g monobasic sodium phosphate and 3.5 g dibasic sodium phosphate for each dose of 66.5 mL. Adult Fleet® enema has twice the volume (118 mL) at the same concentration, resulting in twice the amount of phosphate. The adult size enema is not recommended for children younger than 12 years of age, according to the manufacturer's leaflet.

Hyperphosphatemia with hypocalcemia, sometimes at potentially fatal levels, has been reported following the administration of phosphate-containing enemas. Animal studies have shown that the enema solution may be lethal if retained in doses exceeding 20 mL/kg, the equivalent of four pediatric-size enemas in a 2-year-old child. Phosphate enemas should be used with particular caution in patients who are in renal failure and, thus, are at higher risk of developing hyperphosphatemia. Lack of evacuation of a phosphate enema by patients who have organic constipation or partial bowel obstruction leads to increased absorption of the phosphate, putting these patients at higher risk of metabolic derangement.

The sodium content of these enemas may lead to hypernatremia, hypernatremic dehydration, and acidosis. The associated dehydration results in poor renal excretion of absorbed phosphate and prolongation of hypocalcemia. Hypocalcemia and hyperphosphatemia also have been reported in children who are severely dehydrated for other reasons and might be due to redistribution of calcium into cells and phosphorus from the intracellular to the extracellular space.

An oral sodium phosphate regimen of one dose or two doses several hours apart, designed to clean the bowel before colonoscopy, has not been found to induce clinically significant hypovolemia or hypocalcemia. The oral phosphate-containing laxatives, however, still have the potential to induce hyperphosphatemia and hypocalcemia if they are used in high doses; repetitively; or for patients who have renal failure, bowel obstruction, or ileus. Clinicians should not prescribe more than two doses of oral phosphate-containing laxative and should allow several hours between doses.

Lesson for the Clinician

This case illustrates the potential danger of phosphate-containing enemas in inducing hyperphosphatemic hypocalcemia. The risk is increased in the presence of ileus or partial bowel obstruction and is higher among patients who have dehydration or renal dysfunction. Fluid and electrolyte imbalances and hypocalcemia must be corrected vigorously. Parents should be made aware of these complications and instructed not to exceed the prescribed dosage.

Hyperphosphatemia due to phosphate laxatives or enemas always should be considered when seeking an explanation for the sudden development of hypocalcemia.

Hassib Narchi, MD, Mohammed El Jamil, MD, Saudi Aramco-Al-Hasa
Health Center, Mubarraz, Saudi Arabia

Rash and Joint Pains

PRESENTATION

A 10-year-old boy is brought to the office in late spring because of an erythematous rash on his arms and legs that has been present for 4 days and because he is having joint pains. The rash first appeared after he had been playing outdoors for several hours in the sun. His father had applied a new commercial sunblock lotion to his skin before he went outdoors. The father is concerned because even though the rash is less pronounced, the boy has been experiencing stiff and painful knees and ankles upon awakening for the past 2 days. The joint discomfort improves with movement during the day. The boy has had no other symptoms and has been free of fever.

Results of a physical examination, including an extensive joint evaluation, are normal except for a faint, lacy rash on his thighs. The appearance of the rash leads to a specific blood test that reveals the etiology of this boy's joint symptoms.

What is your differential diagnosis at this point?
Are there any elements of history or physical examination that would help you?
What additional diagnostic studies would you like performed?

DISCUSSION

The characteristic lacy pattern of the rash on this boy's thighs suggested erythema infectiosum, and detection of serum immunoglobulin (Ig) M antibodies to parvovirus B 19 confirmed the diagnosis. The father later recalled noticing his son's unusually red cheeks 3 days before the rash appeared on his arms and legs, which he had ascribed to sun exposure.

Presentation

Human parvovirus B 19 is known to cause an infection called erythema infectiosum (EI), otherwise known as fifth disease. This illness is characterized by an erythematous facial rash—described as a "slapped cheek" appearance—followed by a more extensive maculopapular rash on the trunk and limbs that can form a lacy, reticular pattern. Other signs and symptoms include pruritis, headache, fever, sore throat, anorexia, abdominal pain, coryza, and joint pain.

Occasionally, joint symptoms will be the presenting feature. Knees, ankles, and proximal interphalangeal joints are involved most commonly, and symptoms may persist for months. Adults are plagued by joint involvement more often than are children. Establishing the diagnosis in a child who has a rash and joint pain can be difficult, especially if an epidemic is not present in the community. The timing of this boy's illness is consistent with EI; most epidemics occur in late winter and spring and can last through the summer.

Once the rash of EI has appeared, a child is unlikely to be contagious. The presence of some children who have the typical rash, however, may be a harbinger of more to come, which would have relevance to certain individuals, such as schoolteachers who might be pregnant.

Diagnosis

The diagnosis of EI can be confirmed by detecting IgM antibodies to parvovirus B 19 in the serum of the affected individual. This antibody is most likely to be present during the first month after the onset of illness. Confirmation of EI by measuring IgM antibodies to parvovirus is not always necessary, but it should be performed if the clinical course is confusing or if a pregnant woman has been exposed.

Groups at Risk

Although EI is a benign condition, parvovirus infection in a pregnant woman can spread to her fetus and cause hydrops fetalis, spontaneous abortion, and fetal death, with the highest risk occurring during the second trimester. Parvovirus infection has not been associated with an increased risk of congenital malformation.

Another group at special risk from parvovirus infection comprises patients who have hemolytic anemia, including sickle cell disease, thalassemia, hereditary spherocytosis, and enzymatic red blood cell defects. Because parvovirus infection infects erythrocyte precursor cells and depresses erythrocyte production markedly, these individuals may suffer severe anemia and require transfusion. After the infection has resolved, red blood cell production returns to normal. In the immunocompromised patient, the infection may become chronic, causing an ongoing anemia. Intravenous immunoglobulin appears to be effective therapy for this condition.

Treatment

EI in an otherwise healthy child is a benign condition, and there is no specific treatment for the infection. Analgesics can be used for the joint discomfort, and antipruritics such as diphenhydramine or hydroxyzine as well as topical oatmeal baths may relieve the itching.

Differential Diagnosis

The differential diagnosis of joint pain with rash is extensive; a thorough history and physical examination, with particular attention to the appearance of the rash, are essential for diagnosis. Collagen-vascular conditions that need to be considered include juvenile rheumatoid arthritis, systemic lupus erythematosus, and Henoch-Schönlein purpura. Infection with viruses such as coxsackie or rubella and bacteria such as *Staphylococcus aureus* can cause both joint pain and rash. Other illnesses associated with infection, such as rheumatic fever and Lyme disease, as well as hypersensitivity reaction must be included in the differential diagnosis.

Linda S. Nield, MD, West Virginia University School of Medicine, Morgantown, WV; Jonette E. Keri, Georgetown University School of Medicine, Washington, DC

Testicular Pain and Swelling

PRESENTATION

A 14-year-old boy comes to the emergency department because of testicular pain and swelling. Four days ago he began to experience crampy bilateral abdominal pain associated with vomiting and fever as high as 39.4°C (103°F). After 2 days of worsening pain, nausea, and vomiting, he was seen by a physician, diagnosed as having a viral illness, and given promethazine and intravenous fluids, which provided temporary relief. Since then, the abdominal pain has continued, and he has experienced stabbing pain and increasing swelling in his right scrotal area. He denies trauma, sexual activity, dysuria, frequency, hematuria, upper respiratory tract symptoms, constipation, or diarrhea. His immunizations are current.

On physical examination, he is sleeping but is easily arousable and pleasant. His temperature is 38.6°C (101.5°F), and his pulse is 117 beats/min. His abdomen is soft and nondistended, and bowel sounds are normoactive. Bilateral abdominal tenderness and rebound tenderness are present, as are psoas and obturator signs. No guarding is noted. The right hemiscrotum is swollen, tense, and exquisitely painful to light palpation but not reddened. The swelling prevents palpation of the testicle, and the scrotum does not transilluminate. The left hemiscrotum is normal, and no hernias or penile discharge are noted.

Results of all laboratory studies are normal, including a white blood cell count of 8.4 x 10^9/L (8.4 x 10^3/mcL). Color Doppler ultrasonography reveals echogenic fluid in the right scrotum without evidence of vascular compromise. An imaging study reveals the diagnosis.

What is your differential diagnosis at this point?
Are there any elements of history or physical examination that would help you?
What additional diagnostic studies would you like performed?

DISCUSSION

A computed tomographic (CT) scan of the patient's abdomen and pelvis demonstrated a periappendiceal abscess with peritoneal free fluid and air and a communicating right pyocele of the scrotum. In the operating room, he was found to have a perforated appendicitis with purulent peritoneal fluid.

Differential Diagnosis

Patients who present with acute scrotal swelling and pain should be considered first as possibly having testicular and spermatic cord torsion, which occurs most commonly in pubertal males. The torsion results from a high attachment of the tunica vaginalis to the spermatic cord, which allows the freely mobile testis to twist on the cord. Testicular torsion presents classically as acute testicular pain with associated nausea and vomiting. On physical examination, a transverse lie of the uninvolved testis may be noted. The affected testis generally is situated higher in the scrotum than the other testis because the torsion shortens the spermatic cord. The cremasteric reflex on the affected side often is missing, and the lower pole of the testis usually is extremely tender and swollen. Less obvious cases of testicular torsion can be diagnosed by using high-resolution ultrasonography with color Doppler technique. Diagnosis of testicular torsion and treatment with nonsurgical or surgical detorsion and orchiopexy are imperative within the first few hours after the onset of pain to prevent testicular infarction.

Acute scrotal pain and swelling also occur when there is torsion of the testicular or epididymal appendage. Affected patients present with nausea and vomiting, but they have much less pain, which they may tolerate for days before seeking attention. The pain is localized to the upper pole of the testis, and a bluish nodule on the upper pole sometimes can be seen through the scrotal skin (the "blue dot" sign).

Infectious diseases that can cause acute scrotal swelling and pain include orchitis, epididymitis, and epididymo-orchitis. These conditions cause fever and symptoms that mimic a urinary tract infection. Mumps orchitis should be considered in adolescent males who have not been immunized. It presents gradually, with testicular pain and swelling 4 to 8 days after the appearance of parotitis. These patients may have fever and suffer from diffuse testicular tenderness and swelling for 4 to 10 days.

A history of trauma leads to consideration of a testicular hematoma or ruptured tunica albuginea. A ruptured albuginea causes increasing pain, often of a severity out of proportion to the findings on physical examination. Hydroceles and varicoceles, which are dilated and tortuous veins in the spermatic cord, present less acutely with scrotal swelling that usually is painless. Henoch-Schönlein syndrome can cause acute pain and swelling of the scrotum, but these patients usually have a purpuric rash, abdominal pain, joint pain, and signs of nephritis.

Finally, acute appendicitis is a rare cause of acute scrotal swelling and pain. Perforation of the appendix and pus formation in the presence of a patent process vaginalis are required for this unusual presentation to occur. Purulent fluid descends from the peritoneum into the scrotum by gravity through the patent processus vaginalis.

Presentation

Appendicitis presents typically with periumbilical pain that moves into the right lower quadrant over a matter of hours. The pain is followed in sequence by anorexia, nausea, vomiting, and fever. Children may manifest all or none of these symptoms and signs, and they can have additional clinical features not typically associated with appendicitis. For example, vomiting can occur before abdominal pain begins in some; in others, parents do not notice that the child is in pain until the vomiting begins. Diarrhea occurs in 15% of children who have appendicitis because an inflamed, low-lying appendix can irritate the sigmoid colon. The incidence of diarrhea is increased among patients who have appendiceal perforation.

The pain of appendicitis can be located in the flank area and give the impression of a ureteral calculus when the inflamed appendix is in a retrocecal position. Atypical presentations can lead to erroneous diagnoses of gastroenteritis, sepsis, urinary tract infection, septic arthritis of the right hip, testicular torsion, bowel obstruction, inflammatory bowel disease, and cholecystitis.

Laboratory and Imaging Studies

Results of all laboratory studies are nonspecific in cases of acute appendicitis. An elevated white blood cell count is present in 90% of patients. White blood cells can be seen on urinalysis because of irritation of the bladder or ureter that is caused by a nearby inflamed appendix.

An appendicolith seen on a plain radiograph of the abdomen can support the diagnosis of appendicitis, but this occurs in fewer than 10% of cases. Plain radiographs are recommended only in cases in which the diagnosis is not evident and where signs of other pathologic processes, such as free air, may be revealed. Ultrasonography of the abdomen may be useful when the diagnosis is equivocal. A noncompressible appendix is a specific ultrasonographic finding in acute appendicitis; periappendiceal fluid may indicate a rupture or abscess. In the pubertal female, ultrasonography is useful in differentiating appendicitis from a gynecologic condition.

CT scan of the abdomen and pelvis can help the clinician to diagnose early appendicitis, an unusually located appendix, or a perforated appendix with or without abscess formation. In the present case, the presence of an abdominal condition requiring surgery was determined by physical examination, but the abdominal CT scan clarified the connection between the patient's peritoneal signs and his scrotal swelling and pain.

Jerald DeLaGarza, MD, Holly D. Smith, MD, University of Texas Medical School, Houston, TX

Seizures During a Dental Procedure

PRESENTATION

While undergoing a dental procedure, a previously healthy 5-year-old girl develops generalized tonic-clonic seizure activity. She appears markedly cyanotic, and basic life support is initiated, followed by intubation. She is transported to a local emergency department and receives intravenous diazepam (0.15 mg/kg), which results in cessation of the seizures. The dentist reports that she had received prilocaine and nitrous oxide by inhalation.

On physical examination, the child is lethargic, but no focal neurologic deficits are noted. Her breathing is assisted by bag ventilation at 25 breaths/min with 100% oxygen, and she appears cyanotic. Pulse rate is 150 beats/min, blood pressure is 108/70 mm Hg, temperature is 38.6°C (101.4°F) rectally, breath sounds are clear, heart rate and rhythm are regular, and pulses are strong in all extremities. Arterial blood gases reveal pH, 7.35; Pco_2, 47 torr; Po_2, 329 torr; HCO_3, 25 mmol/L; and oxygen saturation, 99%. Bedside pulse oximetry is 87%.

What is your differential diagnosis at this point?
Are there any elements of history or physical examination that would help you?
What additional diagnostic studies would you like performed?

DISCUSSION

The finding of cyanosis unresponsive to oxygen in the presence of a normal cardiopulmonary examination suggests an abnormal hemoglobin oxygen transport state, such as methemoglobinemia. Methemoglobin is hemoglobin that contains iron in the ferric (Fe^{+++}) instead of the normal ferrous (Fe^{++}) state. Ferric iron is not capable of binding oxygen. It is formed continuously under normal conditions, but its concentration is maintained at low levels (1% to 2%) by active enzymes (NADH- and NADPH-dependent reductase). In pathologic states, as the level increases above 15%, cyanosis and the characteristic chocolate brown discoloration of blood occur.

Laboratory Tests

The appropriate test for detecting such a condition is an arterial blood gas determination that measures the actual oxygen saturation, a procedure that commonly is referred to as co-oximetry. Routine analysis of blood gas measures the partial pressure of oxygen (Po_2) and calculates the oxygen saturation by the oxyhemoglobin dissociation curve. In the presence of abnormal hemoglobin, the calculated oxygen saturation is overestimated. In addition to methemoglobin, the co-oximeter also measures carboxyhemoglobin, a determination that is useful in managing patients who have carbon monoxide poisoning. In patients who have methemoglobinemia, pulse oximetry is useless, displaying levels in the 80% to 85% range regardless of the true oxygen saturation.

This patient's co-oximetry results were: pH, 7.3; Pco_2, 48 torr; Po_2, 279 torr; HCO_3, 23 mmol/L; oxygen saturation, 76%; methemoglobin, 24%; and carboxyhemoglobin, 0.2%. These findings were consistent with results of her physical examination.

Etiology

Methemoglobinemia usually is an acquired disorder, but there are rare hereditary diseases that involve either abnormal hemoglobin (M hemoglobinopathy) or a deficiency of one of the reducing enzymes. The acquired type results from exposure to drugs or toxins. Nitrates that contaminate well water are a well-known cause of methemoglobinemia. The numerous drugs that have been implicated include dapsone, sulfonamides (sulfamethoxazole), amyl nitrite, nitroglycerin, phenazopyridine, and local anesthetics.

In this case, the prilocaine that the patient received caused the methemoglobinemia. Several other local anesthetics, such as benzocaine, tetracaine, cetacaine, and lidocaine, have been reported to cause this condition when administered intravenously, topically, or subcutaneously.

Another important condition that has been reported in infants is methemoglobinemia resulting from diarrheal illness. Infants have low levels of the reducing enzyme NADH-reductase. This physiologic state in combination with nitrates that are produced by intestinal bacteria results in the methemoglobinemia. Infants also have high levels of fetal hemoglobin, which is oxidized more easily to the ferric state than is normal hemoglobin.

Presentation

Symptoms of methemoglobinemia are determined by the concentration of the abnormal hemoglobin and the presence of any underlying medical condition, such as anemia, acidosis, or cardiopulmonary dysfunction. In healthy individuals, levels of methemoglobin lower than 15% produce no symptoms. At levels of 15% to 20%, cyanosis occurs. Dyspnea, weakness, syncope, and headaches are present at levels of 20% to 50%. High levels of 50% to 70% can result in seizures, coma, and dysrhythmias, and a concentration of greater than 70% is lethal.

Treatment

Treatment involves removal of the offending agent, if possible, and supportive care. Indications for pharmacologic treatment are hypoxia or methemoglobin levels greater than 30%. Methylene blue is the agent of choice; it uses the NADPH-reducing system to convert iron from the ferric to the ferrous state. The dose is 1 to 2 mg/kg intravenously, with a positive effect usually seen within 30 to 60 minutes. A second dose may be given if no response is seen within 1 hour.

Because this child had central nervous system manifestations and hypoxia, she received 1 mg/kg methylene blue. A repeat methemoglobin level 2 hours later was 6%. Her mental status improved, and she was extubated and observed overnight in the hospital.

Lesson for the Clinician

Patients who have unexplained cyanosis should have a co-oximeter blood gas performed to determine the presence of abnormal hemoglobin. Pediatricians who use local anesthetics should be aware of this condition.

Bonnie C. Desselle, MD, Louisiana State University School of Medicine,
New Orleans, LA

Heart Murmur in Down Syndrome

PRESENTATION

A 16-year-old girl who has Down syndrome is evaluated by a pediatric cardiologist because of a recently noted heart murmur. Eight years ago, another murmur was heard that sounded innocent and eventually disappeared. Results of electrocardiography (ECG) and chest radiography at that time were normal.

Although she is a participant in the Special Olympics, this girl is not an active person; her mother is concerned that she has gained too much weight in the past year. Findings on physical examination include a weight of 58 kg (128 lb) (75th percentile on Down syndrome growth chart; was 50th at last examination 3 years ago) and a height of 142.2 cm (56 in) (40th percentile; was 75th). Her blood pressure is 90/60 mm Hg and pulse is 52 beats/min, she is at sexual maturity rating (Tanner) stage 5 in breast maturity, and her face is mildly puffy. Her lungs are clear. Cardiac findings include a normal apical impulse, heart sounds of normal intensity with a split second sound that closes on expiration, and peripheral pulses of normal amplitude. A grade I/VI systolic ejection murmur is audible along the left sternal border, radiating across the precordium. No neck masses, neck vein distension, or hepatomegaly are noted.

Results of an ECG show sinus bradycardia, borderline low voltage, and nonspecific T-wave flattening. A chest radiograph shows normal heart size and pulmonary vascular markings. Limited echocardiography reveals a significant abnormality. Blood chemistries are ordered that explain her clinical findings.

What is your differential diagnosis at this point?
Are there any elements of history or physical examination that would help you?
What additional diagnostic studies would you like performed?

DISCUSSION

The limited echocardiography on this girl demonstrated a moderate pericardial effusion but no evidence of cardiac tamponade. Thyroid function tests revealed a free thyroxine (T4) level of less than 5.2 pmol/L (0.4 ng/dL) (normal range, 9.1 to 24.7 pmol/L [0.7 to 1.9 ng/dL]), a triiodothyronine (T3) level of 858 pmol/L (66 ng/dL) (normal range, 1,040 to 1,196 pmol/L [80 to 92 ng/dL]), and a thyroid stimulating hormone (TSH) level of 168 mIU/mL (normal range, 0 to 5.5 mIU/mL). Antithyroid peroxidase, antithyroglobulin, and antithyroid microsomal antibody determinations all were negative. Complete echocardiography showed no structural abnormality. Her pericardial effusion was a result of hypothyroidism, and therapy was started with L-thyroxine.

Etiology

Down syndrome is associated with both congenital and acquired hypothyroidism. Pericardial effusion may be the presenting clinical problem in both situations. Congenital hypothyroidism is approximately 28 times more common in infants who have Down syndrome than in the general population. The cause of the thyroid failure in these patients is unknown; it does not appear to be caused by autoimmune disease, and most patients have normal results on a thyroid scan, which excludes the possibility of ectopic glands or athyrosis.

After the newborn period, the prevalence of thyroid disease in individuals who have Down syndrome is about 3%, which is appreciably higher than that seen in the general population. Evidence of autoimmune disease frequently is detectable in affected patients. When T3 and T4 levels are measured serially over the first 3 decades of life in longitudinal studies, people who have Down syndrome show significantly greater declines than do control populations.

Presentation

Acquired hypothyroidism is associated with a number of clinical signs, the most important of which is growth failure. Constipation, low body temperature, and myxedema can occur. Physical activity may slow, and mental capacities may be impaired. The clinical picture can be subtle and easy to overlook. Many people who have Down syndrome tend to be relatively inactive and are heavy as well as developmentally delayed, making the detection of hypothyroidism even more difficult. As demonstrated by this patient, the significance of the anthropomorphic data that suggest thyroid dysfunction—growth delay and excessive weight gain—may be less apparent if changes in a patient's growth pattern are not recognized and if growth charts specific for individuals who have Down syndrome are not used. The American Academy of Pediatrics recommends that thyroid function tests be performed periodically in patients who have Down syndrome.

Pericardial effusion can be demonstrated by echocardiography in about 50% of infants and 75% of children who have hypothyroidism. The effusion usually is asymptomatic and rarely leads to cardiac tamponade. When the diagnosis of hypothyroidism is delayed, as it may be in patients who have Down syndrome, very large effusions may develop.

Lesson for the Clinician

Use of appropriate growth charts and regular monitoring of thyroid function may allow earlier diagnosis and prevention of effusions as well as other effects of hypothyroidism.

Thomas C. Bisett, MD, Sol Rockenmacher, MD, Lahey Hitchcock Clinic,
Manchester, NH

Diarrhea, Fever, and Abdominal Pain

PRESENTATION

A 2-year-old girl is brought to the clinic because of diarrhea, fever, and abdominal pain that started yesterday. The pain appears to be constant and primarily periumbilical; the diarrhea is described as mucoid, with small amounts of blood. She has continued to feed without vomiting. There is no history of family illness, foreign travel, or ingestion of uncooked meat. She has been healthy and has developed well.

On physical examination, she appears fussy and mildly dehydrated. All vital signs are normal, including temperature. Her abdomen is soft and nontender, without palpable organs or masses; bowel sounds are normal. Rectal examination reveals no fissures, impacted feces, or polyps. The stool is green, loosely formed, and mixed with mucus and blood.

Results of initial laboratory studies are as follows: white blood cell count, 12.9 x 10^9/L (12.9 x 10^3/mcL) with 66% neutrophils, 6% bands, and 23% lymphocytes; hemoglobin, 1.89 mmol/L (12.2 g/dL); platelet count, 150 x 10^9/L (150 x 10^3/mcL); and normal peripheral blood smear. Results of coagulation studies, electrolyte levels, blood urea nitrogen (BUN), and creatinine are normal. Her urine is concentrated but otherwise normal. Abdominal and chest radiographs are normal.

The child is admitted for intravenous hydration and observation. Cultures show no growth from blood and no evidence of Salmonella, Shigella, Yersinia, or Campylobacter in stool, which also has no detectable rotavirus antigen. She develops a fever to 38.3° C (101° F) and continues to pass bloody stools. Repeat laboratory values on the third hospital day are as follows: sodium, 125 mmol/L (125 mEq/L); potassium, 5.0 mmol/L (5.0 mEq/L); bicarbonate, 16 mmol/L (16 mEq/L); BUN, 12.14 mmol urea/L (34 mg/dL); creatinine, 221.43 mcmol/L (2.5 mg/dL); hemoglobin, 1.40 mmol/L (9.0 g/dL); and platelet count, 28 x 10^9/L (28 x 10^3/mcL). The peripheral blood smear shows fragmented red blood cells. Urinalysis reveals moderate levels of protein and blood but no casts.

What is your differential diagnosis at this point?
Are there any elements of history or physical examination that would help you?
What additional diagnostic studies would you like performed?

DISCUSSION

The child was diagnosed as having hemolytic-uremic syndrome (HUS), based on the acute development of microangiopathic hemolytic anemia, renal failure, and thrombocytopenia. The presentation of an irritable child who has gastroenteritis supported this diagnosis. Further validation came in the form of a microbiology report showing growth of *Escherichia coli* 0157:H7 from a stool sample that was sent to an outside laboratory for special culturing techniques.

Epidemiology and Etiology

HUS is the most common cause of acute renal failure in young children, with an incidence in the United States ranging from 0.3 to 10 cases per 100,000 children. It most commonly affects children between the ages of 7 months and 4 years.

There are two subtypes of HUS: diarrhea-associated and nondiarrhea-associated. As the name implies, diarrhea-associated HUS typically is initiated by enteric bacterial infection. The incidence of diarrhea-associated HUS peaks in summer and early fall and afflicts patients of all races and both genders equally. Diarrhea-associated HUS can occur in epidemic form. The subset of HUS that is not related to enteric bacterial infection does not show a seasonal variation.

The usual offending organism in diarrhea-associated HUS is an enterohemorrhagic strain of *E coli* of the serotype 0157:H7. The reservoir for this pathogen is the intestinal tract of domestic animals; thus, it can be transmitted in undercooked meat or unpasteurized milk. Other reported sources include contaminated apple cider, vegetables, and swimming pools. Infected individuals can transmit the infection to others.

The 0157:H7 strain of *E coli* causes HUS via a bacterial toxin (verotoxin). After being absorbed by the intestine, this toxin presumably initiates glomerular endothelial cell injury, which is the inciting event in the pathogenesis of HUS. *Shigella* sp also produce a toxin that has many structural similarities to the *E coli* toxin, which is why the term Shiga-like toxin often is used. Various other viruses and bacteria have been linked to HUS, but the causal relationship has not been proven. The only pathogens definitely shown to cause HUS are *E coli* (including some non-0157 forms), *Shigella*, and *Streptococcus pneumoniae*. *S pneumoniae* causes a nondiarrhea-associated version of the syndrome, at least theoretically due to the presence on its surface of neuraminidase, which directly damages platelets, erythrocytes, and glomerular endothelium. Rarer causes of nondiarrhea-associated HUS include pregnancy, oral contraceptives, cyclosporine, and malignancy. Multiple cases in single families have prompted speculation about a genetic cause, although none has been identified definitively.

In diarrhea-associated HUS, when the bacterial toxin damages the glomerular endothelium, the cells swell and fibrin clots form in response. The result is vessel occlusion and ultimately sclerosis of glomeruli. The narrowing of these channels leads to mechanical damage of erythrocytes and a microangiopathic hemolytic anemia. The swollen and damaged endothelial cells also cause intrarenal platelet adhesion, which leads to localized coagulation and thrombocytopenia. An increase in circulating platelet aggregating factors also may play a role. Endothelial cell prostacyclin normally prevents platelets from adhering to endothelium, but this factor is depleted as the endothelial cells are damaged by the bacterial toxin, contributing further to platelet aggregation. Renal insufficiency results from decreased glomerular filtration due to reduced blood flow through the stenotic vessels.

Presentation

These pathologic changes cause the typical presentation of HUS. The disorder generally follows an acute gastroenteritis that is characterized by abdominal pain and diarrhea. Fever and vomiting may be present, although *E coli* 0157 is less likely to cause fever than are other enteric pathogens. *E coli* is more likely, however, to be associated with visible blood in the stool. From 3 to 12 days after the onset of gastroenteritis, the patient suddenly develops pallor, irritability, weakness, lethargy, and oliguria. Physical examination reveals a dehydrated, irritable child who may have edema, pulmonary congestion, hypertension, petechiae, purpura, or hepatosplenomegaly.

Diagnosis

Diagnosis is based on the clinical pattern of microangiopathic hemolytic anemia in conjunction with thrombocytopenia and acute renal failure. The hemoglobin level declines typically to 0.76 to 1.4 mmol/L (5 to 9 g/dL). The peripheral smear shows evidence of erythrocyte destruction in the form of helmet cells, burr cells, and schistocytes. As with other hemolytic anemias, the plasma hemoglobin level is elevated and the plasma haptoglobin level is decreased. The direct Coombs test is negative, and the reticulocyte count is mildly elevated, as are the total bilirubin and lactate dehydrogenase levels. The white blood cell count may increase to as high as 30 x 10^9/L (30 x 10^3/mcL). Platelet levels as low as 20 x 10^9/L (20 x 10^3/mcL) can occur. Most patients have oliguria or anuria, but the urine output may remain normal. Low-grade microscopic hematuria and mild-to-severe proteinuria may occur, and the urine sediment may contain dysmorphic erythrocytes and cellular casts. The degree of renal failure ranges from mild to severe, necessitating dialysis in some cases.

Standard techniques for performing stool cultures are ineffective in detecting *E coli* 0157. Unlike most human fecal flora, *E coli* 0157 does not ferment sorbitol rapidly. When grown on sorbitol-MacConkey agar plates, the 0157 colonies are colorless. The presence of 0157 antigen in these colonies can be detected with antiserum directed at the antigen. The H-type must be identified in reference laboratories, although 0157:H7 can be identified presumptively once the somatic (0) antigen is identified.

Differential Diagnosis

When considering the diagnosis of HUS, other potential causes of microangiopathic hemolytic anemia and acute renal failure, such as systemic lupus erythematosus and malignant hypertension, should be excluded. Renal biopsy is indicated only if the renal failure persists longer than 2 weeks. The presence of thrombocytopenia may preclude performing the procedure. HUS can be difficult to distinguish from bilateral renal vein thrombosis. Both conditions often are preceded by gastroenteritis and are characterized by pallor, dehydration, thrombocytopenia, acute renal failure, and microangiopathic hemolytic anemia. Hypertrophy of the kidneys is typical of renal vein thrombosis and may be evident on ultrasonographic examination, but angiography may be the only way to distinguish between the two conditions.

Complications

Complications of untreated HUS include acidosis, hyperkalemia, hyponatremia, fluid overload, ascites, congestive heart failure, hypertension, and uremia. Serum phosphorus, uric acid, and triglyceride levels also may be increased. Central nervous system manifestations include irritability, seizures, coma, ataxia, cerebral swelling, and hemiparesis. Enteric sequelae are rare but may include melena, bowel perforation, intussusception, infarction, and colitis. The pathogenesis of all these complications is unknown but may be intravascular thrombosis in locations other than the kidney. Even after recovery, the development of hypertension or chronic renal disease is possible, so long-term follow-up is mandatory.

Management

Management of the syndrome depends primarily on assessing the severity of the renal failure and addressing alterations in volume status and electrolyte imbalance. Dialysis is indicated for oliguria or anuria accompanied by volume overload and severe hyponatremia or hyperkalemia. Peritoneal dialysis has been shown to be as effective as hemodialysis. Management of the microangiopathic process is mostly supportive, with transfusions of blood and platelets as indicated. In diarrhea-associated HUS, no benefit has been demonstrated from infusing fresh frozen plasma or performing plasmapheresis. Nondiarrhea-associated forms of HUS may respond to plasma infusion or exchange.

More than 90% of patients who have HUS survive when acute renal failure is managed aggressively; 65% to 85% recover normal renal function. A poor prognosis is associated with the nondiarrhea-associated form of HUS. Familial and nondiarrhea-associated forms of HUS tend to be more severe and are more likely to lead to hypertension, relapses of microangiopathy, and end-stage renal disease.

In this child, when the acute renal failure was recognized, she was treated with intravenous infusion of normal saline and furosemide. In spite of effective diuresis, the acidosis and azotemia worsened. She was transferred to a tertiary care center for peritoneal dialysis and eventually recovered fully.

John A. Horiszny, MD, St. Joseph Hospital, Chicago, IL

Sudden Drooling and Increasing Confusion

PRESENTATION

A previously healthy 3-year-old boy is playing outdoors when he suddenly shrieks loudly. His parents run to his side and find him frightened, drooling out of the right corner of his mouth, and unable to respond verbally to questions, although he appears alert. As he walks into the house, his gait is clumsy and ataxic. Over the next 10 to 15 minutes he appears increasingly confused. He continues to drool and develops a vacant, glassy-eyed gaze. As he attempts to get up, his right arm and leg appear weak and he falls onto his right side.

He is taken to the emergency department where he is noted to be still drooling and confused. He can speak, but his speech is garbled and nonsensical. His blood pressure is 90/60 mm Hg and his heart rate is 120 beats/min. Neurologic examination reveals right-sided weakness. A complete blood count, electrolyte levels, and renal and liver function test results all are normal. A urine toxicology screen is negative. Over the next 4 hours his signs and symptoms resolve completely and he is sent home.

The boy does well until 9 days later, when he awakens in the morning and is noted to have drooling from the right corner of his mouth, ataxia, expressive aphasia, and confusion. His right side again is weak, and he stumbles and falls toward that side. He is taken to his pediatrician's office and observed for 2 hours, at which point he had returned to normal except for mild right lower extremity weakness. A diagnostic procedure performed later that day reveals the reason for his alarming episodes.

What is your differential diagnosis at this point?
Are there any elements of history or physical examination that would help you?
What additional diagnostic studies would you like performed?

DISCUSSION

The boy underwent a computed tomographic (CT) scan of the head, which revealed a high-density area in the region of the left caudate and putamen consistent with a recent hemorrhage in the distribution of a branch of the left middle cerebral artery. He was transferred to a tertiary care center, where an exhaustive evaluation failed to find a specific cause for his stroke. The most likely explanation was that he had experienced the rupture of a small arteriovenous malformation (AVM). He had no obvious neurologic sequelae from the stroke.

Presentation

Although stroke occurs infrequently in children, this young boy exhibited one sign that might have made the clinician suspect this diagnosis. The most common clinical feature in children older than 1 year who have strokes is the sudden onset of hemiparesis or weakness. In trying to reconstruct the chain of events in this boy's clinical course, the clinicians caring for him postulated that he may have had a small bleeding episode—perhaps a small leak from which he quickly recovered—that caused the first episode. The bleeding is believed to have stopped spontaneously but recurred in a more catastrophic form to cause the second episode. His complete recovery speaks to the resilience and adaptability of the brain.

Transient ischemic attacks, in which cerebral perfusion is compromised but a true stroke does not occur, can cause temporary neurologic deficits, followed by complete recovery within 24 hours. These episodes may precede both thrombotic and embolic strokes.

Etiology

Strokes in older children have myriad etiologies that can be categorized as embolic, thrombotic, and hemorrhagic. Congenital heart disease is a common cause of embolic stroke in children. Cyanotic lesions pose the greatest risk. Patent foramen ovale and other defects involving right-to-left-side shunting also are common causes. Thus, echocardiography is an essential part of the evaluation of most children who suffer a stroke.

Hemorrhagic strokes frequently are associated with coagulation disorders. The possible existence of X-linked hemophilia A or B should be investigated in any male child who has a hemorrhagic stroke by obtaining levels of factors VIII and IX. Severe thrombocytopenia is the cause of intracranial hemorrhage in a small number of patients and may be due to idiopathic thrombocytopenic purpura, malignancy, or severe infection.

AVM is the most common cause of hemorrhagic stroke in preadolescent children and occurs more often in boys. Intracranial aneurysms are found more commonly among adolescents than preschool children and usually are due to vascular developmental abnormalities.

Subarachnoid hemorrhage occurs most frequently in children who have incurred trauma and is manifested by severe headache, altered mental status, and focal neurologic deficits. Sickle cell disease is associated with cerebral infarction more often than with other forms of stroke, but it also can cause subarachnoid or intraparenchymal hemorrhage.

Thrombosis can follow vascular dysplasia, which occurs in moyamoya disease, fibromuscular dysplasia, neurofibromatosis, and other disorders. Thrombosis can result from vasculopathies or vascular injuries; vasculitis, as occurs in autoimmune disorders such as systemic lupus erythematosus; and hematologic abnormalities. Therefore, determining the presence or absence of various anticoagulants or clotting factors usually is an appropriate part of the evaluation of a child who has had a stroke.

Imaging Studies

Both CT scan and magnetic resonance imaging (MRI) will document the structural changes that occur in a stroke at any age. CT imaging can be performed more rapidly, but MRI will provide greater resolution and allow detection of smaller infarctions. An electroencephalogram (EEG) often is performed in the newborn who has focal seizures. Localized abnormalities on the EEG may raise the suspicion of stroke and lead to imaging studies.

Cerebral arteriography must be considered for the child who has a stroke in which the cause is not evident from other forms of imaging. If the patient has an AVM or an aneurysm, surgery may correct it. Even if a small AVM is present, it may be obscured transiently by acute hemorrhage, leading some clinicians to repeat the arteriography a few months after the acute hemorrhage has resolved in search of a malformation.

William E. Wear, MD, Staunton, VA

Poor Feeding and Hypotonia in an Infant

PRESENTATION

A 4-month-old boy has been feeding poorly and has appeared weak for 2 days; the initial impression is that he has a viral syndrome. Because of hypotonia that appears to be worsening, tachypnea, weak cough, and a lack of feeding activity for more than 12 hours, he is brought to the hospital. Previously, he had nursed well, gained weight appropriately, and passed one stool every 4 to 5 days. He had achieved normal developmental milestones. After arriving at the hospital, the baby has a prolonged apneic episode that requires positive pressure ventilation; he is transferred to the intensive care unit.

On physical examination, the baby's temperature is 35.6°C (96°F) axillary, pulse is 170 beats/min, respiratory rate is 68 breaths/min, blood pressure is 100/59 mm Hg, and pulse oximeter reading is 98% in room air. He appears ill and has dry mucous membranes but is alert. He does not cry. Mild respiratory distress is evident, and coarse crackles are heard on inspiration and expiration throughout the lung fields. These findings improve after the infant receives nebulized albuterol, chest physical therapy, and suctioning. His capillary refill time is 3 sec. Neurologic evaluation demonstrates a lack of extraocular movements, absence of facial movements and gag reflex, and significant hypotonia of all extremities. Although deep tendon reflexes are present initially, they disappear overnight. The infant is intubated and placed on mechanical ventilation.

Additional history leads to further investigations and a diagnosis.

What is your differential diagnosis at this point?
Are there any elements of history or physical examination that would help you?
What additional diagnostic studies would you like performed?

DISCUSSION

Differential Diagnosis

The differential diagnosis of hypotonia in a 4-month-old who is afebrile and in respiratory distress that progresses to respiratory failure can be extensive and includes infant botulism, Werdnig-Hoffman syndrome (spinal muscular atrophy), sepsis (bacterial or viral), postinfectious neuropathy, toxic ingestion (specifically, organophosphates), myasthenia gravis, and Guillain-Barré syndrome.

Diagnosis

The additional history revealed in this case was that the infant had been exposed to dust and dirt when he was carried through a construction site. Also, his grandparents were squeezing grape juice from single grapes into his mouth. This family lives near the Delaware River, where botulism is endemic. Ingestion of honey or corn syrup was denied. The diagnosis of infant botulism was confirmed by obtaining a stool sample that was found to contain botulinum toxin.

Infantile botulism should be considered in any baby who is younger than 6 months of age and demonstrates weakness, poor feeding, constipation, a weak cry, and listlessness. It is caused by a neurotoxin produced by *Clostridium botulinum.* After the spores are ingested, the neurotoxin is produced and released into the infant's colon. The toxin is absorbed and enters the circulation where it causes a flaccid paralysis by binding irreversibly to the ganglionic and postganglionic parasympathetic synapses. The toxin affects the peripheral and cranial nerves and causes autonomic instability. Recovery occurs only when new receptors are generated in the neuromuscular junctions.

The risk factors for acquiring botulism are age younger than 12 months, exposure to honey or corn syrup, exposure to dust and dirt, and geographic factors (the disorder is common in eastern Pennsylvania, California, and Utah). Whether breast-feeding or bottle-feeding is a risk factor is controversial.

Evaluation

Stool from this patient was obtained and sent to the laboratory of the New Jersey Department of Health, where an extract was injected into four rats. The procedure involves injection of an unaltered extract into one rat that serves as a positive control. The second rat is injected with a heat-treated sample; because botulinum toxin is heat-labile, the heating serves to inactivate both A and B toxin. The third rat is treated with antitoxin A before being injected. The fourth rat is treated with antitoxin B before being injected. Rats 1 and 4 (positive control and antitoxin B) were dead by 24 hours after being injected. Rats 2 and 3 (negative control and recipient of antitoxin A) remained alive 3 days after being injected. These results established the diagnosis of infantile botulism, serotype A.

Spores of *C botulinum* can be isolated from the stool as another method of diagnosis, although such an investigation was not carried out in this case. Electromyographic studies also can be useful in diagnosing infantile botulism. The typical pattern is brief, small, abundant motor-unit potentials.

Treatment

Traditional treatment of infantile botulism has been supportive care. Endotracheal intubation may be necessary to protect the airway if the gag reflex is lost and is required until the gag reflex returns. Mechanical ventilation also may be needed to support gas exchange. Antibiotic therapy is not useful and actually may aggravate the disease. Aminoglycosides should be avoided in treating secondary bacterial infections because they are known to block the neuromuscular junction. The syndrome of inappropriate secretion of antidiuretic hormone is a common complication and should be watched for and treated appropriately.

An exciting new therapeutic tool is botulism immune globulin (BIG), which is a human-derived botulinum antitoxin. A recent study demonstrated that this agent is safe and can reduce the mean hospital stay by 50% to approximately 2.5 weeks. BIG should be given to affected infants as early as possible.

Infantile botulism is a self-limited disease, and the overall prognosis is good. Even before the availability of BIG, children generally have recovered with minimal complications. Aggressive management of the pulmonary tract to avoid the development of atelectasis, pneumonia, and tracheitis minimizes morbidity.

Howard Kornfeld, MD, Overlook Hospital, Summit, NJ

Update: Although the case for implicating honey as a risk factor for the development of infant botulism is strong, available data about corn syrup do not support an etiologic role for that product.

Worsening Pain in the Foot

PRESENTATION

A 2-year-old boy presents with pain in his right foot that has worsened over the past 2 days to the point that he refuses to walk or bear weight and only will crawl. When asked what is bothering him, he points to his right ankle and states, "It hurts." Administration of acetaminophen has had no effect. There is no history of trauma, but he has had a low-grade fever, cough, and clear rhinorrhea. He has been irritable for a few days, and his appetite is decreased. The child has been healthy otherwise, as have his three older siblings, and the mother reports he has had no recent contact with ill people.

Physical examination reveals a well-developed, friendly boy whose rectal temperature is 37.6°C (99.8°F), pulse is 130 beats/min, respiration rate is 24 breaths/min, blood pressure is 105/65 mm Hg, and pulse oximetry level is 98% saturation. A complete examination yields normal findings except for evaluation of his extremities. Although the boy has a full passive and active range of motion of his right hip and knee, he refuses to move his right ankle or foot. Moderate tenderness is noted over the right midfoot, but there is no warmth, erythema, or swelling. He refuses to walk and complains of pain in the right foot.

Radiographs of the right ankle and foot appear completely normal, and a bone scan is read as negative. Further testing suggests a diagnosis.

What is your differential diagnosis at this point?
Are there any elements of history or physical examination that would help you?
What additional diagnostic studies would you like performed?

DISCUSSION

Diagnosis

Foot pain is not an unusual complaint in children, and the cause usually can be determined from results of the history and physical examination. In most cases, the pain resolves spontaneously without treatment and without determination of a specific etiology. In children younger than 6 years, the differential diagnosis includes poorly fitting shoes, a foreign body, an occult fracture, osteomyelitis, and leukemia.

In this boy, acute leukemia was suggested by the results of a complete blood count that showed: hemoglobin, 0.82 mmol/L (5.3 g/dL); hematocrit, 0.159 (15.9%); platelet count, 20 x 10^9/L (20 x 10^3/mcL); and white blood cell (WBC) count, 4.8 x 10^9/L (4.8 x 10^3/mcL). Examination of the peripheral smear demonstrated the presence of blast cells. A bone marrow biopsy confirmed the diagnosis of acute lymphoblastic leukemia (ALL).

Acute leukemia is the most common cancer of childhood, accounting for nearly one third of all malignancies in the pediatric population. It is diagnosed in nearly 3,000 children annually, and the incidence seems to be increasing. ALL represents approximately 80% of cases of acute leukemia; acute myeloid leukemia (AML) represents 15% to 20%. The disease most often affects children between the ages of 3 and 5 years and is more common among boys than girls (1.2:1) and among white than nonwhite children (1.8:1).

The cause of acute leukemia has yet to be determined, but like most childhood cancers, it has a strong genetic component. Siblings of children who have ALL are at an increased risk of developing the disease. Children who have chromosomal abnormalities and fragility syndromes, such as trisomy 21, Bloom syndrome, Fanconi anemia, ataxia-telangiectasia, and neurofibromatosis, also are at increased risk. Certain environmental factors, such as exposure to radiation, also may play a role, although a recent study has shown that exposure to electromagnetic fields, such as living near power lines, does not increase a child's risk of developing leukemia.

Presentation

ALL can present with relatively subtle, nonspecific symptoms, such as anorexia, malaise, irritability, and weight loss. More often, the child who has ALL presents with signs and symptoms associated with the failure of normal hematopoiesis, which results from the replacement of normal marrow cells by malignant cells. The child may exhibit fatigue, pallor, and decreased activity due to anemia; easy bruising and bleeding associated with thrombocytopenia; or fever and infection secondary to neutropenia. Lymphadenopathy and hepatosplenomegaly indicate the presence of extramedullary disease. Finally, as in this case, the child may present with bone pain, which is caused by the rapid expansion of leukemic cells within the marrow space. Young children may present with a limp or refuse to walk, as this child did.

Differential Diagnosis

The differential diagnosis of leukemia includes infection, rheumatologic disease, and other hematologic diseases, such as aplastic anemia. Other pediatric cancers involving the bone marrow may present with similar signs and symptoms, especially lymphoma and neuroblastoma. The diagnosis usually can be made on the basis of findings from the history, physical examination, and careful laboratory testing.

Evaluation

Laboratory evaluation of the child who is suspected of having leukemia should include a complete blood count; peripheral blood smear; reticulocyte count; and levels of serum electrolytes (including phosphorous and calcium), uric acid, and lactate dehydrogenase. Anemia and thrombocytopenia are noted in nearly two thirds of patients. The WBC count is normal in about 50% of cases, but approximately 20% of patients have a WBC count greater than 50×10^9/L (50×10^3/mcL). A WBC count greater than 100×10^9/L (100×10^3/mcL) is found in nearly 10% of patients and usually indicates a poor prognosis. Hyperuricemia, hyperkalemia, and hyperphosphatemia with subsequent secondary renal failure indicate the presence of tumor lysis syndrome, which occurs primarily in patients who have high WBC counts reflective of an increased tumor load.

Many patients have evidence of extramedullary disease at the time of diagnosis. In addition to hepatosplenomegaly, a mediastinal mass may be detected on chest radiography in 5% to 10% of these children. Further laboratory tests that might be helpful include a test for human immunodeficiency virus and viral titers (cytomegalovirus, varicella, Epstein-Barr virus). Blood typing and cross-matching may be needed, especially when the patient requires transfusion with blood products.

Definitive diagnosis of ALL requires a bone marrow biopsy. The presence of greater than 5% lymphoblasts is considered abnormal, but most laboratories require the presence of a minimum of 25% lymphoblasts to establish the diagnosis of leukemia. Morphologic assessment is performed with special staining techniques. Immunocytochemical and cytogenetic testing should be performed and may assist in establishing a prognosis.

Treatment

The initial treatment of a child who has ALL includes aggressive intravenous hydration, alkalinization, and therapy with allopurinol to minimize or prevent tumor lysis syndrome, which may occur either before or during the first 5 days of chemotherapy. Blood products should be used with caution; when possible, cytomegalovirus-negative, irradiated products should be used. If the child is febrile and appears ill, blood cultures should be obtained and treatment with systemic antibiotics started.

In the past few decades, advances in the treatment of ALL have improved the overall prognosis greatly. Patients are placed into high-, intermediate-, or low-risk groups, and their chemotherapy protocols are adjusted accordingly. With available management, long-term disease-free survival has improved to approximately 60% to 70%.

Derek S. Wheeler, MD, United States Naval Hospital, Guam

Fever, Irritability, and Refusal to Breastfeed

PRESENTATION

A 6-day-old girl is brought into the clinic having a 12-hour history of fever to 101° F (38.3° C), irritability, and refusal to breastfeed. The child's mother is a bright, articulate woman who is very concerned about providing the best for this baby, her first, and is dedicated to breastfeeding. She notes that the child previously had been "a very good baby"—quiet, pleasant, and nondisruptive. Since birth, the child has slept for much of the day and night, awakening every 5 to 7 hours to feed. The baby usually wets her diapers after each feeding. However, her mother says that the last wet diaper was noted 6 hours ago, and it was barely wet.

Upon physical examination, the child appears quiet but awake. She is forceful in refusing to feed when her mother attempts to nurse her. Her oral mucous membranes are dry and tears are absent; skin turgor is decreased. Blood is drawn for a complete blood count and electrolyte levels, and an evaluation for sepsis is initiated.

What is your differential diagnosis at this point?
Are there any elements of history or physical examination that would help you?
What additional diagnostic studies would you like performed?

DISCUSSION

At the time of evaluation, the baby weighed 2,300 g, which was 555 g (19%) below her weight at discharge 4 days ago. Her serum sodium level was 159 mmol/L (159 mEq/L), and her blood urea nitrogen was 14.28 mmol urea/L (40 mEq/L), with a serum creatinine level of 53.14 mcmol/L (0.6 mg/dL). Results of the complete blood count were normal.

Presentation

This case demonstrates how hypernatremia may be mistaken for sepsis. Poor feeding in an infant is a nonspecific complaint. Closer examination of this case, however, reveals details typical of hypernatremia of infancy. These babies usually are affected before 20 days of age and lack a history of prenatal or early neonatal problems. The mother often is a primigravida who is intelligent and strongly motivated to breastfeed. The mother may observe low milk secretion or, as in this case, she may be misled into believing that her child is receiving adequate nutrition. The infant's sleepy behavior frequently is mistaken for contentment; only a perceived change in her baby's behavior may lead the mother to suspect that something is amiss. Weight loss and poor skin turgor suggest dehydration; the child not being near shock despite such marked weight loss suggests hypernatremia.

The apparent discrepancy between the infant's appearance and her degree of dehydration can be accounted for by the distribution of sodium in the body. Extracellular fluid and plasma contain a higher concentration of sodium than does intracellular fluid. When hypernatremia is due to loss of or inadequate consumption of free water, the volume of extracellular fluid and plasma is maintained at the expense of intracellular fluid. The skin, thus, takes on a characteristic "doughy" feel, and shock is infrequent.

Loss of intracellular volume in brain cells causes central nervous system (CNS) dysfunction and may result in permanent sequelae. CNS involvement is manifested early as lethargy or irritability and may progress to coma, spasticity, seizures, and death. Brain hemorrhage may result from shrinkage of brain cells and engorgement of cerebral vessels caused by fluid shifts.

Therapy

Therapy for hypernatremic dehydration is aimed at repletion of fluid deficits and prevention of brain cell overdehydration. If rehydration is too rapid, cerebral edema may result. Thus, repletion of fluid deficits should be slow, at least over a 48-hour period and not exceeding 50 mL/kg per 24 hours.

Etiology

In the case of this infant, hypernatremia was caused primarily by insufficient fluid intake. Another contributing factor was the relatively high sodium content of the mother's milk, which was measured at 64 mmol/L (64 mEq/L). An increased sodium concentration in maternal milk usually is the result of insufficient lactation. The sodium content of maternal milk typically drops as breastfeeding progresses, with colostrum reported to average 22 mmol/L (22 mEq/L) and mature milk averaging 7 mmol/L (7 mEq/L) at 2 to 3 weeks. When maternal milk is salty because of insufficient lactation, frequent pumping may lower the sodium content, allowing resumption of lactation.

This case illustrates both causes of hypernatremia: excess ingestion of sodium and insufficient intake of water. Hypernatremia is more common in the newborn infant, who is slower to excrete the sodium load. Among children and adults, excess ingestion of sodium most commonly is iatrogenic, the result of improperly prepared formula or rehydration solution or of excessive sodium bicarbonate administration in the course of a resuscitation. Hypernatremia due to water deficit is more common and may result from diabetes insipidus, diabetes mellitus, excessive sweating, or water losses secondary to primary renal disease or diarrhea. In all cases, correcting the electrolyte disturbance slowly is the rule.

Lesson for the Clinician

This unusual complication of breastfeeding often can be avoided by careful monitoring of a baby's weight and the mother's history and should not discourage mothers from full breastfeeding.

Mary D. Dvorak, MD, Loring Air Force Base, ME

Imcomprehensible Mumbling and Inability to Follow Commands

PRESENTATION

A 9-year-old Native American boy is brought to the emergency department because of bizarre behaviors. He was acting normally at dinner, but at 10:00 PM he was found wandering, picking at things in the air, mumbling incomprehensibly, and unable to follow commands.

On physical examination, the child is unable to engage in meaningful conversation and cannot give any reliable information. His oral temperature is $37.6°C$ ($99.6°F$), pulse is 129 beats/min, respiratory rate is 24 breaths/min, and blood pressure is 141/90 mm Hg. There are no signs of head trauma. Neurologic examination is limited by his lack of cooperation. His pupils are equal in size, round, and reactive to light. He moves all extremities spontaneously and symmetrically, but his gait is unsteady. Patellar and biceps reflexes are 1+ bilaterally. Following discovery of dried perianal blood, examination reveals a dilated anus with decreased sphincter tone and a deep perianal tear. A stool sample is guaiac-positive.

Normal test results are found on measurement of serum electrolyte and blood glucose levels, blood chemistry screen, urine screen for drugs that affect the central nervous system, and complete blood count. Arterial blood gases on 2 L/min of supplemental oxygen are: pH, 7.34; Po_2, 143 torr; and Pco_2, 42.6 torr. Serum levels of salicylate, acetaminophen, and alcohol are 2.8 mg/dL, 2 mcg/mL, and 1 mg/dL, respectively. A computed tomographic scan of the head reveals no abnormalities. Cerebrospinal fluid is normal. Subsequent laboratory studies and additional history reveal the cause of his clinical condition.

What is your differential diagnosis at this point?
Are there any elements of history or physical examination that would help you?
What additional diagnostic studies would you like performed?

DISCUSSION

Differential Diagnosis

The differential diagnosis of this patient's acute mental status changes includes intracranial processes (encephalitis, hemorrhage, infarction), metabolic disturbances (hypoglycemia, hyperammonemia, hyperthyroidism), psychiatric disorders (schizophrenia, drug withdrawal), and drug ingestion (sympathomimetics, lysergic acid, anticholinergics). In the emergency department, he was given 25 g of activated charcoal, intravenous fluids, and lorazepam. The boy had three episodes of jerking movements lasting only 15 sec each that were believed to be seizures. He was given a loading dose of phenytoin, but ketamine also was required to control his movements while he was undergoing the head scan.

Laboratory Evaluation

After admission to the pediatric intensive care unit, a comprehensive urine drug screen performed with thin layer chromatography was reported as being positive for diphenhydramine. The patient admitted to taking 15 25-mg diphenhydramine tablets in an attempt to kill himself after being sodomized by members of a local gang. His mental status gradually returned to normal over the next 12 hours.

Diphenhydramine is a competitive H_1-histamine receptor blocker that has multiple effects on the central and peripheral nervous systems. It is an active ingredient in many over-the-counter (OTC) medications, including antiallergy, sedative, hypnotic, and sleep preparations. Diphenhydramine is absorbed rapidly from the gastrointestinal tract without any gastric irritation. Peak blood and tissue levels are achieved within 2 hours of ingestion.

Presentation
The most common adverse reaction to diphenhydramine at therapeutic doses is impaired consciousness. The predominant features in an overdose are anticholinergic effects, which include fever, mydriasis, blurred vision, dry mouth, constipation, urinary retention, tachycardia, dystonia, and confusion. Other common symptoms of diphenhydramine poisoning include catatonic stupor, anxiety, and visual hallucinations. Among rare presentations are respiratory insufficiency, rhabdomyolysis, cardiac rhythm disturbances, and seizures. Some complications, such as hyperpyrexia, seizures, arrhythmia, rhabdomyolysis, and coma, can develop quickly. This patient demonstrated many symptoms of diphenhydramine toxicity, including hypertension, tachycardia, tachypnea, confusion, seizures, and hallucination.

Treatment
In approximately 90% of cases of diphenhydramine overdose, anticholinergic signs and symptoms and seizures are the predominant features, and general supportive measures form the mainstay of therapy. If there is a strong clinical suspicion that a patient has taken an overdose of an anticholinergic agent, a single dose of physostigmine can be given. If symptoms resolve with this treatment, the clinician might be able to spare the patient a computed tomographic scan or lumbar puncture because trauma or infection would be far less likely causes of those symptoms.

Anticholinergic signs due to other causes, such as encephalitis, may improve marginally following the administration of physostigmine. Consequently, clinical improvement following physostigmine administration is not pathognomonic of overdose with an anticholinergic agent. Because physostigmine may cause cholinergic toxicity, including arrhythmia and seizures, it should be used only in a controlled, monitored setting.

There is the potential for severe cardiovascular collapse following massive intentional overdoses, and one of the manifestations is a wide QRS complex, as seen in patients who take overdoses of tricyclic antidepressants.

Induced emesis and gastric lavage usually do not play significant roles in treatment. Activated charcoal may be very effective in lowering serum levels of diphenhydramine and should be administered. The extent to which serum levels are reduced depends on a number of factors, including the effect of diphenhydramine on slowing gastric emptying, and can vary from 0 to 100% in a given patient.

Follow-up
Most diphenhydramine overdoses among adolescents and adults are intentional.

Accidental overdoses are more common in younger patients. Nonetheless, it is important to question children as young as 5 years of age carefully about suicidal intent if they have taken an excessive amount of medication. This patient admitted to attempting suicide after being molested. Although he later denied being raped by gang members, the boy failed to identify anyone else as the perpetrator. Law enforcement agents and the Child Protective Services (CPS) were contacted to investigate the sexual abuse. The child's family had had contact with both the police and CPS. A psychiatric consultant in the hospital felt that the child would be traumatized further by foster care. Although the perpetrator remains at large, the boy was discharged home, to be followed by CPS. Psychological counseling was offered to the child, but his parents refused the service.

Lesson for the Clinician

Because diphenhydramine is a common component of many OTC medications, the possibility of overdose with this drug should be considered whenever a patient presents with acute mental status changes.

Cindy Duke, MD, Mary Rimsza, MD, Maricopa Medical Center, University of Arizona College of Medicine, Phoenix, AZ

Abrupt Syncope Leading to a Car Crash

PRESENTATION

While driving to work, a 17-year-old high school senior who has been in good health has an abrupt syncopal episode that results in a head-on collision at 40 mph. She is alert and oriented right after the accident, but complains of sternal pain as well as pain in her left chest, left shoulder, and the right side of her jaw. Evaluation in the emergency department reveals slight tachypnea at 26 breaths/min, blood pressure of 90/60 mm Hg, a midsternal abrasion, a left pneumothorax, and nondisplaced fractures of the left clavicle and right mandible. Results of her neurologic examination, including mental status, are normal.

She denies the use of any medication, street drugs, or alcohol, but she does report a 9-month history of brief spells of lightheadedness, diaphoresis, nausea, and visual blackouts, with one previous episode proceeding to complete syncope. The episodes can be terminated by lying down. She reports neither presyncopal palpitations nor confusion after the events. These spells typically occur only during the 24-hour period preceding the onset of her menses, which are irregular but not heavy. Her last menstrual period was 35 days before the present event. Her mother had similar spells as a teenager, but there is no family history of arrhythmias or sudden unexpected premature cardiovascular death. The entire family eats a low-fat diet and uses very little salt.

A chest tube is inserted, and the jaw is fixed in place with arch bars. Further evaluation reveals a hematocrit of 0.38 (38%), normal electrolyte levels, normal findings on electrocardiography and Holter cardiac monitoring, negative results on a urine toxicology screen and pregnancy test, and normal findings on electroencephalography. Her menses begin 16 hours after the accident.

What is your differential diagnosis at this point?
Are there any elements of history or physical examination that would help you?
What additional diagnostic studies would you like performed?

DISCUSSION

Diagnosis

Six weeks after her accident, this young woman underwent a head-upright tilt study. Nine minutes into the procedure, she developed bradycardia, hypotension, and syncope, supporting the diagnosis of neurally mediated syncope (NMS), otherwise known as vasovagal or vasodepressor syncope.

As many as 30% of people experience at least one fainting episode at some time in their lives. NMS is the leading etiology of fainting in the pediatric age group, and variations in the clinical pattern occur. Fainting frequently causes anxiety in patients, their families, and practitioners, partly because syncope may be perceived as a harbinger of sudden death.

The common faint usually is benign. If, however, the prodrome (lightheadedness, a sensation of warmth, diaphoresis, nausea, visual and auditory changes) is brief or absent, there is insufficient warning to allow the patient to alter his or her posture. As a consequence, injuries may occur to the patient or others, especially if the patient is driving. The shorter the presyncopal phase, the greater the likelihood of injury. Most syncope in young people occurs in adolescents who are in an erect, relatively stationary position. However, at least 5% of syncopal episodes develop while the patient is sitting, most commonly in the classroom but occasionally behind the wheel of a car.

The diagnosis of NMS usually can be established by a detailed history of events and symptoms immediately prior to, during, and following the episode. It is important to know what position the patient was in at the time of syncope, in what activity he or she was engaged, and how long he or she was doing it. Lightheadedness, a sensation of warmth, diaphoresis, nausea, visual darkening or loss, and either a diminution in hearing or a roaring sound are frequent presyncopal symptoms, indicating the need to assume a supine position. Failure of these symptoms to abate when the patient lies down should increase the suspicion of arrhythmia, another important cause of syncope. In general, palpitations, especially a forceful tachycardia, are uncommon in pediatric NMS. Bystanders usually report marked pallor.

Differential Diagnosis
Occasionally, brief tonic-clonic movements with or without incontinence may occur, particularly if the affected person does not assume a supine position quickly. Such findings may raise the suspicion of a seizure disorder. The best discriminating feature between syncope and a seizure is the status of the patient immediately following the event. Although complaints of fatigue, nausea, and headache are common after syncope, fainting victims invariably are immediately alert and oriented, in contrast to the typical postictal state of confusion seen in individuals who have just had a generalized seizure.

Evaluation
To investigate further the possibility of a cardiac rhythm disturbance, a comprehensive family history should be obtained in anyone who faints, focusing especially on the occurrence of sudden death in young relatives, arrhythmias, and atypical syncope. In as many as 30% of patients who have NMS, there is a history of similar fainting episodes in a first-degree relative.

A complete physical examination should be performed, but typically results are normal, including the absence of orthostatic changes in vital signs. When an adolescent patient stands, findings of an erect diastolic blood pressure of less than 80 mm Hg, a decrease in systolic pressure of greater than 30 mm Hg, or an increase in pulse rate of greater than 30 beats/min may indicate the presence of mild dehydration or, less likely, acute anemia. An electrocardiogram should be obtained to rule out prolongation of the QT interval, left ventricular hypertrophy, Wolff-Parkinson-White syndrome, or a high grade of atrioventricular block. A pregnancy test and drug screen should be considered. Electroencephalography and cranial computed tomography have extremely low yields in the presence of a normal neurologic examination. Blood glucose determinations are of no value unless the patient remains obtunded or the prodrome is markedly prolonged.

On the other hand, if a prodrome is absent, if significant injury has occurred, if syncope occurs during (not immediately after) exercise, or if there is a family history of unexpected and early sudden death, referral to a pediatric cardiologist is appropriate. Further investigation might include Holter monitoring, event recording, or tilt table testing. Occasionally, echocardiography is indicated. Rarely, an electrophysiologic study or coronary angiography will be appropriate. A gold standard test for NMS is not available, but head-upright tilt table testing may reproduce the patient's symptoms and help confirm the diagnosis. Tilt studies should be interpreted cautiously because false-positive results do occur, especially when isoproterenol is used to evoke syncope.

Orthostatic stress (standing, sitting) is a more common provocative stimulus for adolescent NMS than stressful events such as phlebotomy or minor injury. Typically the teenager has been standing or sitting for several minutes before syncope develops. A subclinical degree of dehydration, as may occur after exercise, with mild dieting, or after estrogen withdrawal, may enhance the tendency to faint. Children and teenagers now are following their parents' example of limiting their salt intake, but for active adolescents, such habits may result in a marginal sodium intake, which could be a cause of syncope. This concept is supported by the fact that most orthostatically induced NMS responds readily to transient augmentation of salt intake.

Treatment

Appropriate initial therapy of NMS is, in fact, an increase in dietary sodium (1 g/d or 500 mg BID), usually in the form of salt tablets, because many adolescents find table salt unpalatable. If symptoms improve but do not resolve when salt is added, fludrocortisone acetate (0.1 mg/d) may be added to enhance sodium retention. Blood pressure should be measured weekly for 1 month. It is not necessary to increase fluid intake because increased drinking automatically will follow augmentation of dietary salt. An alternative approach is the use of beta-adrenergic blockers, which should be discussed in consultation with a pediatric cardiologist.

The young woman described in this report did have a low sodium intake. Diuresis following estrogen withdrawal was thought to be an additional factor causing her symptoms, all of which occurred immediately prior to menstruation. She was treated with sodium tablets and fludrocortisone acetate, but also was put on low-dose estrogen oral contraceptives to regulate her menstrual cycles, so that her period of risk could be defined more accurately. No further episodes of presyncope or syncope have occurred during 2 years of follow-up. Six months after her accident she resumed driving. Her fludrocortisone has been discontinued, but she continues to take salt tablets.

J. Peter Harris, MD, Carol J. Buzzard, MD, University of Rochester School of Medicine and Dentistry, Rochester, NY

Bleeding Spider Angioma on Face and Elevated Liver Enzyme Levels

PRESENTATION

An 8-year-old Norwegian girl is seen by a dermatologist because of a bleeding spider angioma on her face and similar lesions on her neck and arm. Further evaluation reveals elevated levels of liver enzymes, and he refers her to you. The child has lost weight recently and has seemed weak to her parents. She is not taking medication and has traveled only in southern Europe. There is no family history of liver disease.

Findings on physical examination include the spider angiomas, mild jaundice, several enlarged cervical lymph nodes, a palpable liver edge 5 cm below the right costal margin, and a palpable spleen edge 4 cm below the left costal margin. There are no signs of ascites or impaired mental status.

Results of laboratory evaluation are: hemoglobin, 1.55 mmol/L (10 g/dL); erythrocyte sedimentation rate, 40 mm/h; albumin, 45 g/L (4.5 mcg/dL); total bilirubin, 47.6 mcmol/L (2.8 mg/dL); unconjugated bilirubin, 13.6 mcmol/L (0.8 mg/dL); aspartate aminotransferase, 759 U/L; alanine aminotransferase, 659 U/L; lactic dehydrogenase, 533 U/L; alkaline phosphatase, 560 U/L; gamma glutamyl transferase, 115 U/L; and immunoglobulin G, 35 g/L (350 mg/dL) (upper limit of normal, 15.5 g/L [1,550 mg/dL]). Ceruloplasmin, copper, and alpha-1-antitrypsin levels are normal. Serologic tests for hepatitis A, B, and C yield negative results, as does testing for antinuclear and antimitochondrial antibodies. Anti-smooth muscle antibodies are present.

The diagnosis is established by a biopsy.

What is your differential diagnosis at this point?
Are there any elements of history or physical examination that would help you?
What additional diagnostic studies would you like performed?

DISCUSSION

Diagnosis

Liver biopsy showed moderate-to-severe portal, periportal, and lobular inflammation; periportal and septal fibrosis; and early changes of cirrhosis. The portal areas showed dilatation and infiltration by lymphocytes, plasma cells, and granulocytes. Areas of piecemeal necrosis were noted in portal areas. The histologic changes in the liver, positive titers of anti-smooth muscle antibodies, and blood chemistry changes confirmed the diagnosis of chronic autoimmune hepatitis.

Chronic autoimmune hepatitis is a rare condition that occurs most commonly in adult women. Although relatively rare in the first decade of life, it can affect individuals of both genders from infancy to old age. A genetically determined defect in immunoregulation involving suppressor T cells is believed to play a part in the pathogenesis.

Presentation

This child presented a common clinical picture, experiencing weight loss, weakness, jaundice, and hepatosplenomegaly. Spider angiomas can develop, as in her case, but it is unusual for them to bleed. Palmar erythema also can occur. She had elevated liver enzyme concentrations, which is typical, as is hypergammaglobulinemia. Levels of immunoglobulin G often exceed 20 g/dL (2,000 mg/dL) in this condition; total globulin levels usually are greater than 4 g/L (400 mg/dL).

Patients who have chronic autoimmune hepatitis may develop anti-smooth muscle antibodies, as this child did, or anti-liver-kidney microsomal antibodies, which are associated with a poorer prognosis. Thyroid antibodies may be present, and thyroiditis can be part of the syndrome. Rheumatoid factor also can be found, and some patients present with arthritis, which can precede the liver disease (see Index of suspicion. *Pediatr Rev.* 1999;20:29-31). Coombs-positive hemolytic anemia may occur. Vasculitis, nephritis, amenorrhea, and acne may be associated extrahepatic conditions.

In addition to appreciating the specific features of autoimmune hepatitis, the clinician making this diagnosis must rule out other hepatic disorders, including viral infections and extrahepatic causes of biliary obstruction. It should be noted that a similar clinical picture may result from therapy with certain drugs, including nitrofurantoin, isoniazid, and methyldopa.

Some patients who have autoimmune hepatitis can be in an asymptomatic phase, and the condition might be detected only on the basis of abnormal liver function tests, making it important to take seriously the presence of elevated liver enzymes discovered during the clinical evaluation of any condition. The interval between the development of initial symptoms and diagnosis can be long because the clinical manifestations can be so vague.

Treatment

Treatment of autoimmune hepatitis should begin as soon as the diagnosis is confirmed. Immunosuppressive therapy reduces morbidity and prolongs survival. The primary therapeutic principle is to suppress or eliminate inflammation with a minimum of adverse effects. Prednisone is administered initially at a dosage of 2 mg/kg per day (not to exceed 60 mg/d), then is reduced slowly, to minimize side effects, to a level that will maintain normal levels of transaminases. Azathioprine may be added to achieve control and keep the steroid dosage to a minimum. In some cases, cyclosporine has been used when other therapy has not been satisfactory.

For patients in whom the process has become inactive, gradual withdrawal of drug therapy should be attempted while monitoring liver enzyme and autoantibody levels. It is a very rare patient, however, who will tolerate complete withdrawal of immunosuppressive therapy without a clinical or biochemical flare-up. Once cirrhosis develops, liver enzyme levels may revert to normal; at that point, therapy is of questionable value.

Prognosis

The prognosis for patients who have autoimmune hepatitis depends on whether cirrhosis has developed at the time of diagnosis. The 10-year survival for those who have cirrhosis when diagnosed is 65% compared with 98% among those who do not have cirrhosis. As many as 80% of patients will relapse despite adequate treatment and eventually may develop cirrhosis. Liver transplantation is indicated in those who progress to end-stage liver disease.

Chandra S. Devulapalli, MD, University Hospital of Trondhiem, Trondheim, Norway

Fever, Diarrhea, and Vomiting

PRESENTATION

A 4 ½-year-old boy is brought to the emergency department because of fever and diarrhea. Three weeks ago he returned from Pakistan, where he had experienced a week of diarrhea. Watery diarrhea recurred 2 weeks ago and contained neither blood nor mucus. One week ago, the diarrhea diminished in frequency, but he began to have diffuse abdominal pain that later localized to the right upper quadrant. Fever has been present for 12 days, peaking at 38.8°C (101.8°F). He has eaten poorly and has lost 1.8 kg in 2 weeks. In the last 24 hours he has experienced chills, nausea, and nonbilious vomiting.

On physical examination, the boy appears hydrated and does not look toxic. His oral temperature is 41°C (105.8°F), pulse rate is 108 beats/min, respiratory rate is 40 breaths/min, and blood pressure is 100/50 mm Hg. His throat is slightly hyperemic, and cervical and inguinal lymph nodes smaller than 2.0 cm are noted. His abdomen is soft and nondistended with normal bowel sounds. No abdominal masses or organs are felt.

Results of laboratory studies include: white blood cell count, 4.8 x 10⁹/L (4.8 x 10³/mcL) with 57% neutrophils and 37% lymphocytes; hematocrit, 0.35 (35%); platelet count, 120 x 10⁹/L (120 x 10³/mcL); serum sodium, 144 mmol/L (144 mEq/L); potassium, 3.2 mmol/L (3.2 mEq/L); chloride, 98 mmol/L (98 mEq/L); bicarbonate, 21 mmol/L (21 mEq/L); creatinine, 35.4 mcmol/L (0.4 mg/dL); bilirubin, 5.13 mcmol/L (0.3 mg/dL); alanine aminotransferase, 98 U/L; and erythrocyte sedimentation rate, 61 mm/h. Results of urinalysis and abdominal radiography are normal.

A blood test confirms the diagnosis.

What is your differential diagnosis at this point?
Are there any elements of history or physical examination that would help you?
What additional diagnostic studies would you like performed?

DISCUSSION

Diagnosis

The child was admitted to the hospital, where further testing was performed. Stool examination revealed no ova or parasites. Blood smears for malaria and serologic testing for hepatitis were negative. Two days after admission, a blood culture was growing *Salmonella typhi*. The organism was reported to be sensitive to ampicillin, which was administered to the boy. His temperature began to decline after 2 days of therapy and was back to normal on the sixth day of treatment. His symptoms improved, and he was discharged 9 days after admission on oral amoxicillin for a total course of 14 days.

Typhoid fever is an acute systemic illness characterized by prolonged fever, sustained bacteremia, and multiplication of bacteria within the mononuclear phagocytic cells of the liver, spleen, lymph nodes, and Peyer patches. Although encountered in all parts of the world, the infection is found primarily in developing countries. The organism is acquired by ingestion of contaminated food or water.

Presentation

The incubation period of typhoid fever usually is 7 to 14 days, with a range of 3 to 30 days. At the beginning of the incubation period, 10% to 20% of patients will have transient diarrhea. The diarrhea this boy experienced in Pakistan most likely was due to this phenomenon, shortly after he had ingested the bacteria. At the end of the incubation period, other signs and symptoms become manifest and include fever, headache, malaise, sore throat, anorexia, nausea, diarrhea, abdominal pain, and myalgias. Diarrhea is a more common occurrence in young children than in adults. Constipation also may be present in the early part of the illness.

A relative bradycardia, in which the pulse rate is lower than would be expected for the height of the fever, is a common physical finding that occurred in this patient. A maculopapular rash on the upper abdomen and chest (rose spots) is present in 50% of patients; this boy did not have a rash.

At the time of admission, most patients will have normocytic, normochromic anemia, an elevated erythrocyte sedimentation rate, and a platelet count in the range of 150 x 10^9/L (150 x 10^3/mcL). The white blood cell count frequently is low. Mild hyponatremia and hypokalemia also can occur, and the alanine aminotransferase and aspartate aminotransferase levels commonly are elevated. Blood cultures are positive in about 80% of patients, and culture of bone marrow identifies the organism in 85% to 90% of individuals, making bone marrow aspirate the very best source of culture material if the blood culture is negative. The classic Widal test, a serologic test for *Salmonella* agglutinins, is reported to have many false-positive and false-negative results and should not be used as a diagnostic test for typhoid fever.

Treatment

Antibiotics often shorten the course of typhoid fever and reduce the rate of complications, although clinicians should realize that the fever generally will begin to abate only after 2 days of therapy, and a normal temperature is not reached for 5 to 7 days. Chloramphenicol remains the antibiotic used most widely, but ampicillin, trimethoprim-sulfamethoxazole (TMP-SMX), third-generation cephalosporins, and quinolones also are effective. A 14-day course of treatment usually is recommended. Ampicillin-resistant strains have been documented worldwide, and *Salmonella* organisms resistant to ampicillin, chloramphenicol, and TMP-SMX have been isolated from individuals visiting the Indian subcontinent. For these patients, third-generation cephalosporins or quinolones offer optimal therapy.

Complications of typhoid fever include intestinal perforation and hemorrhage. Some patients evolve into a carrier state. In 5% to 15% of those who have typhoid fever, a relapse will occur about 1 week after therapy is completed. These patients respond well to a second course of therapy; the relapse does not mean that the original selection of antimicrobial agent was inappropriate.

Lesson for the Clinician

In this case, the presence of unremitting fever in a child who recently had been in a developing country was a pattern that suggested typhoid fever as a potential diagnosis.

Luis Arturo Batres, MD, Ronald Marino, DO, MPH, Winthrop-University

Cough, Progressive Shortness of Breath, and Weight Loss

PRESENTATION

A 7-year-old boy is admitted to the hospital because of a 2-month illness consisting of cough, progressive shortness of breath, loss of appetite, and weight loss. Two years ago he was admitted for a similar illness, which was diagnosed as miliary tuberculosis and was treated with four drugs. Both symptoms and radiographic findings resolved completely. There had been a possible previous exposure to tuberculosis on a visit to Pakistan.

On physical examination, the child looks well and is afebrile.

Auscultation reveals bilateral wheezing and diffuse rales. Cardiac and abdominal examinations yield normal findings. The boy requires 28% oxygen by mask to maintain pulse oximetry readings above 95%.

Results of a complete blood count are normal, but his erythrocyte sedimentation rate is 25 mm/h. A radiograph of his chest shows diffuse bilateral interstitial infiltrates and a normal cardiac silhouette. Computed tomography of the chest shows fine micronodularity and interstitial infiltrates. A purified protein derivative skin test and anergy panel yield negative results, but an enzyme-linked immunosorbent assay (ELISA) test for human immunodeficiency virus (HIV) is positive. Immunoglobulin levels are: IgG, 22.23 g/L (2,223 mg/dL) (normal, 6.3 to 15.5 g/L [630 to 1,550 mg/dL]); IgE, 27.98 g/L (2,798 mg/dL) (normal, 0.058 to 2.16 g/L [5.8 to 216 mg/dL]); IgA, 2.07 g/L (207 mg/dL) (normal, 0.68 to 3.79 g/L [68 to 379 mg/dL]); and IgM, 2.76 g/L (276 mg/dL) (normal, 0.46 to 2.68 g/L [46 to 268 mg/dL]).

Additional laboratory findings and history lead to the diagnosis.

What is your differential diagnosis at this point?
Are there any elements of history or physical examination that would help you?
What additional diagnostic studies would you like performed?

DISCUSSION

Differential Diagnosis

On admission, the differential diagnosis of this child's illness included atypical pneumonia (viral or mycoplasmal) and lymphoid interstitial pneumonia (LIP). Antibodies to *Mycoplasma* were not found, and the prolonged course of the disease made an atypical pneumonia unlikely. LIP is a condition found in patients who are infected with HIV. The characteristic radiograph seen in LIP shows bilateral interstitial infiltrates, as in this child. The positive ELISA test raised the suspicion of LIP even further, and the results of an open biopsy of the lung also were read as being consistent with that condition. However, a Western blot test for HIV was negative.

Because the serum immunoglobulin levels were elevated, the possibility of a hypersensitivity pneumonitis was considered. The child was treated with corticosteroids and improved dramatically. He was discharged from the hospital and on follow-up examination 2 weeks later was completely asymptomatic. His chest radiograph showed marked improvement as well.

While chatting with the physician, the child's father mentioned that the next door neighbor breeds pigeons and keeps about 200 birds. The child goes there every day to play. Serum from the patient was analyzed, and antibodies against pigeon serum were found. Six months later, no antibodies to pigeon serum were detectable. In retrospect, the child's improvement during his first hospitalization appears to have been related to his removal from the pigeons.

Diagnosis

Hypersensitivity pneumonitis, or extrinsic allergic alveolitis, is uncommon in children. A detailed description of the environment, a history of exposure to antigens, distinct clinical features, characteristic radiologic findings, and the presence of antibodies in the serum are the critical elements in making the diagnosis. Hypersensitivity pneumonitis is caused by an immunologically mediated reaction to inhaled antigenic particles of less than 10 microns in diameter. These antigens include mold spores, bacterial products, avian droppings, and other proteins of animal origin.

Presentation

The acute stage of the disease is characterized by cough, fever, a tight feeling in the chest, and body aches. Symptoms appear 4 to 8 weeks after exposure to the offending antigen, and the illness can be mistaken for influenza or atypical pneumonia. Histologically, the alveolar wall is infiltrated with inflammatory cells, neutrophils, plasma cells, and macrophages. The alveolar spaces are filled with proteinaceous exudate and inflammatory cells.

A subacute stage can follow in which the patient manifests cough, dyspnea, anorexia, and weight loss. In this stage, noncaseating granulomas are found scattered throughout the lung parenchyma, and there is interstitial infiltration by lymphocytes, plasma cells, and histiocytes. As in the case of the child presented, the patient may improve after admission to the hospital because he or she has been removed from the antigen exposure.

The disease may progress to a chronic state in which the granulomatous alveoli are replaced by interstitial fibrosis. The normal lung architecture is destroyed, and the lungs take on a honeycomb appearance. The patient may develop cor pulmonale, manifesting progressive dyspnea, cyanosis, and clubbing.

An interesting feature of this child's clinical situation was the positive ELISA test for HIV. False-positive ELISA tests are seen in patients receiving hemodialysis and in those having autoimmune disorders, multiple myeloma, and hemophilia. The finding has not been documented previously in patients having hypersensitivity pneumonitis.

In the face of the positive test for HIV, consideration of the possibility of LIP is very reasonable. Although the histopathology may be consistent with a number of predominantly interstitial processes, hypersensitivity pneumonitis is characterized by positive immunofluorescence of immunoglobulin and complement in addition to the mixed lymphocytic cellular infiltrate and alveolar proteinaceous fluid.

LIP, on the other hand, is not associated with an alveolar component or positive immunofluorescence, but with an intensely lymphocytic interstitial infiltrate, as well as the rare presence of histiocytes, plasma cells, and giant cells.

Treatment
Treatment of hypersensitivity pneumonitis consists of removal from the offending agent and short-term corticosteroid therapy.

*Melodi Karakurum, MD, Brinda Doraswamy, MD, S. Sagar Bennuri, MD,
The Brooklyn Hospital Center, Brooklyn, NY*

Dull Back Pain and Difficulty Playing

PRESENTATION

A 9-year-old boy is brought to your office with a 6-week history of dull, nonradiating back pain and difficulty in play; there is no history of trauma.

He says that he has had trouble running the bases and riding his bicycle. Two weeks ago he began having urinary incontinence; last week he started having fecal incontinence. Because his parents recently were divorced, he was taken to a psychologist for counseling. He has been afebrile with no other constitutional symptoms.

Physical examination reveals a well-nourished boy who is anxious but in no acute distress. Deep tendon reflexes are diminished in his knees and absent in his ankles. He has difficulty walking on his toes and heels, and his hip extension is weak. Gastrocnemius muscle strength is graded at 3/5, anterior tibialis at 4/5, and gluteus maximus at 3/5. Sensation to touch on his sole and lateral left foot is diminished. His upper extremities have normal strength and reflexes. An anal wink cannot be elicited. Over the sacrum he has a sacral dimple with a patch of hyperpigmented skin and slight tenderness; there is no apparent scoliosis or lordosis. His white blood cell count, differential count, and erythrocyte sedimentation rate are all normal.

What is your differential diagnosis at this point?
Are there any elements of history or physical examination that would help you?
What additional diagnostic studies would you like performed?

DISCUSSION

Differential Diagnosis

Although pain, loss of interest in usual activities, and incontinence all can be attributed to stressful life events, other etiologies should be considered. Lower extremity weakness can occur with diseases of the muscles, peripheral nerves, spinal cord, or brain. Although "upper motor neuron" lesions of the brain and spinal cord ultimately are associated with hyperreflexia and hypertonia, they often present initially with a flaccid, areflexic pattern. This child's fecal and urinary incontinence with absent anal wink and diminished reflexes make diseases of the muscle (such as acute postviral myositis) less likely. His back pain increases the likelihood that the problem is in the spine.

Infection, trauma, tumors, and congenital malformations of the spinal column all can lead to the signs and symptoms shown by this child. Vertebral osteomyelitis, including that caused by mycobacteria, diskitis, ankylosing spondylitis, and spondylolisthesis cause back pain, but these conditions usually are not associated with weakness or loss of sensation. Inflammatory and "toxic" conditions, such as Guillain-Barré syndrome, tick-bite paralysis, peripheral neuritis, transverse myelitis, and poliomyelitis, cause paralysis, although the time course in this child is longer than would be expected with these conditions.

Masses of the spinal column can cause paralysis and back pain. These masses may be intramedullary, such as astrocytoma or ependymoma, or extramedullary. Extramedullary lesions may occur in the meninges (eg, arachnoid cyst), the nerve root (eg, neurofibroma), the epidural space (eg, neuroblastoma), the disk space (eg, herniated disk), or the bone (eg, bone cysts and osteogenic sarcoma). Congenital anomalies that may produce the symptoms described include diastematomyelia, in which a bony or cartilaginous septum divides the spinal cord; a tethered cord, in which a scar or tumor stretches the spinal cord, preventing normal movement; and an arachnoid cyst.

Diagnosis and Treatment
The sacral dimple and hyperpigmented patch make an occult neural tube defect likely in this child. Neural tube defects are associated with spinal cord tethering and tumors that include lipomas, dermoids, and epidermoids. A magnetic resonance imaging scan of this child's lumbosacral region revealed a lipoma with spina bifida occulta and tethering of the spinal cord. Following surgery, his symptoms resolved except for some weakness of hip extension.

Early diagnosis and treatment of children suspected of having a spinal cord lesion are critical to preventing progressive neurologic damage and increasing the likelihood of reversibility. The single most useful test is the magnetic resonance imaging scan with or without intravenous gadolinium. This diagnostic procedure should be followed by prompt referral to a neurosurgeon.

Gregory S. Liptak MD, University of Rochester School of Medicine and Dentistry, Rochester, New York

Terror, Screaming, and Seeing Rats

PRESENTATION

A 2-year-old boy is brought to the emergency department at 4 AM because of a fever and a 6-hour history of intermittent fits of terror and screaming, with complaints of seeing rats. He has had clear rhinorrhea for 3 days. The boy is cared for by his father, who had put him to bed that night, at which time he was acting normally. The child awoke at 11 PM, screaming in terror and pointing to the floor. The father saw nothing where the boy was pointing and found it difficult to console the child.

The boy lives with his father and is visited by his mother daily, having spent the previous afternoon with her. The only medication in the father's house is an oral hypoglycemic agent; the mother is not on any medications. The father is unaware of exposure to any medications or other substances.

On physical examination, the boy's oral temperature is 40°C (104°F), pulse is 190 beats/min, respiratory rate is 28 breaths/min, and blood pressure is 120/80 mm Hg. The child has a fluctuating mental status, at times appearing alert, calm, and playful, then displaying fits of terror, screaming and pointing at the floor. His pupils are 6 mm in diameter and constrict to 3 mm with light. There is a copious clear nasal discharge. His neck is supple without adenopathy. Cardiac examination reveals tachycardia with a normal rhythm. Neurologic evaluation documents the variable mental status and symmetric neuromuscular irritability, with myoclonic jerks noted at rest and on intentional movement.

What is your differential diagnosis at this point?
Are there any elements of history or physical examination that would help you?
What additional diagnostic studies would you like performed?

DISCUSSION

Differential Diagnosis

For any child who has fever and altered mental status, the clinician must consider an infectious etiology such as viral encephalitis or bacterial meningitis. This child's white blood cell count was 21.5×10^9/L (21.5×10^3/mcL), but his cerebrospinal fluid was normal, and a central nervous system (CNS) infection appeared unlikely. An electrocardiogram (ECG) showed only sinus tachycardia. He was given antipyretics pending the results of additional laboratory tests.

A toxic ingestion also would be part of the differential diagnosis. Diphenhydramine, antidepressants (tricyclics and serotonin reuptake inhibitors), anticholinergic agents, H_2 histamine blockers, lysergic acid diethylamide (LSD), meperidine, amphetamines, and cocaine have been reported to cause fever and psychosis when given in excess. This patient's diagnosis was established when his urine toxicology screen was reported to be positive for cocaine. When confronted, the father admitted to having stored crack cocaine in a dresser drawer.

Presentation

The toxic effects of cocaine relate primarily to the cardiovascular system and the CNS. All routes of administration—intranasal, oral, rectal, intravenous, and passive inhalation of crack cocaine—are associated with toxicity.

Initial cardiovascular symptoms include tachycardia and hypertension, which can proceed to hypotension and shock in severe cases. Arrhythmias, as well as sinus tachycardia, can occur, and an ECG is recommended in all cases of exposure to cocaine. Infarction, ischemia, hemorrhage, and vasculitis also can occur as a result of the vasoactive properties of the drug.

Mental status changes can consist of excitement, restlessness, anxiety, delirium, psychosis, tonic-clonic seizures, and coma. As demonstrated by this patient, cocaine can elevate temperature significantly.

Other effects from acute exposure include respiratory failure or arrest due to bronchospasm and pulmonary edema, gastrointestinal irritation or ischemia, hepatic dysfunction, and renal failure secondary to rhabdomyolysis and myoglobinuria.

Treatment

Treatment varies with the degree of symptomatology, ranging from supportive care to more aggressive interventions. Beta-blocking agents are not recommended for routine use because of their potential for exacerbating cardiac ischemia, but they may be used to treat life-threatening arrhythmias. Benzodiazepines, especially diazepam, may help to counter the effects of CNS excitation. Hyperpyrexia that is unresponsive to antipyretics can be life-threatening and should be treated aggressively with mechanical cooling.

Cocaine is known to have a short biologic half-life. In this patient, the suspected time of ingestion was more than 8 hours prior to presentation. His duration of symptoms led to the concern that he may have swallowed cocaine rocks that still were being absorbed from his intestinal tract. For this reason, he was given oral charcoal in the emergency department.

The boy then was admitted to the hospital and observed on a cardiac monitor. For the next 12 hours he continued to have hallucinations as well as fever to 41°C (105.8°F) that responded only minimally to antipyretics. His sinus tachycardia gradually resolved, as did his fever and mental status changes. A child protective investigation was begun while he was in the hospital. He was discharged 2 days after admission in good condition without any clinical evidence of organ damage or ischemia.

Lesson for the Clinician

One additional clinical point worth noting is that children who have high fever, even if the etiology is an infectious illness that is not serious, can have hallucinations. These children, however, should revert quickly to a normal mental status when the fever is reduced and should not have the prolonged effects seen in a child who has a CNS infection or who has ingested a toxic substance. Often, the children are more lucid by the time they reach medical care. The clinician always must consider the more serious conditions first when evaluating a febrile child who manifests changes in mental status.

Margaret Colpoys, MD, University of Rochester School of Medicine and Dentistry, Rochester, NY

Developing Clumsiness in a Toddler

PRESENTATION

A mother is concerned because her 2-year-old son is "not as sure on his feet as he used to be." In the past 2 weeks she has noticed that he seems clumsy and is falling more than usual when playing or walking. His babysitter also has noticed this change in abilities, which has heightened the mother's concern. No other neurologic impairment is noted, and his play does not seem to be disrupted.

The boy's medical history is unremarkable. Recently, he had a persistent middle ear infection that finally resolved after 1 month of treatment with three different antibiotics. He also has been having 6 to 12 loose stools a day. Clostridium difficile *toxin has been isolated from his stool.*

Findings on physical examination, including neurologic evaluation, are normal except for otoscopic findings consistent with bilateral middle ear effusions.

What is your differential diagnosis at this point?
Are there any elements of history or physical examination that would help you?
What additional diagnostic studies would you like performed?

DISCUSSION

Diagnosis
Middle ear disease with associated eustachian tube dysfunction is the most likely cause of the recent balance disturbance in this boy, whose incidental gastrointestinal problem was a complication of antibiotic therapy. The presence of middle ear infection or effusion with eustachian tube dysfunction is known to be associated with frequent falls and unsteady gait in a patient who has otherwise normal findings on physical examination.

Differential Diagnosis
Vertigo is the subjective feeling of movement of self or environment and may be accompanied by nystagmus. Problems with balance can accompany vertigo. Because younger children are unable to describe their sensations, the clinician cannot know whether vertigo is present and, thus, must consider the causes of vertiginous and nonvertiginous balance disturbances in a child such as the one described in this case.

Idiopathic benign paroxysmal vertigo causes brief episodes (lasting minutes) of unsteadiness and nystagmus and is believed to be a migraine variant. Other middle ear and vestibular disorders, such as labyrinthitis, vestibular nerve inflammation, middle-to-inner ear fistula, cholesteatoma, and Ménière disease, also can cause vertigo. Central nervous system (CNS) disorders such as posterior fossa tumor, migraine, seizures, demyelinating disease (such as multiple sclerosis), infection (such as meningitis and brain abscess), and toxic ingestion can present with a balance disturbance.

Although all of these conditions can cause balance disturbances, the majority of these diagnoses typically have specific symptoms or signs. For instance, the middle ear and vestibular disorders generally are associated with nystagmus, hearing impairment, or tinnitus. A CNS tumor can cause headaches, early morning vomiting, and neurologic deficits. Migraine and seizures usually are of longer duration; migraine commonly causes headache, and seizures usually cause changes in mental status. Multiple sclerosis is very unusual in this age group and requires at least two neurologic deficits for diagnosis. Infection is associated with fever and also causes other physical findings, as does toxic ingestion.

Evaluation

The evaluation of a balance disturbance must include a detailed medical history. Ideally, the patient can describe subjective feelings, such as dizziness or sensations of motion or spinning; in younger children, parental observations are critical. Children who have true vertigo often are very reluctant to move at all, lying quite still and resisting any attempted movement by caregivers. A detailed physical examination, with emphasis on evaluation of the ears and CNS, will narrow possible causes. Pneumatic otoscopy will help detect middle ear effusion and eustachian tube dysfunction. Abnormal findings on audiometric evaluation in a cooperative child may lead to the detection of middle ear disease, Ménière disease, or a tumor.

The child's gait should be observed for signs of unsteadiness. An experienced observer may be able to distinguish the wide-based cerebellar gait from the staggering vestibular gait. Coordination tests, such as finger-to-nose, heel-to-shin, and rapid alternating movement evaluations, and testing for a Romberg sign should be done when possible to detect cerebellar disease. Nystagmus should be sought and may be elicited by a maneuver in which the patient's head is lowered 45 degrees below the level of the body on the examination table. Keep in mind that the balance disorder may be evident only at certain times, as in this child, and that neurologic function at the time of examination might be completely normal.

Other evaluations, such as caloric testing and electronystagmography, are difficult to perform on younger patients in an office. Neurologic findings may suggest the need for computed tomography, magnetic resonance imaging, electroencephalography, or lumbar puncture. Certain institutions are specially equipped to test children who have vertigo and balance disorders.

Treatment

Treatment of a balance disorder is directed at the specific cause. Consultation with an otolaryngologist or neurologist may be appropriate. Symptoms of vertigo may be relieved with rotational exercises and vestibular suppressants such as dimenhydrinate.

Linda S. Nield, MD, West Virginia University School of Medicine,
Morgantown, WV

Development of New, Different Seizure Activity

PRESENTATION

A 9-year-old boy is admitted to the hospital after having a generalized, afebrile, tonic-clonic first convulsion. He has been well except for a history of learning disabilities, otitis media, and mastoiditis. He is one of 10 children in an impoverished family. His seizure is controlled with phenytoin and he is discharged on this medication.

He is readmitted several times with complaints of dizziness, drowsiness, fears of dying, weakness, and leg pains. The only abnormal finding on physical examination is a mild right-sided ptosis that does not increase on upward gaze. Electroencephalography (EEG), magnetic resonance imaging of the brain, and all laboratory studies yield normal results. He is believed to have a paroxysmal seizure disorder with basilar migraine. The seizures recur when he has acute illnesses but are controlled eventually with valproic acid and gabapentin.

After several months, the boy develops a different type of seizure in which he sinks to the floor and apparently becomes unresponsive for about 10 minutes. His breathing is shallow, but his vital signs and pulse oximetry remain normal. He is sleepy for 10 more minutes, then acts normal.

After he recovers from what appears to be an episode of status epilepticus, he undergoes 24-hour video EEG monitoring, which reveals the diagnosis and leads to a rapid cure.

What is your differential diagnosis at this point?
Are there any elements of history or physical examination that would help you?
What additional diagnostic studies would you like performed?

DISCUSSION

Diagnosis

Over 2 weeks of monitoring, during which the boy experienced daily atonic episodes, no EEG activity consistent with seizures was seen. He was told that his video games would be taken away if he had another seizure, and the episodes ceased.

This boy was experiencing psychogenic seizures, also called pseudoseizures, which is a diagnosis of exclusion. Such seizures occur frequently among older children and adults who, like this boy, already are taking several anticonvulsants for a true seizure disorder. A pseudoseizure may resemble true generalized or partial complex seizures, but it often includes grimacing, unusual or bizarre movements, verbalizations, or other nonstereotypic activity. There is no cyanosis, incontinence, or loss of pupillary responsiveness. When this boy sank to the floor, he never injured himself, which is typical of psychogenic seizures.

An EEG during a pseudoseizure will show no electrical evidence of seizures. Unlike true seizures, serum prolactin levels are not elevated by pseudoseizures.

Associated Findings

Pseudoseizures have been compared with conversion disorders and hysteria. Patients who have pseudoseizures are likely to have other behavioral or emotional disorders. Girls are affected more often than boys. One study of adults who had pseudoseizures revealed that almost 50% of the women had been sexually abused.

Patients often achieve secondary gain from their "seizures." This patient often had his atonic spells on the school bus, making it necessary for the driver to stop the bus and come to his aid. Eventually he was provided with a home tutor. Patients who have pseudoseizures may be able to stop them on request. Studies indicate the effectiveness of behavioral approaches to pseudoseizures by using operant conditioning techniques or hypnotherapy. Patients who have pseudoseizures are suggestible to hypnosis, but the same tendency has been shown among those experiencing bona fide partial complex seizures.

Treatment
After the initial period of freedom from spells, this boy again began to have atonic episodes, which continued despite several counseling sessions, consultation with a traditional Puerto Rican healer, and a trial of relaxation mental imagery (self-hypnosis). A consulting psychiatrist suggested a trial of antidepressant medication, but the family refused. The boy continued to complain of leg and chest pains in school and walked as if out of balance, although he acted normally when greeted by his classmates.

Lesson for the Clinician
This case demonstrates the tremendous disruption that pseudoseizures can bring to the lives of a child and his family, along with unnecessary medical expense and consequent risks to the child because of inappropriately extensive evaluation and treatment. It also illustrates the difficulties in treating this disorder, with its complex linkages of mind and body. If pseudoseizures are diagnosed, psychiatric consultation usually is required. Many of these events represent conversion reactions and even if the spells stop, the patient will develop another type of symptom if the underlying emotional problems are not addressed.

When faced with a child who appears to have refractory epilepsy, the clinician should think of pseudoseizures, especially when the characteristics of the spells do not seem to fit known seizure patterns.

David Gottsegen, MD, Holyoke Pediatrics Associates, Holyoke, MA

Swollen, Erythematous Conjunctival Membranes and Discharge

PRESENTATION

A 6-week-old girl is brought to the emergency department with a 3-day history of decreased oral intake, clear rhinorrhea, and drainage from both eyes. She has been free of fever, cough, vomiting, and diarrhea. Her parents and four siblings, including her twin, all have been well.

The baby was born prematurely at 33 weeks' gestation. Her mother received little prenatal care, and the pregnancy was complicated by preterm labor and oligohydramnios. She and her twin spent approximately 3 weeks in the neonatal intensive care unit; neither developed any documented infection.

On physical examination, the baby is afebrile and does not look ill. Her weight is in the 10th percentile when corrected for her gestational age. The conjunctival membranes of both eyes are markedly swollen and erythematous. Purulent, yellow-green discharge is noted in both eyes. Slight nasal drainage is present. Red reflexes are elicited bilaterally. The remainder of the physical examination is normal.

Results of a complete blood count are normal. Careful study of the baby's conjunctival drainage yields unexpected findings.

What is your differential diagnosis at this point?
Are there any elements of history or physical examination that would help you?
What additional diagnostic studies would you like performed?

DISCUSSION

Gram stain of the baby's conjunctival drainage revealed abundant polymorphonuclear leukocytes and moderate numbers of intracellular and extracellular gram-negative diplococci, suggesting *Neisseria* sp. With the mother's history of poor prenatal care, *N gonorrhoeae* infection was suspected. Blood, urine, and cerebrospinal fluid cultures were obtained. The baby was hospitalized and started on intravenous cefotaxime and ocular saline irrigations.

Surprisingly, the conjunctival drainage grew *N meningitidis*; the blood, urine, and cerebrospinal fluid cultures were sterile. Because the *N meningitidis* isolate was beta-lactamase-negative, therapy was changed to intravenous ampicillin; she received a total course of 7 days of antibiotics. The baby also was given rifampin 10 mg/kg orally every 12 hours during the last 2 days of ampicillin therapy. Her recovery was complete. Her parents and siblings received a 2-day course of rifampin prophylaxis and remained well.

Differential Diagnosis

Conjunctivitis is the most common acute eye disease in children. When it occurs in the first month of life, it is termed ophthalmia neonatorum. The most frequent cause of neonatal conjunctivitis is chemical irritation from antimicrobial prophylaxis against ocular gonorrheal infection. This conjunctival inflammation is sterile, usually occurs on the first day of life, and resolves spontaneously within 2 to 4 days.

In contrast, infectious conjunctivitis may occur throughout the neonatal period and is associated with discharge and edema that worsen until appropriate antimicrobial therapy is initiated. Important infectious etiologies of neonatal conjunctivitis include *N gonorrhoeae*, *Chlamydia trachomatis*, and herpes simplex virus. These agents are transmitted most frequently by direct inoculation of the baby's conjunctival sac during passage through the birth canal. The conjunctiva also may be inoculated before birth by an ascending infection.

Etiology

N gonorrhoeae no longer is a major cause of ophthalmia neonatorum in the United States because of prenatal screening and treatment of maternal gonorrhea as well as the mandated use of ophthalmic prophylaxis in newborns. This prophylaxis typically consists of either silver nitrate solution in single-dose ampules or single-use tubes of ophthalmic ointment containing erythromycin or tetracycline. An infant born to a woman who has untreated gonococcal infection should receive a single dose of ceftriaxone intravenously or intramuscularly in addition to topical prophylaxis. Gonococcal conjunctivitis may present within the first few days of life or may be delayed, owing to partial suppression by ophthalmic prophylaxis. It also may occur beyond the neonatal period in infants following inoculation from the contaminated fingers of adults, providing another good reason for scrupulous hand washing by people who handle infants. *N gonorrhoeae* conjunctivitis, if not treated properly, can lead to corneal perforation, blindness, and even septicemia.

With the declining incidence of gonococcal neonatal conjunctivitis, *C trachomatis* has become the most common organism causing ophthalmia neonatorum in the United States. Silver nitrate solution is not adequate prophylaxis for neonatal chlamydial conjunctivitis, providing a rationale for the use of antibiotic ointment. Chlamydial conjunctivitis, also referred to as inclusion blennorrhea, usually begins 5 to 14 days after birth and is characterized by a mucopurulent exudate with occasional pseudomembrane formation. The tarsal conjunctivae primarily are involved; rarely are the corneas affected.

Herpes simplex virus may cause neonatal conjunctivitis associated with corneal epithelial changes and dendritic keratitis. The majority of neonates who have herpes simplex keratoconjunctivitis have infection at other sites, such as the skin and mucous membranes, or have disseminated disease. Conjunctivitis may be the first abnormality noted. A vesicular rash may be present.

A variety of other pathogens have been reported to cause ophthalmia neonatorum, including *Staphylococcus aureus*, *Streptococcus pneumoniae*, *Haemophilus influenzae*, and *Pseudomonas aeruginosa*. These bacteria usually are inoculated into the conjunctival sac postnatally from an exogenous source.

This baby had primary meningococcal conjunctivitis. Although conjunctivitis is a well-described secondary manifestation of systemic meningococcal disease, primary meningococcal conjunctivitis occurs rarely. In a recent literature analysis of 84 reported cases, 9 of the patients were neonates and 55 were children beyond the neonatal period. The source of the meningococcus in cases occurring within the first week of life is likely to be the maternal genital tract. In cases arising later, the organism probably is acquired from an exogenous source, possibly by way of hands contaminated with nasopharyngeal secretions from an individual who is a pharyngeal carrier of meningococci. Meningococcal ophthalmia presents similarly to gonococcal ophthalmia, with intense conjunctival erythema and purulent discharge. If proper therapy is delayed, systemic meningococcal disease may occur.

Diagnosis
All neonates and young infants who have conjunctivitis should undergo a prompt and thorough evaluation to determine the etiologic agent and to guide therapy decisions. Gram stain and culture always should be obtained to look for gram-negative intracellular diplococci that suggest *Neisseria* sp. Many laboratories use antigen detection assays for the diagnosis of *C trachomatis*. The glues in cotton or calcium alginate-tipped wooden swabs can be toxic to *C trachomatis*; therefore, Dacron® fiber wire shaft swabs should be used to collect specimens for these assays. If herpes simplex virus is suspected, conjunctival scrapings should be obtained on a swab (not a calcium alginate-tipped wooden swab) and submitted in viral transport media. Fluorescent antibody tests, if available, can allow for more rapid diagnosis but always should be confirmed by viral culture. A dendritic pattern on fluorescein staining of the cornea indicates presumptive herpes simplex virus keratitis.

Treatment
Systemic antimicrobial therapy is indicated for the treatment of infectious conjunctivitis in neonates and young infants. The baby also should be evaluated for possible infection elsewhere, including sepsis, meningitis, and pneumonia. For gonococcal and meningococcal ophthalmia, initial therapy should be ceftriaxone or cefotaxime, along with frequent ocular saline irrigations. If the isolate is sensitive to penicillin, intravenous aqueous penicillin G can be substituted. The duration of therapy usually is 7 days for uncomplicated ophthalmia and 10 to 14 days if meningitis is present. In cases of gonococcal conjunctivitis, parents should be evaluated for gonococcal infection and treated appropriately.

Babies who have meningococcal conjunctivitis should receive rifampin near the end of therapy to eradicate the carrier state. Established guidelines for meningococcal prophylaxis should be followed in managing family members and close contacts of an infant who has meningococcal conjunctivitis.

The treatment of choice for neonatal *C trachomatis* conjunctivitis is a 14-day course of oral erythromycin. Parents also should be treated with erythromycin or tetracycline, erythromycin being the drug of choice for lactating mothers. Neonates and young infants who have herpes simplex conjunctivitis should receive a topical ophthalmic drug—specifically, 1% to 2% trifluridine, 1% iododeoxyuridine, or 3% vidarabine—as well as intravenous acyclovir. Consultation with an ophthalmologist and an infectious diseases specialist should be considered.

Conjunctivitis in neonates and young infants has an excellent prognosis if treated appropriately. However, potential life- and sight-threatening complications may occur if therapy is delayed.

Lesson for the Clinician
This case illustrates that laboratory investigations are essential in determining a specific etiology and selecting appropriate therapy for conjunctivitis in neonates and

young infants. It also makes clear the importance of careful hand washing when caring for an infant who has an infectious secretion and reinforces the need for proper isolation techniques in a hospital, where other patients are at risk.

Rebecca C. Brady, MD, University of Cincinnati Medical Center, Cincinnati, OH

Intermittent Headache and Lethargy

PRESENTATION

A 12-year-old boy is brought to the office with a 3- to 4-day history of intermittent headache and lethargy. He has had no fever and denies vomiting, diarrhea, cough, or congestion. When asked about illness contact, his mother reports that the entire family has been ill with flu-like symptoms of nausea, mild headache, myalgias, and malaise. When asked about pets, she mentions that the family dog died last week of unknown causes.

On physical examination, the patient appears slightly ill, but is oriented and cooperative. His temperature, taken rectally, is 37.2°C (99°F). Pulse is 110 beats/min. Other vital signs are normal, as is the remainder of the general physical examination. A neurologic examination reveals normal cranial nerve, motor, and sensory function. Deep tendon reflexes are 3+ throughout; plantar reflexes are normal. The results of blood tests, including a complete blood count, monospot, electrolyte concentrations, and liver function test, are normal.

What is your differential diagnosis at this point?
Are there any elements of history or physical examination that would help you?
What additional diagnostic studies would you like performed?

DISCUSSION

Diagnosis

Carbon monoxide (CO) intoxication has been referred to as the great mimic because its presenting clinical features are generally nonspecific. CO is generated from the incomplete combustion of carbonaceous materials. Therefore, CO poisoning generally occurs during winter months, resulting from faulty furnaces, gas or wood stoves, space heaters, and automobile exhaust. Once absorbed, CO binds to hemoglobin, where it forms carboxyhemoglobin. It also will attach to myoglobin and cytochromes or remain dissolved in plasma. Nonsmokers typically have a carboxyhemoglobin concentration of 5%, while concentrations in smokers may be as high as 10%.

Presentation

Symptoms of mild CO poisoning are similar to those of a viral illness, with predominant features of headache, nausea, and malaise, as described for this boy. With more significant exposure, life-threatening symptoms and signs, including severe headache or frank coma, may result. Severe CO poisoning (carboxyhemoglobin of 50%) often is associated with death. Survivors of significant CO poisoning frequently have long-term neuropsychiatric sequelae.

Evaluation

The diagnosis of CO poisoning first requires suspicion on the part of the examiner. Risk factors associated with the diagnosis of CO exposure are occurrence during the winter months, symptoms of viral illness in the absence of significant fever, and headache as a prominent presenting complaint. As in this case, the history also may be remarkable for other family members having identical symptoms. Laboratory evaluation is of limited utility because oxygen saturation by pulse oximetry is normal (due to the inability of pulse oximeters to detect abnormal hemoglobins), and arterial blood gas levels may be normal if oxygen saturation is calculated rather than measured directly by co-oximeter. Oxygen saturation measured by the co-oximeter represents oxyhemoglobin divided by the sum of reduced hemoglobin plus carboxyhemoglobin plus methemoglobin plus other hemoglobins, rather than oxyhemoglobin divided by reduced hemoglobin alone. The definitive diagnostic test for CO poisoning is measurement of circulating carboxyhemoglobin.

Treatment and Prevention

Because of the potential sequelae of CO poisoning, carboxyhemoglobin concentrations of 10% in a child should be treated. Treatment of mild-to-moderate intoxication consists of administration of 100% oxygen. Patients suffering from severe intoxication (defined as either a carboxyhemoglobin concentration of 40% or coma, seizures, or arrhythmias, regardless of carboxyhemoglobin concentration) should be referred for hyperbaric oxygen therapy.

Prevention of CO poisoning includes careful inspection of heating systems each winter. Inexpensive colorimetric CO detectors are available and may aid in reducing the rate of this serious intoxication.

Michael Shannon, MD, Frederick H. Lovejoy, Jr, MD, Children's Hospital,
Boston, MA

Persistent Wrist Pain After an In-line Skating Fall

PRESENTATION

A 14-year-old boy comes to the office complaining of right wrist pain. He was in-line skating in the park, not wearing any protective gear, and fell onto his outstretched hands. Examination of his wrist reveals no swelling, bruising, or deformity, but he does complain of pain and tenderness in the dorsal radial portion of his wrist. He also has discomfort when making a firm grip. A radiograph of his wrist reveals no fracture, and he is put into a plastic thumb splint with instructions to return in 10 days.

When the boy returns, physical examination reveals increased tenderness over the same dorsal radial area of the wrist. Repeat routine anteroposterior and lateral radiographs again are read as normal. An orthopedic colleague suggests an expanded physical examination and ordering of an unusual radiograph. Results of those procedures reveal the diagnosis.

What is your differential diagnosis at this point?
Are there any elements of history or physical examination that would help you?
What additional diagnostic studies would you like performed?

DISCUSSION

Diagnosis

When evaluating a patient who experiences wrist pain after falling onto outstretched hands, the clinician should consider the high likelihood of fracture involving the distal radius and ulna. However, another potential site of fracture is the scaphoid bone. The scaphoid, also called the carpal navicular, is the carpal bone fractured most frequently in both adolescents and adults. Fracture through the waist of this bone, because of the unique blood supply, is associated with a high rate of nonunion and subsequent wrist arthrosis if not treated promptly and properly. In addition, a fracture through the waist of the scaphoid carries a high risk of avascular necrosis involving the proximal fragment. Because of the potential for these complications, it is important to make the diagnosis as early as possible to provide definitive treatment. Fortunately, waist fractures are relatively uncommon among children and adolescents; fractures occur more commonly through the distal third of the bone.

Presentation

Scaphoid fractures are notorious for yielding negative radiographs on routine views of the wrist, so clinical findings provide the clues to diagnosis. A major finding is tenderness in the anatomic snuffbox, located in the dorsal radial area of the wrist, just radial to the extensor pollicis longus tendon (a tendon easily found by hyperextending the thumb in a "thumb's up" fashion). Ulnar deviation of the wrist may help in eliciting tenderness within the anatomic snuffbox. Besides snuffbox tenderness, there also may be tenderness over the volar radial aspect of the wrist at the distal flexor crease because this area corresponds to the distal pole of the scaphoid. Finally, scaphoid compression tenderness has been shown to be even more sensitive and specific for scaphoid fracture than the classic anatomic snuffbox tenderness. It can be elicited by holding the patient's thumb and applying pressure along the axis of its metacarpal toward the scaphoid bone. Other more subtle findings include pain while trying to grip and a symptom pattern in the untreated patient of lessening pain that gives way ultimately to worsening discomfort.

Evaluation
The patient presented here initially had posterior-anterior and lateral radiographs taken of his wrist, which failed to reveal any fracture. At his return visit, a special scaphoid view radiograph, which is an anteroposterior view of the wrist held in 30 degrees of supination and ulnar deviation, was obtained. Many times this special scaphoid view will aid in diagnosis. However, if all repeat radiographs remain negative after several weeks, but the patient continues to complain of scaphoid area tenderness, many orthopedists will obtain a bone scan or magnetic resonance imaging to pursue the diagnosis further and, if the imaging yields positive results, initiate proper treatment.

Treatment
Because of the high risk of avascular necrosis, nonunion, and subsequent wrist arthrosis, an injury suspected to be a fracture of the scaphoid must be treated as such until it is confirmed radiographically or a treatment course has been completed under the supervision of an orthopedic specialist. Proper treatment includes placement in a thumb spica splint or cast (a cast is more appropriate for this age group). If the diagnosis is confirmed, immobilization for 8 to 12 weeks for fractures through the waist and 6 to 8 weeks for distal pole fractures typically is required. Open reduction may be necessary if there is displacement, instability, or dislocation of the scaphoid or other carpal bones as a result of navicular fracture. Because of these perils, timely referral of the patient to an orthopedic physician is warranted for a suspected fracture of the scaphoid bone.

Santos Cantu, Jr, MD, Gregory P. Connors, MD, MPH, University of Rochester Medical Center, Rochester, NY

Recurrent Fever and Rash

PRESENTATION

A 7-year-old Caucasian girl is evaluated for recurrent episodes of fever and rash. Since the age of 1 year, she has developed intermittent tender pink patches, papules, and nodules on her face and lower extremities. These eruptions typically follow episodes of fever.

On physical examination, the girl is afebrile and does not appear ill. Her height and weight are at the 50th percentile. There is no lymphadenopathy or organomegaly. She has a minimal degree of effusion in both knees, and there is a Baker cyst in her right popliteal fossa. Reddish-pink, nummular, tender lesions of variable size are scattered diffusely over her arms, legs, chest, back, and face. The older lesions are purplish, scaly papules. Ophthalmologic evaluation reveals bilateral iritis and patchy retinal choroiditis. Results of the rest of her examination are unremarkable.

Laboratory results are as follows: hemoglobin, 1.53 mmol/L (9.9 g/dL); hematocrit, 0.303 (30.3%); white blood cell count, 5 x 10^9/L (5 x 10^3/mcL) with a normal differential count; platelet count, 243 x 10^9/L (243 x 10^3/mcL); erythrocyte sedimentation rate, 45 mm/h; serum immunoglobulin levels (IgG), 14.9 g/L (1,490 mg/dL) (normal, 5.95 to 12.75 g/L [595 to 1,275 mg/dL]); and angiotensin-converting enzyme level, 77 mU/mL (normal, 14 to 44 mU/mL). The following laboratory studies yield normal or negative results: urinalysis; blood urea nitrogen; serum electrolytes, calcium, creatinine, uric acid, and liver enzymes; C3 and C4 complement; antinuclear antibodies; rheumatoid factor; purified protein derivative and Candida skin tests; and chest radiography.

Skin histopathology reveals epidermal interface changes suggestive of erythema multiforme as well as panniculitis, both septal and lobular, that is consistent with erythema nodosum. A biopsy of the conjunctival lacrimal gland reveals the specific diagnosis.

What is your differential diagnosis at this point?
Are there any elements of history or physical examination that would help you?
What additional diagnostic studies would you like performed?

DISCUSSION

Diagnosis

The diagnosis of early-onset sarcoidosis in this patient was based on the clinical findings of papular skin rash, arthritis, and iritis and the histologic results of a conjunctival lacrimal gland biopsy that showed the classic appearance of noncaseating granulomata. The diagnosis was supported further by the presence of elevated angiotensin-converting enzyme (ACE) levels, negative stains and cultures for fungi and mycobacteria, and a negative purified protein derivative tuberculin skin test.

Sarcoidosis is a multisystem granulomatous disease of unknown etiology, most frequently affecting young adults and occurring relatively rarely in children. Among older children and young adults, the disease is most common in African-American females. Sarcoidosis generally presents with bilateral hilar lymphadenopathy, pulmonary infiltration, skin lesions, and eye lesions. The clinical spectrum can vary, depending on the organs involved. The disease typically involves the lungs, lymph nodes, eyes, skin, liver, and spleen. Facial nerve palsy may occur in older patients. Organ involvement may be symptomatic or silent.

There appear to be two distinct forms of childhood sarcoidosis. Older children usually present with multisystem disease similar to that observed in adults that includes frequent pulmonary involvement, lymphadenopathy, and systemic signs and symptoms, such as fever and malaise. In contrast, early-onset childhood sarcoidosis is a unique form of the disease characterized by the triad of skin rash, arthritis, and uveitis in patients who present before age 4 years. Hilar lymphadenopathy, the leading feature of late-onset disease, is rare in early-onset sarcoidosis. Uveitis, which occurs in about 90% of early-onset disease cases, is relatively less common among patients who have later-onset disease.

Presentation
Early-onset sarcoidosis frequently presents in the first year of life. The fever pattern and joint symptoms initially might suggest systemic-onset juvenile rheumatoid arthritis (JRA), but the two disorders are distinguished readily when all disease manifestations are considered. Skin changes can help to distinguish between sarcoidosis and JRA at the onset. The rash of JRA is pink, evanescent, and macular; the skin lesion of sarcoidosis is classically a papule or a plaque with scaling. The uveitis of sarcoidosis is characterized by firmly edged keratic precipitates, preferentially in the limbus; conjunctival nodules; and focal synechiae related to nodule formation. The arthritis of sarcoidosis is characterized by painless, boggy effusions of the synovium without limitation of range of movement. However, painful, destructive polyarthritis accompanied by functional impairment that is indistinguishable from JRA has been described in early-onset sarcoidosis.

Laboratory Evaluation
No laboratory test is diagnostic of sarcoidosis. Laboratory evaluation may reveal anemia, leukopenia, eosinophilia, or an elevation of the erythrocyte sedimentation rate or other acute-phase reactants. Immunologic abnormalities include hypergammaglobulinemia and impaired delayed hypersensitivity on skin testing. Hypercalcemia or hypercalciuria may be found. The serum level of ACE typically is elevated in as many as 80% of children who have late-onset sarcoidosis.

The diagnosis of sarcoidosis is confirmed by demonstration of a typical non-caseating granuloma on a biopsy specimen. To support the diagnosis, infectious granulomatous conditions (such as histoplasmosis, blastomycosis, and tuberculosis) must be excluded by special stains and cultures.

Treatment
The current treatment of childhood sarcoidosis that has multisystem involvement is corticosteroids. Long-term treatment with high doses may be required to achieve satisfactory responses, and patients usually become steroid-dependent. They may develop a course of chronic relapses, and serious complications due to chronic corticosteroid therapy may occur. Accordingly, steroid-sparing agents are needed.

Recent reports suggest that immunosuppressive agents, such as methotrexate, given orally in low doses, are effective and safe and have steroid-sparing properties. Methotrexate is given weekly, whereas prednisone is administered daily.

Prognosis
The overall prognosis of childhood sarcoidosis is reported as good compared with that for adults; most children experience considerable improvement in clinical manifestations, chest radiographic findings, and pulmonary function test results. Early-onset sarcoidosis that involves the eyes, joints, and skin suggests a guarded prognosis with the likelihood of a chronic progressive course and even life-threatening complications. Approximately 80% to 100% of these children develop uveitis, polyarthritis, and other organ involvement. Periodic ophthalmologic evaluations are essential in all cases of childhood sarcoidosis to identify ocular disease and to prevent further morbidity. Currently, serial clinical examinations to monitor disease severity in affected organs, with appropriate treatment when indicated, remain the best approach to management.

Avinash K. Shetty, MD, Abraham Gedalia, MD, Louisiana State University Medical Center, New Orleans, LA

Sudden Onset of Sharp Abdominal Pain

Presentation

A 9-year-old Arabic boy is seen because of pain in his right lower abdomen that started abruptly about 24 hours ago. He describes a sharp, constant pain that varies in intensity. For the past 2 hours the pain has been severe, and he has been nauseated. He has had no fever, chills, jaundice, vomiting, or diarrhea.

His parents describe him as a healthy child who has had occasional vague abdominal pain in the past. He experienced two episodes of "red urine" 3 years ago; each time the urine cleared spontaneously over 1 week. There is no family history of hematuria, renal disease, urinary tract infection, or kidney stones, and he does not eat excessive calcium- or sodium-rich foods.

On physical examination, the boy has a temperature of $37°C$ (98.6°F) orally, a pulse rate of 142 beats/min, and a blood pressure of 110/70 mm Hg. His weight is 25 kg (10th percentile), and his height is 130 cm (50th percentile). He is thin and well-hydrated, with good color and pink mucous membranes, but he is anxious and in pain. He reports tenderness in the right lower quadrant and right groin. There is no rebound tenderness, but the pain seems worse during deep palpation. Bowel sounds are present, and no masses or enlarged organs are felt. There is questionable tenderness on percussion of his costovertebral areas. Rectal examination yields brown, guaiac-negative stool. Findings on the remainder of the physical examination are normal.

What is your differential diagnosis at this point?
Are there any elements of history or physical examination that would help you?
What additional diagnostic studies would you like performed?

DISCUSSION

Diagnosis

Diagnosing the cause of acute abdominal pain is challenging. The clinician must be aware of a broad differential diagnosis that includes acute appendicitis, mesenteric adenitis, gastroenteritis, intussusception, hernia, pyelonephritis, pneumonia, and vasculitis, among myriad other, less common entities. As is so often the case, the history allowed rapid focusing on the likely cause of the pain in this case.

The sudden onset of pain in the right abdomen, which varied in intensity and radiated to the right groin, together with the history of previous episodes of "red urine" prompted further studies. His urinary sediment contained 100 erythrocytes per high-power field; the erythrocytes were eumorphic, and no casts were seen. A plain abdominal radiograph revealed a 4-mm radiopaque stone in the area of the right ureter.

Etiology

Calcium oxalate and calcium phosphate are the most common components of urinary stones. These calculi may be associated with hypercalciuria, with or without hypercalcemia. Idiopathic childhood hypercalciuria implies normocalcemia and is responsible for about one third of calcium stones. Characteristic pain and hematuria, either gross or microscopic, may be present in patients who had idiopathic hypercalciuria years before the first stone is detected. Other factors associated with calcium stones are hyperuricosuria, hyperoxaluria, high urine pH, and the use of furosemide. Uric acid stones are associated with a low urine pH and hyperuricosuria; cystine stones also are associated with acid urine and with cystinuria. Struvite (magnesium ammonium phosphate) stones may develop as the result of foreign bodies in the urinary tract, urine stasis, high urine pH, and urinary tract infections caused by urea-splitting organisms, such as *Proteus* sp. Xanthine stones are extremely rare.

The genesis of urolithiasis often is multifactorial, and the urinary tract should be evaluated completely for obstruction, infection, anatomic malformations, stasis, and metabolic abnormalities. Analysis of the chemical structure of the stone after passage or surgical removal gives valuable information about the pathogenesis of that stone's formation. Unfortunately, stones are not always recovered.

Evaluation

Intravenous urography or ultrasonography should be considered to detect any obstruction and radiolucent stones. A comprehensive laboratory evaluation should include analysis of the blood for serum electrolyte levels, carbon dioxide, blood urea nitrogen, creatinine, calcium, phosphorus, and uric acid. Urine should be obtained for culture, urinalysis (including pH), spot creatinine and spot calcium measurements, and a urine metabolic screen for cystinuria. Twenty-four hour collections are not needed initially. Spot samples can be used to determine the fractional excretion of calcium, phosphorus, oxalate, and uric acid. A spot calcium/creatinine ratio greater than 0.2 with normal serum calcium concentrations suggests idiopathic hypercalciuria. A timed urine collection (12 to 24 hours) is confirmatory, with normal calcium excretion being less than 4 mg/kg per 24 hours.

Treatment

Children who have urolithiasis and obstruction of the urinary system should be hospitalized for pain management and possible surgical intervention. If obstruction is not present, most children can be managed as outpatients. Treatment consists of medical management of any underlying condition that contributed to stone formation and, in selected cases, removal of the stone by surgery, percutaneous nephrolithotomy, or extracorporeal shock wave. Regardless of the stone's chemical composition, the most effective way to prevent recurrence is to increase fluid intake to maintain adequate hydration. A dilute urine decreases the likelihood of supersaturation with and precipitation of the solutes involved in stone formation.

Other general measures include avoidance of excessive sodium and calcium intake, avoidance of unnecessary immobilization, and education of the parent and child about the need to minimize risks for recurrence of stone formation by these measures.

Alexandre T. Rotta, MD, Children's Hospital of Michigan, Detroit, MI

Anuria and Vomiting in a Neonate

PRESENTATION

A 4-day-old boy is brought to the emergency department because of anuria and vomiting. Born vaginally after an uneventful pregnancy, the baby was discharged from the nursery at 24 hours of age but developed increasingly severe nonbilious vomiting. He had passed meconium on the first day of life and a dark stool yesterday. He wet several diapers earlier, but his urine output has decreased. His family history reveals a maternal uncle who had a congenital hydronephrosis.

On physical examination the infant appears comfortable and in no distress. He has a respiratory rate of 50 breaths/ min, heart rate of 156 beats/min, blood pressure of 75/59 mm Hg, and temperature of 36.6°C (97.9°F). He weighs 2.88 kg (4.3 kg below his birthweight) and is mildly jaundiced. His abdomen is soft, and bowel sounds are present; no hepatosplenomegaly is noted. The remainder of the physical examination is normal.

Blood chemistry values are as follows: sodium, 143 mmol/L (143 mEq/L); potassium, 7 mmol/L (7 mEq/L); ionized calcium, 0.82 mmol/L (0.82 mEq/L); phosphate, 14 mmol/L (14 mEq/L); magnesium, 2 mmol/L (2 mg/dL); blood urea nitrogen, 12.9 mmol urea/L (36 mg/dL); and creatinine, 283.4 mcmol/L (3.2 mg/dL). Catheterization of the bladder results in a small amount of urine, which reveals: specific gravity, 1.015; pH, 8.5; and no protein. Microscopic examination shows 2 to 3 erythrocytes, 5 to 8 white blood cells, and 1 to 2 finely granular casts per high-power field. The baby's urinary sodium is 70 mmol/L (70 mEq/L); potassium is 53.5 mmol/L (53.5 mEq/L); chloride is 31 mmol/L (31 mEq/L); and creatinine is 0.42 mmol/kg (49 mg/kg) body weight. Results of renal ultrasonography are normal.

A simple radiographic procedure leads to the correct diagnosis.

What is your differential diagnosis at this point?
Are there any elements of history or physical examination that would help you?
What additional diagnostic studies would you like performed?

DISCUSSION

Diagnosis

An abdominal radiograph revealed a double-bubble sign and the absence of bowel gas, which are hallmark findings of complete duodenal obstruction. The infant, who was anuric on arrival at the emergency department, underwent aggressive rehydration. His urine output, serum electrolyte levels, and renal function normalized rapidly over fewer than 48 hours. A duodenostomy was performed subsequently, and the baby did well. Although the neonate had experienced some minor regurgitation before discharge at birth, its significance was not apparent. Had he not been discharged at 24 hours of age, but been allowed to stay longer, it is likely that the diagnosis would have been made sooner and subsequent renal problems avoided.

Presentation

Duodenal atresia occurs in 1 of every 10,000 births. In 70% to 85% of cases, the atresia is located in the second or third portion of the duodenum, distal to the ampulla of Vater. Infants who have this anomaly usually present with polyhydramnios and bilious vomiting that starts shortly after birth. The presence of bilious secretion in the amniotic fluid often is mistaken for meconium. In 15% to 30% of cases, the atresia is proximal to the ampulla of Vater, and neonates present with nonbilious vomiting and dark stools, as in this case.

Three types of duodenal atresia have been described. Type 1 takes the form of an intact membrane of mucosa and submucosa. Type 2 consists of a short fibrous cord connecting two blind ends of duodenum. In type 3, there is a gap between blind duodenal ends. The defect is believed to be caused by a failure of recanalization of the duodenal lumen, which begins between 8 and 10 weeks of gestation. Atresias of the jejunum and ileum are caused by intrauterine vascular anomalies or accidents that occur later in pregnancy than the events leading to duodenal atresia.

Of all patients who have duodenal atresia, 10% to 30% also have Down syndrome. Other congenital anomalies frequently associated with duodenal atresia include esophageal atresia, malrotation, congenital heart disease, and anorectal malformations. Jejunal and ileal atresias usually are not associated with other anomalies.

The abdomen of an infant who has duodenal atresia usually is scaphoid, with localized epigastric distention caused by a dilated stomach. Many conditions will cause significant vomiting in a newborn, including a number of disorders that cause obstruction. Certain clinical findings will help the clinician to localize an obstruction. Nonbilious vomiting indicates an obstruction proximal to the ampulla of Vater, as in this infant, whereas the presence of bile points to a more distal obstruction. When the obstructed area is in the ileum, jejunum, or colon, abdominal distention occurs, in contrast to a scaphoid abdomen. Delay in the passage of stool beyond 48 hours suggests a lesion in the distal small intestine or colon, although the passing of meconium does not rule out a complete intestinal obstruction.

Evaluation
Plain radiographs of the abdomen can be helpful in many ways, such as by indicating the extent to which the intestinal tract is filled with air. Sometimes a specific pattern can lead to a diagnosis. The double-bubble sign associated with duodenal atresia is caused by air-fluid levels in the gastric antrum and the duodenum.

Differential Diagnosis
Another cause of congenital duodenal obstruction, which is less common than duodenal atresia, is compression of the second portion of the duodenum by an annular pancreas (associated with other anomalies in 70% of cases), a preduodenal portal vein, a mesenteric band, or a malrotation of the gut with volvulus. In patients who have findings of duodenal obstruction, it is extremely important to rule out malrotation with midgut volvulus. In as many as 50% of these cases, results of the physical examination are normal. Other patients present with distention, abdominal tenderness, or signs of peritonitis and shock. If the patient has malrotation, an upper gastrointestinal series will show that the duodenojejunal junction is located to the left of the spine. A barium enema may identify an abnormally positioned cecum. In 5% to 20% of patients who have malrotation, however, the cecum is in a normal position. Ultrasonographic examination by an experienced radiologist sometimes is helpful in identifying an inversion of the mesenteric artery and vein.

Malrotation with volvulus must be considered to be present until proven otherwise because it requires immediate surgical correction.

Treatment

The infant who has duodenal atresia should have a nasogastric tube placed and be given nothing by mouth. Intravenous fluids should be administered. Once the diagnosis of malrotation with midgut volvulus has been ruled out, dehydration and electrolyte abnormalities should be corrected prior to surgery.

If duodenal atresia is not diagnosed rapidly, the patient will develop hypochloremic metabolic alkalosis because of the emesis of gastric secretions and hypokalemia from the shift of potassium ions into cells as a response to the alkalosis. Another reason to defer surgery until correction of electrolyte disturbances is that the hyperventilation associated with intubation and anesthesia can aggravate the alkalosis acutely, worsening hypokalemia and inducing hypocalcemia, which can lead to arrhythmias. Advanced degrees of dehydration can lead to prerenal failure and subsequent hyperkalemia, which can be a misleading sign in the presentation of duodenal atresia.

Lesson for the Clinician

A challenging feature of this infant's clinical course was his renal involvement. He had a blood urea nitrogen/creatinine ratio of 11.25 and a fractional excretion of sodium of 3.2% (< 2.5% in prerenal failure versus > 2.5% in intrinsic renal failure), both of which suggest intrinsic renal failure. His physicians were faced with a dilemma: a dehydrated baby who has prerenal failure requires aggressive fluid therapy, whereas one who has true intrinsic renal failure could be seriously harmed by fluid overloading. The fact that this patient had lost considerable weight was informative. In any case, it is safe to administer one initial bolus of 20 mL/kg of intravenous fluid and monitor the patient for response. Clinical improvement and the passage of urine indicates that it is safe to administer more fluid. The normalization of this baby's renal function and electrolyte concentrations over the next 2 days indicated that most of his problem was prerenal, although a literal interpretation of the indices raises the question of whether he had sustained some renal damage. The important lesson is that clinicians must interpret indices of renal function with great care in newborns.

Isabelle G. De Plaen, MD, The Childrens Memorial Hospital, Chicago, IL

Daily Coughing for Two Months

PRESENTATION

*A 13-year-old boy comes to your office for the first time because he has been cough-
ing for 2 months, both day and night. One month ago he was treated for presumed
sinusitis with a 10-day course of clarithromycin and inhaled albuterol, but his
symptoms improved only slightly. He has had no fever, chills, ear pain, sinus pain,
or night sweats. He is a nonsmoker and generally feels well. His medical history
reveals only an increased number of respiratory infections during the past winter.*

*You notice that the boy appears withdrawn and somewhat depressed. On fur-
ther questioning, he tells you that he has been feeling "down in the dumps" since
his mother died 6 months ago. His grandmother, who brought him, says he has a
poor appetite and has lost weight.*

*On physical examination, the boy is alert, afebrile, and has normal vital signs.
Height and weight both are in the 75th percentile for his age. Mucoid nasal discharge
is noted bilaterally, and "shotty" lymph nodes are present in his neck. The remainder of his examination, including evaluation of heart and lungs, yields normal results.*

*A radiograph of his chest shows normal findings, but sinus radiographs reveal
bilateral ethmoid and maxillary sinus opacification. A purified protein derivative
tuberculin skin test is negative. He is treated for sinusitis and asked to return 2 weeks
later, at which time further information about his family leads to the performance
of a laboratory test that reveals an underlying diagnosis.*

What is your differential diagnosis at this point?
Are there any elements of history or physical examination that would help you?
What additional diagnostic studies would you like performed?

DISCUSSION

Diagnosis

By the time the boy returned 2 weeks later, records had arrived from his previous
physician. Although there were no data to substantiate concerns of weight loss (his
weight was between the 25th and 50th percentiles 3 years ago), he did experience
"severe cellulitis with vesicles" 1 year previously and herpes zoster infection in a
different dermatome 5 years previously. A thorough and direct inquiry into the family history revealed that the boy's mother died of acquired immunodeficiency syndrome (AIDS) and that a younger half-brother had human immunodeficiency virus
(HIV) antibody at birth but became seronegative later. At the follow-up visit, the
boy's sinusitis had resolved and his weight had not changed.

After counseling the patient and his grandmother, blood was drawn for HIV antibody testing, which yielded a positive result. A Western blot study also was positive, confirming the presence of HIV infection.

Subsequent studies revealed a CD4 lymphocyte count of 682 cells/mm^3 and a viral
load of 23,000 copies/mL. These data, together with relatively few symptoms, put
him into the Centers for Disease Control and Prevention (CDC) category N1 (no evidence of immunosuppression; not symptomatic). He was given antiretroviral ther-

apy employing two different nucleoside analog reverse transcriptase inhibitors. Three months later, his viral load was undetectable and he was asymptomatic.

Pathogenesis
The prevalence of HIV infection among adolescents and young adults has been increasing in recent years, paralleling the overall increase nationwide. In 1994, this disease was the sixth leading cause of death among youth between the ages of 15 and 24 years. Adolescents who are members of minority groups and those from lower socioeconomic groups are at particularly high risk, and the risk is spreading from urban areas into suburban and rural locations. Although the majority of adolescents who have HIV infection have one or more recognized risk factors for the disease, a few have no reported risk factors, suggesting that the infection in some children who are infected through maternal-infant transmission may not be detected until they are adolescents. This was believed to be the case with this patient. A small but significant percentage of patients who have hemophilia and were known to be infected in the early 1980s are still healthy despite not receiving antiretroviral therapy, which makes the mechanism of congenital infection with delayed symptoms appear more plausible.

Presentation
Although suspecting the diagnosis of AIDS is relatively straightforward in patients who have such typical manifestations as *Pneumocystis carinii* infection, lymphoid interstitial pneumonia, failure to thrive, encephalopathy, or recurrent bacterial infections, diagnosing HIV infection in its earlier stages can be difficult. A thorough history that focuses on frequency and especially on severity of infections, on growth parameters, and on chronic symptoms is essential. For example, although frequent episodes of sinusitis do not necessarily raise a "red flag," frequent or prolonged episodes of sinusitis that are unresponsive to the usual courses of antibiotics or sinusitis with suppurative complications on more than one occasion should arouse suspicion. Further, a single episode of herpes zoster or recurrent mild herpes simplex infections may not suggest HIV infection, but herpes zoster infection occurring in multiple dermatomes or a severe case of herpes simplex infection in an unusual location should alert the clinician to the possibility of immune system dysfunction.

Evaluation
Elucidation of risk factors for HIV infection may take time, but it is important. Risk factors for the acquisition of HIV infection by adolescents include those noted in adults, such as unprotected homosexual or heterosexual activity, especially with multiple partners, and exposure to blood. Because HIV infection typically takes years to become apparent clinically, it also is important to determine if there has been sexual abuse in the past. These risk factors frequently are difficult to ascertain in an adolescent, especially on an initial visit.

A careful physical examination is important because subtle skin findings, lymphadenopathy, and mild hepatosplenomegaly can be missed easily. Although children and adolescents do not present typically with Kaposi sarcoma, nonspecific skin findings such as eczema and widespread or recurrent tinea infections may aid in diagnosis. Many children and adults who are well otherwise will have mild-to-moderate generalized lymphadenopathy or hepatosplenomegaly as their only manifestation of HIV infection. Assessing the patient's mental status also is important. Depression can be both a risk factor for and a consequence of HIV infection. Cognitive losses and other neurobehavioral problems typically occur later in the course of the disease and usually are not present at the time of the diagnosis.

Treatment

After HIV infection has been diagnosed, management can vary, depending on the progression of disease in the patient and the availability of resources in the community. The patient may be referred to a regional HIV program for consultation or for comprehensive care, depending on the comfort level of the primary care clinician. Over time, success in controlling HIV infection has increased, and the disease has gone from being regarded as a rapidly progressive illness to a disorder with the potential for long-term survival. Thus, the role of the primary care clinician in dispensing comprehensive care has expanded, and with this responsibility has come the need for greater knowledge of HIV infection on the part of the generalist.

On the other hand, dedicated HIV programs often can provide specialized drug and dietary management, social services, and psychological support for families affected by HIV infection that primary practitioners cannot. Multidrug regimens now are recommended for all patients who have HIV infection, and such management frequently requires special expertise. Nonetheless, the proximity of most primary care clinicians to the families they serve, combined with the special relationship many families have with their practitioners, make generalists important partners in the care of patients who have HIV infection.

Christopher J. Stille, MD, Connecticut Children's Medical Center, Hartford, CT

Bilious Vomiting With Abdominal Pain

PRESENTATION

A 15-year-old girl presents to the emergency department having a 1-day history of 11 episodes of bilious vomiting with abdominal pain. There is no history of fever, diarrhea, dysuria, trauma, vaginal discharge, suspicious foods, or illness contacts. The patient is finishing her regular menstrual cycle. She is sexually active and uses condoms inconsistently.

On physical examination, the girl appears alert but experiences frequent episodes of forceful bilious emesis. Her abdomen is soft and nondistended. Her upper abdomen is tender, especially in the epigastric area, and no bowel sounds are audible. There is no costovertebral angle tenderness. The liver edge is palpable 2 cm below the costal margin. Rectal examination yields normal findings and guaiac-negative stool.

The white blood cell count is 3.2 x 10^9/L (3.2 x 10^3/mcL). Hemoglobin and platelet levels are normal, as are concentrations of liver enzymes, bilirubin, and pancreatic enzymes. A urine pregnancy test is negative. Urinalysis yields normal results. An abdominal radiograph is consistent with ileus. Computed tomography of the abdomen with contrast shows normal findings.

The girl is admitted to the hospital for hydration and monitoring, and ranitidine is prescribed. The next day, 30 mL of brown, guaiac-positive fluid containing small, bright red blood clots drains from her nasogastric tube. Endoscopy reveals esophagitis, duodenitis, and gastric erosions but no active bleeding. Repeat blood levels are: alanine aminotransferase (ALT), 2,697 U/L; aspartate aminotransferase (AST), 251 U/L; total bilirubin, 18.7 mcmol/L (1.1 mg/dL); amylase, 181 U/L; and lipase, 515 U/L. The prothrombin time is prolonged at 14.1 seconds. No aspirin or acetaminophen is detectable in the blood.

The next day, the patient contributes information that reveals her diagnosis.

What is your differential diagnosis at this point?
Are there any elements of history or physical examination that would help you?
What additional diagnostic studies would you like performed?

DISCUSSION

Diagnosis

The teenager revealed that at 1:30 AM on the day of admission, she had taken approximately 15 extra-strength Tylenol® tablets (7.5 g or 100 mg/kg of acetaminophen) as well as approximately 1.5 oz of a hydrocodone cough suppressant. She stated that it was her birthday and she was disappointed that she did not get to go out with her mother and siblings to celebrate because her mother had just returned from a vacation. She said that she was angry, was unable to sleep, and had a headache. She took the acetaminophen and cough medicine "to sleep."

The minimum acute toxic dose of acetaminophen in adults is 5 to 15 g. The acute lethal dose ranges from 13 to 25 g. In children, ingestion of greater than 150 mg/kg is associated with liver toxicity. Children younger than 12 years of age demonstrate less hepatotoxicity than adults despite equivalent toxic plasma acetaminophen levels, perhaps because different metabolic pathways are used. Acetaminophen absorption is rapid and complete. When normal doses are taken, peak therapeutic concentrations occur in 1 hour. In cases of overdose, the concomitant use of other drugs that delay gastric emptying may delay peak concentration up to 4 hours. In these cases, blood levels should not be drawn before 4 hours have elapsed since ingestion.

The liver transforms 90% of acetaminophen by conversion to sulfate or glucuronide. The sulfate pathway predominates in children younger than 12 years of age, whereas adults primarily use the glucuronide pathway. A small portion (5% to 15%) of the acetaminophen dose is metabolized by the p450 pathway to a toxic metabolite that undergoes glutathione conjugation to mercapturic acid metabolites. This toxic metabolite, postulated to be N-acetyl-imidoquinone, is believed to cause hepatocyte damage in cases of acetaminophen overdose.

At therapeutic doses, the half-life of acetaminophen is about 2 to 3 hours. In overdose situations, the half-life increases. When the time of ingestion is not known, calculating the half-life is a useful method of predicting hepatic toxicity. When two successive acetaminophen levels are measured, the half-life can be calculated by using a formula. A half-life of greater than 4 hours suggests that liver toxicity will occur; a half-life of greater than 12 hours indicates the likelihood of hepatic coma. When the time of ingestion is known, the likelihood of hepatic toxicity can be predicted by plotting the acetaminophen level on the Rumack-Matthew nomogram. This nomogram is useful only when the patient has ingested a single dose of acetaminophen, when the precise time of that ingestion is known, and when that ingestion time is within 24 hours of the level being drawn.

The clinical course of acetaminophen toxicity can be divided into four stages. The initial stage occurs in the first 24 hours after ingestion. During this stage, the child experiences gastrointestinal irritation, including anorexia, nausea, and vomiting, although some patients may be asymptomatic. Mental status changes are rare. During the second stage (24 to 48 h postingestion), the patient may appear well. The gastrointestinal symptoms resolve, but biochemical evidence of hepatic dysfunction begins to appear approximately 36 hours after ingestion.

The third (hepatic) stage occurs 3 to 4 days after ingestion. In this stage, manifestations of hepatic necrosis develop and include nausea, anorexia, vomiting, hypoglycemia, and right upper quadrant pain. Fulminant liver failure is rare, but when it does occur, it can manifest as jaundice, bleeding, confusion, lethargy, asterixis, and coma. In the most severely affected individuals, death from fulminant hepatic necrosis occurs 4 to 18 days after ingestion. The patient may develop some of the nonhepatic toxicities of acetaminophen, including renal failure, myocardial necrosis, and pancreatic inflammation.

In patients who recover, the fourth stage — the recovery stage — begins about 5 days postingestion, with normalization of liver function tests, and lasts 7 to 8 days. Hepatic architecture returns to normal within 3 months.

Treatment

The treatment of acetaminophen overdose is dictated by when the patient begins to receive medical care and by the acetaminophen level at the time of presentation. The mainstay of treatment is the antidote N-acetyl-cysteine (NAC). Patients who present within 4 to 6 hours of ingestion should receive syrup of ipecac, unless contraindicated by the absence of a gag reflex. Gastric lavage should be used if the induction of emesis is contraindicated. The use of activated charcoal is controversial because charcoal adsorbs NAC. Activated charcoal may be useful in overdoses of more than one drug. If charcoal is used, the subsequent NAC dose should be increased by 30%.

NAC is a glutathione precursor that prevents accumulation of the toxic intermediary compound. It provides effective protection against hepatotoxicity when administered within 10 hours of the acetaminophen ingestion. Treatment with NAC should start immediately for patients in whom hepatotoxicity is a possibility, as judged by a history of dose ingested or blood levels. Beyond 15 to 24 hours, NAC does not appear to be as effective an antidote. However, NAC therapy should be started even if more than 24 hours have passed since the ingestion if liver enzymes continue to be elevated or if it is anticipated that the liver enzymes will become elevated based on the quantity of acetaminophen ingested or the levels of drug in the blood.

The dosage for oral NAC is a loading dose of 140 mg/kg, followed by 70 mg/kg every 4 hours for 17 additional doses. If the acetaminophen clears rapidly and there is no hepatotoxicity, treatment until 36 hours after ingestion may be sufficient. Longer courses of therapy (until recovery or death) are appropriate if hepatic failure occurs. Although 18 doses is the standard course, modification based on clinical and biochemical parameters is appropriate. The intravenous form of NAC is associated with a risk of anaphylaxis and is not approved for use in the United States. In cases of serious hepatic injury, however, major tertiary care centers do use the intravenous form.

This patient received NAC through a nasogastric tube every 4 hours for a total of 13 doses. Her liver enzymes peaked on the third hospital day and normalized by the 25th hospital day. (Her AST and ALT levels had begun to decline even prior to the first dose of NAC.) Pancreatic enzyme levels fluctuated in a high range for more than 4 weeks, and she required partial parenteral nutrition for 12 days. She was evaluated by psychiatry, and once she was cleared medically, she was transferred to the inpatient psychiatric unit.

Lesson for the Clinician
In this case, the diagnosis was not obvious because the patient was not forthcoming in her admission of having taken an overdose of drugs. By the time an acetaminophen level was obtained, the drug was undetectable, and the test could not offer any diagnostic clues. The differential diagnosis prior to her admission included the following: viral gastroenteritis, food poisoning, peptic ulcer disease, gallstone disease, Wilson disease, toxic ingestion, hepatitis (A, B, and C), cytomegalovirus infection, Epstein-Barr virus infection, and a Reye-like syndrome. Detecting acetaminophen toxicity early, when the patient is manifesting the common presentation of severe gastritis and emesis, remains a clinical challenge.

This case demonstrates that the clinician faced with a patient who has abdominal pain and vomiting should include in the broad differential diagnosis an overdose of toxic substances that cause those symptoms, particularly acetaminophen, which is ingested very commonly.

Julie Isaacson, MD, New York Hospital-Cornell Medical Center, New York, NY

Painful Urination Leading to Acute Urinary Retention

PRESENTATION

A 13-year-old girl presents with painful urination that has caused the development of acute urinary retention. Over the past 6 months she has had recurrent mild abdominal cramps; exactly 1 month ago she experienced a similar episode of dysuria. At that time she was able to urinate and was diagnosed by positive culture as having a urinary tract infection, for which she was treated.

While preparing to catheterize her, you notice that this young woman is at sexual maturity rating (SMR)(Tanner) stage 5 in breast and pubic hair development, yet she states that she has never had a menstrual period. Her mother recalls that her own menarche occurred at age 11 years. Observations during the procedure allow you to determine the underlying cause of her problems.

What is your differential diagnosis at this point?
Are there any elements of history or physical examination that would help you?
What additional diagnostic studies would you like performed?

DISCUSSION

Diagnosis

Imperforate hymen is a congenital anatomic aberration that causes primary amenorrhea if uncorrected and is diagnosed or excluded easily by physical examination. The incidence of imperforate hymen is approximately 1 in 1,000 girls. In the newborn, careful examination to ensure that all orifices are patent is important and will detect imperforate hymen. Mucus accumulation in the vagina of the newborn who has imperforate hymen causes a condition similar to that of the adolescent woman and is known as mucocolpos.

Most girls will start menstruating when they reach SMR (Tanner) stage 4 or within 2.5 years of the onset of breast development (thelarche). Once the sequential events of puberty have been initiated, a delay of further expected events requires investigation. Consequently, a girl whose breast and pubic hair maturation are advanced and who has not had her first menstrual period should receive an appropriate evaluation.

Presentation

Classic symptoms of imperforate hymen include an absence of menstruation in the presence of monthly abdominal cramps, although many patients are free of discomfort. When sufficient blood has accumulated in the vagina (hematocolpos), a midline lower abdominal mass is formed. The diagnosis is made readily on examination of the introitus, where a bluish, bulging hymen is evident. Complications of hematocolpos can include pressure on the urethra and bladder, resulting in urinary obstruction and stasis, which, in turn, can lead to urinary tract infection.

If hematocolpos remains uncorrected, hematocorpos (blood in the uterus) can develop, resulting in retrograde menstruation, which is the flow of uterine blood through the fallopian tubes and out into the peritoneal cavity. This process can lead to endometriosis.

Treatment
Surgical correction is the treatment for imperforate hymen and is best performed while the tissue is estrogenized, that is, soon after birth or after the onset of breast development.

Lesson for the Clinician
Add imperforate hymen to the list of reasons that girls should have their genitalia examined at birth and on subsequent physical examinations.

Elliott M. Friedman, MD, The Jamaica Hospital, Jamaica, NY

Seizures Associated With Foot Drop and Difficulties Urinating

PRESENTATION

A 14-year-old boy is brought to the emergency department because of seizures. Three weeks ago he began to have headaches with nausea and vomiting. Weakness of his left foot and difficulty in urination also have been present. There is no history of fever, neck pain, or the use of recreational drugs, nor is there a family history of seizures.

The patient is in the midst of a generalized tonic-clonic seizure. His airway is secured, and he is treated with intravenous diazepam and phenytoin. On physical examination in the postictal phase, his blood pressure is 187/117 mm Hg and his temperature is 37.1 °C (98.8 °F). He is oriented and has no meningeal signs. There is paralysis of his right arm and a left foot drop without a sensory deficit. Arteriolar constriction is found on funduscopy, but no papilledema or retinal hemorrhages are evident. A firm abdominal mass is felt on his left side, extending from the level of the umbilicus into the pelvic region. Rectal examination reveals a hard mass on the left side; anal tone is normal. A firm mass measuring approximately 9x6x4 cm is palpated in his left hemiscrotum. No significant lymphadenopathy is noted.

Serum levels of glucose and calcium, serum electrolyte levels, complete blood count, and cerebrospinal fluid (CSF) evaluation are normal. Opening pressure on lumbar puncture is 35 cm of water. Serum creatinine is 141.7 mcmol/L (1.6 mg/dL), and uric acid and lactic acid dehydrogenase levels are elevated. Computed tomography of the head shows generalized decreased cortical and subcortical attenuation, but no evidence of intracranial masses or bleeding. Ultrasonography reveals left hydronephrosis and a left hydrocele. Despite anticonvulsant therapy, the boy continues to have seizures until his blood pressure is controlled.

What is your differential diagnosis at this point?
Are there any elements of history or physical examination that would help you?
What additional diagnostic studies would you like performed?

DISCUSSION

Diagnosis

This boy's seizure was caused by hypertensive encephalopathy, the increased blood pressure resulting from the effect of a neoplasm on his renal system. He was found to have a pelvic-abdominal nonHodgkin lymphoma that was compressing his left ureter, resulting in left hydronephrosis and hydrocele. This structural change likely caused elevation of the serum renin, aldosterone, and angiotensin levels.

A pressure effect on the lumbosacral plexus was believed to explain the left foot drop and the difficulty in micturition. Paralysis of his right arm was transient and thought to be a postictal phenomenon (Todd paralysis). The elevated serum creatinine was due to acute renal insufficiency secondary to obstruction of the left kidney and either tumor invasion or urate nephropathy affecting both kidneys. The elevated uric acid is explained by lysis of the tumor cells, and lactic acid dehydrogenase is a tumor marker.

Differential Diagnosis

The differential diagnosis of seizures in this patient included central nervous system (CNS) lymphoma, which was ruled out by the absence of intracranial masses and malignant cells in the CSF. Meningoencephalitis was unlikely in the absence of fever or signs of meningeal irritation and especially in view of the normal CSF analysis. Hypocalcemia, hyponatremia, and hypoglycemia may precipitate seizures that are refractory to anticonvulsant therapy, but these disorders were ruled out by appropriate studies. In the absence of other causes, his seizures might have represented the onset of idiopathic epilepsy.

Presentation

Hypertensive encephalopathy is a rare cause of convulsions in children. It is defined as a constellation of encephalopathic signs and symptoms, including headache, confusion, drowsiness, stupor, ataxia, blurred vision, nausea and vomiting, and seizures, all of which are associated with a sudden, sustained rise in blood pressure. In as many as 50% of patients, hypertension may not be recognized until CNS symptoms appear. The degree of hypertension required to precipitate encephalopathy is believed to be related to the premorbid blood pressure.

Pathogenesis

The pathogenesis of the encephalopathy is believed to be related to generalized arteriolar vasoconstriction associated with loss of cerebral blood vessel autoregulation. Normally, even with a significant increase in blood pressure, cerebral autoregulatory mechanisms will compensate by constricting the cerebral vessels. When the pressure exceeds the level of the ability of these mechanisms to compensate, transvascular transudation will occur.

Causes of hypertensive encephalopathy include acute glomerulonephritis, renal vascular hypertension, chronic renal failure from any cause, and abrupt elevation in blood pressure in a patient who has chronic hypertension. Imaging studies such as computed tomography (CT) and magnetic resonance imaging (MRI) may be required to exclude a cerebral infarction or intracerebral hemorrhage, both of which can mimic hypertensive encephalopathy or result from it. Findings on CT and MRI scans include reversible changes consistent with generalized or multifocal edema.

Treatment

Hypertensive encephalopathy should be treated promptly with antihypertensive therapy. Nifedipine is the drug of choice for initial therapy, with intravenous diazoxide as an alternative. The aim of therapy is to reduce mean arterial pressure as much as 25% or to lower diastolic pressure to 100 mm Hg, whichever value is higher, in the first hour. An abrupt and profound drop in blood pressure should be avoided; it may result in hypoperfusion of the brain and ischemic brain injury.

Prognosis
The prognosis for children who have CNS symptoms caused by renal hypertension is unclear. Complete neurologic recovery occurs in uncomplicated cases. The primary residual effects are hemiplegia, epilepsy, impaired vision, disturbed cognitive function, and cerebral atrophy.

Lesson to the Clinician
This case should alert the pediatrician to unusual causes of seizures and to the variable presentation of relatively common tumors in children. Careful attention to blood pressure values in all patients, especially those who have seizures, is important.

The clinical manifestations of lymphoma — the second most common solid tumor in children — are protean, but lymphadenopathy and hepatosplenomegaly are common presentations. Systemic constitutional symptoms can include fever, weight loss, and night sweats. Abdominal lymphoma may cause abdominal distension or intestinal obstruction. Acute respiratory distress may be precipitated by mediastinal lymphoma. Other manifestations may be related to pressure on adjacent structures, as seen in this patient.

Nasha't M. Khanfar, MD, Mayo Clinic, Rochester, MN

Update: An additional agent used by some intensive care specialists to control acute hypertension is intravenous sodium nitroprusside.

Rapid Weight Gain and Irritability

PRESENTATION

A 13-month-old girl is being evaluated in a genetics clinic because of rapid weight gain, irritability, and concern that her facial features are dysmorphic. At the 9-month-old health supervision visit, her linear growth had slowed from the 50th to the 10th percentile, while her weight had increased from the 50th to the 75th percentile. Her parents, who were pleased initially with her weight gain, had noted an increase in her appetite and an intake of large amounts of fluids. Evaluation at that time included thyroid studies, a complete blood count, and electrolyte levels, all of which were normal. Since that visit, she has become increasingly fussy and irritable and has been noted to strike her head with her hand and to bang her head against the side of the crib.

Medical history includes a full-term, uncomplicated pregnancy and an unremarkable early infancy. The child sat by herself at 7 months of age and currently is "cruising" with assistance. She has a vocabulary of five words and follows some requests. A 2-year-old brother and the extended family are well.

On physical examination, the child appears markedly obese and irritable. Her length is below the 5th percentile, weight is at the 75th percentile, and head circumference is at the 50th percentile. Her blood pressure is 130/78 mm Hg. She has a very round, plethoric face with dark hair extending down over her forehead, sideburn areas, and upper back, where she has a thick, fleshy pad.

What is your differential diagnosis at this point?
Are there any elements of history or physical examination that would help you?
What additional diagnostic studies would you like performed?

DISCUSSION

Presentation

This infant had clinical signs of Cushing syndrome, including growth arrest, central obesity, buffalo hump, hirsutism, hypertension, and neuropsychiatric changes. Her admission laboratory values included a low serum potassium level of 3.3 mmol/L (3.3 mEq/L), a decreased serum bicarbonate level of 19 mmol/L (19 mEq/L), and a leukocytosis of 17.5 x 10^9/L (17.5 x 10^3/mcL). Spinal radiography showed generalized osteopenia. Additional findings in Cushing syndrome not found in this patient include acne, striae, bruising, clitoral hypertrophy, and hyperglycemia.

Evaluation

The most common cause of Cushing syndrome in children is exogenous steroid therapy, which should be revealed by a careful history. When exogenous sources of steroids are ruled out, laboratory studies should be performed, starting with measurement of the 24-hour urinary free cortisol excretion, which in this child was elevated at 259.4 mmol/24 h (94 mcg/24 h) (normal, 165.6 mmol/24 h [60 mcg/24 h]). Plasma cortisol levels often are elevated, and the normal diurnal variation is lost. In this patient, a morning cortisol level was 1,048.8 nmol/L (38 mcg/dL) (normal, 82.8 to 579.6 nmol/L [3 to 21 mcg/dL]), and an afternoon level was 1,021.2 nmol/L

(37 mcg/dL) (normal, 110.4 to 303.6 nmol/L [4 to 11 mcg/dL]).

After determining that cortisol levels are elevated, the next step is to differentiate adrenocorticotropic hormone (ACTH)-dependent hypercortisolism from hypercortisolism due to autonomous adrenal hyperfunction independent of ACTH secretion. ACTH-dependent states are caused by pituitary gland hypersecretion (Cushing disease), usually due to macro- or microadenomas, or by ectopic ACTH production, which is very rare. ACTH-independent hypercortisolism may be due to adrenal adenoma, adrenal carcinoma, primary adrenocortical nodular dysplasia, or macronodular adrenal hyperplasia. Children older than 10 years usually have Cushing disease; younger children are more likely to have primary adrenal pathology.

The measurement of ACTH and dose-dependent suppression of hypercortisolism by dexamethasone are helpful in determining the etiology of the increased cortisol levels. Low ACTH levels and lack of suppression of cortisol production by the administration of high doses of dexamethasone indicate a primary adrenal etiology without feedback control by the hypothalamic-pituitary-adrenal axis. High levels of ACTH and no response to suppression indicate ectopic ACTH production. Normal levels of ACTH and successful suppression of cortisol production by administration of high-dose dexamethasone indicate Cushing disease.

Treatment

This patient had an ACTH level of 7 ng/L (7 pg/mL) (normal, 20 to 100 ng/L [20 to 100 pg/mL]) in a morning sample. Abdominal ultrasonography and computed tomography (CT) documented a 6.4x5.5x5.0 cm right adrenal mass. Additional studies revealed no local invasion or metastases. Most adrenal lesions that produce Cushing syndrome are of a size unlikely to be missed on CT or magnetic resonance imaging. In this patient, an encapsulated mass was excised that proved to be an adrenal cortical carcinoma. Complete excision of this type of tumor and of any local metastases affords the best chance for cure. Radiation therapy is ineffective in adrenal carcinomas. Medical therapy, if necessary, involves the use of drugs to block steroid biosynthesis (metapyrone, aminoglutethimide) or an adrenolytic agent (o,p'-DDD), which may provide symptomatic relief. Some chemotherapeutic regimens have had limited success in the treatment of metastatic adrenal carcinoma.

Compared with adrenal adenomas, adrenal cortical carcinomas progress more quickly and are associated more often with virilization (due to weak androgens that are produced by the tumor) as well as with hypertension and hypokalemia (due to the mineralocorticoid activity of the high levels of cortisol and its precursors). In some patients, the clinical presentation of an adrenal cortical carcinoma will be determined by the effects of the tumor mass on adjacent structures rather than by hormone excess.

As in all patients whose hypothalamic-pituitary-adrenal axis has been suppressed by high levels of circulating cortisol, patients who have had these tumors removed will require glucocorticoid replacement therapy, which must be tapered gradually. Stress-dose steroid coverage for severe intercurrent illness or surgery is necessary for 6 to 12 months following recovery from hypercortisolism.

Franz E. Babl, MD, Boston University School of Medicine, Boston, MA;
Susan K. Ratzan, MD, University of Connecticut Health Center, Farmington, CT

Delayed Speech Development in a 6-year-old

PRESENTATION

The parents of a 6-year-old boy would like your opinion regarding a tonsillectomy and adenoidectomy for their son. His speech development has been delayed, and even now, despite 2 years of therapy, he is difficult to understand. The child had experienced recurrent ear infections for which pressure equalization tubes were placed 4 years ago.

Physical examination reveals bilateral serous otitis media and a bifid uvula. The tonsils appear normal for his age. His speech has a hypernasal quality. An audiologic evaluation reveals bilateral conductive hearing loss. You see a pattern that suggests an underlying condition with important therapeutic implications.

What is your differential diagnosis at this point?
Are there any elements of history or physical examination that would help you?
What additional diagnostic studies would you like performed?

DISCUSSION

Presentation

Submucous (or submucosal) cleft palate was first described in 1825 by J.P. Roux of Paris, but it was not until 1910 that A.B. Kelly coined the term submucous cleft palate (SMCP). In this condition, the oral and nasal mucosa are intact, but the muscle is attached to the soft palate abnormally. Its incidence is about 1 in 1,200 births.

The triad of bifid uvula, diastasis of the muscles in the midline of the soft palate with intact mucosa, and notching of the posterior border of the hard palate describes the classic SMCP. Not all of these features must be present for the condition to be diagnosed, and occult SMCP has been reported in the absence of a cleft uvula. Conversely, bifid uvula without other physical signs of SMCP or velopharyngeal incompetence is reported to occur in about 0.1% to 10% of the general population, with considerable racial variation in incidence. The notching of the posterior border of the hard palate sometimes can be appreciated by intraoral palpation. Another physical finding present in some patients who have SMCP is visible furrowing of the soft palate in the midline.

Only a small percent of cases of SMCP are symptomatic. During infancy, SMCP may cause slow feeding or nasal regurgitation of feedings and should be considered in babies who have these problems. The most common consequences of symptomatic SMCP are hypernasal speech due to velopharyngeal incompetence and chronic symptomatic serous otitis media. The middle ear symptoms more likely are related to the abnormal muscle attachments, with eustachian tube dysfunction, than to adenoidal hypertrophy. Adenoidectomy is contraindicated in these patients because of the risk of developing hypernasal speech postoperatively or of worsening an already existing speech problem.

Evaluation

Videofluoroscopy with barium contrast and nasopharyngoscopy are the most reliable diagnostic tests for SMCP. These examinations allow visualization of the soft palate and eustachian tube orifices as well as evaluation of any pharyngeal disproportion and assessment of the ability of the soft palate to achieve velopharyngeal closure during speech

Management

Early recognition is important so that appropriate management can be instituted, including speech therapy, careful middle ear examinations, and regular audiometric screening. The anatomic severity of the SMCP will not, by itself, predict which children will develop poor speech. Therefore, surgery to repair the cleft should be delayed until the child is 4 to 6 years old and is mature enough to have adequate speech evaluation and assessment of velopharyngeal competence.

Geeta Berera, MD, Harbor-UCLA Medical Center, Los Angeles, CA

Fever and Facial Swelling

PRESENTATION

A 10-year-old boy seeks care because of a temperature of 38.9°C (102°F) and left facial swelling. For the past few days he had been complaining of malaise, headache, neck pain, and a sore throat. His primary care physician had diagnosed him yesterday as having a viral upper respiratory tract infection. When he awoke today, his mother noted that the left side of his face was swollen; the fever developed later. The child also complains of trismus, pooling of saliva in his mouth, and difficulty swallowing. He has never had facial swelling before. His immunizations are complete.

The physical examination reveals a well-built, well-nourished boy who is cooperative but looks ill. There is nonerythematous swelling of the left side of his face, primarily involving his left cheek and obscuring the lines of the posterior mandible. The swelling extends down to the left anterior neck. The oral examination shows edema of the left side of the pharynx and soft palate. The left tonsil is displaced medially but is not inflamed. No dental caries are present. The opening of the Stensen duct is red and swollen and exudes clear saliva; the left submandibular area also is swollen. No hepatosplenomegaly or scrotal swelling are noted, and results of his neurologic examination are normal.

What is your differential diagnosis at this point?
Are there any elements of history or physical examination that would help you?
What additional diagnostic studies would you like performed?

DISCUSSION

Diagnosis

The preauricular area is occupied primarily by the parotid gland, the preauricular lymph nodes, and the main trunk of the facial nerve. Preauricular swelling is due most commonly to disorders of the parotid gland. Swelling of the parotid gland characteristically fills the space posteriorly, obscuring the angle of the mandible and extending to the mastoid process, displacing the ear upward and outward.

Mumps paromyxovirus infection, or epidemic parotitis, is the most common cause of parotid swelling and is the etiology of this child's illness. Despite the administration of the mumps vaccine, mumps still must be considered as an etiology because the efficiency of the vaccine is between 75% and 90%.

Meningeal signs are common in mumps, and other complications should be kept in mind, such as encephalitis, orchitis, epididymitis, pancreatitis, nephritis, arthritis, thyroiditis, myocarditis, and hearing impairment.

Differential Diagnosis

Rarely, other viruses have been implicated in acute parotitis, including Epstein-Barr, coxsackie, influenza, parainfluenza, echoviruses, and the virus of lymphocytic choriomeningitis.

Another condition that causes parotid swelling is juvenile recurrent parotitis. Although rare, it is the second most common inflammatory salivary gland disease of childhood. It usually starts in a 5- to 7-year-old child who has signs and symptoms similar to those of mumps. The swelling usually is unilateral, but both glands may be involved simultaneously or alternately, and it resolves spontaneously, only to recur periodically up to 10 or more times. After puberty, the condition usually disappears.

Another less common disorder, suppurative parotitis, tends to recur in some children, usually is unilateral, and appears to be due primarily to salivary stasis. Most children who have this condition are otherwise healthy and often appear well during the acute episodes. Expression of pus from the opening of the Stensen duct, with demonstration of bacteria on Gram stain, supports a diagnosis of a suppurative infection, most commonly caused by *Staphylococcus aureus* and *Streptococcus viridans*. Suppurative parotitis in the neonatal period (neonatal sialadenitis) usually is associated with prematurity. Dehydration also has been identified as a predisposing factor.

Stones (sialoliths) obstructing the Stensen duct also can cause parotid swelling. There is pain and swelling before meals and an inability to express secretions from the duct; fever and signs of inflammation of the gland are absent. At times, a stone in the duct can be palpated. More than 90% of parotid gland stones are radiolucent. Sialography should be performed when a sialolith is suspected.

An isolated mass palpable within the substance of the parotid gland suggests a benign tumor; malignant neoplasms are uncommon in children. Benign tumors include congenital salivary gland cysts, such as dermoid, branchial cleft, branchial pouch, and congenital ductal cysts; vascular tumors, such as hemangiomas and lymphangiomas; and pleomorphic adenomas. A firm, painful salivary gland mass associated with facial paralysis suggests malignancy, commonly a mucoepidermoid carcinoma.

Because the preauricular area contains lymph nodes, disorders such as lymphadenitis, lymphoma, and lymphosarcoma should be considered. Pharyngeal and dental abscesses also can cause preauricular swelling.

Evaluation

Serologic tests such as complement fixation and hemagglutination tests can help to distinguish viral infection of the parotid gland. Mumps virus can be cultured from throat washings or urine. Serum amylase usually is elevated in parotitis of any cause.

Nathalie Quion, MD, Thomas G. DeWitt, MD, University of Massachusetts Medical Center, Worcester, MA

Update: Parotid gland enlargement also is a manifestation of human immunodeficiency virus (HIV) infection. Clinicians must consider this disorder in the differential diagnosis of parotitis. Infectious disease consultants point out that although children who have HIV infection are more susceptible to mumps, most of the parotitis seen in these children probably is caused by the HIV agent itself.

Shortness of Breath and Chest Pain

PRESENTATION

A 19-year-old South American woman who is visiting her sister is seen in the emergency department because of mild shortness of breath and moderately severe, sharp chest pain, which have developed over the past 24 hours. Because the young woman speaks no English, it is difficult to obtain a complete history. Her sister, who speaks some English, does not know of any history of cardiac or pulmonary disorders. Apparently she is taking only one medication, a "female hormone."

On physical examination, the patient appears anxious and mildly distressed. Her temperature is 99 °F (37.2 °C), pulse is 120 beats/min, respirations are 22 breaths/min, and blood pressure is 100/55 mm Hg. She is a short, mildly obese person who has a short neck, ears that appear to be set low, and mild hypertelorism. Her skin is pale and she has many nevi. Her hands and feet are cool. She is not tender to palpation along the costochondral junctions. Her precordial activity is increased, and her pulses are bounding. Audible at the left sternal border are a systolic click, a grade 2/6 midsystolic murmur, and a grade 3/6 decrescendo diastolic murmur. Her lungs are clear. A radiograph of the chest reveals prominence of the mediastinum, and an electrocardiogram shows a sinus tachycardia with nonspecific ST-T wave changes.

The physician believes that the patient has a bicuspid aortic valve with mild aortic stenosis and moderate regurgitation and that the chest pain is of pleuritic origin. He also suspects that she has an underlying disorder associated with these findings. An echocardiogram demonstrates that this is partially correct.

What is your differential diagnosis at this point?
Are there any elements of history or physical examination that would help you?
What additional diagnostic studies would you like performed?

DISCUSSION

Diagnosis
The suspicion that the patient had Turner syndrome was borne out when a Spanish interpreter arrived, and the young woman confirmed that she had been diagnosed in infancy. Previously in good health, she had not seen her pediatrician for 6 years. Her only medication was cyclic estrogen-progesterone that was initiated by a pediatric endocrinologist at age 8 years. She recalled that a murmur had been heard by her pediatrician when she was 12 years old, but it was believed to be innocent.

Evaluation and Treatment
Two-dimensional echocardiography with Doppler examination showed a bicuspid aortic valve with mild aortic stenosis (10 mm gradient) and severe aortic regurgitation. Additionally, there was marked aortic root dilation (diameter, 58 mm). Because the echocardiographic window was inadequate to examine the transverse and descending aorta, magnetic resonance imaging (MRI) was performed. The aortic dimension was confirmed, and coarctation of the descending aorta was not seen,

but an intimal flap consistent with ascending aortic dissection was. The patient required emergency aortic valve replacement and reconstruction of the ascending aorta. She had a satisfactory postoperative course and was discharged on coumarin anticoagulation and prophylaxis for subacute bacterial endocarditis.

Etiology and Presentation

Turner syndrome results from a chromosomal abnormality, the most common being a 45,X karyotype, which is found in 50% of affected patients. Less frequently, the karyotype is X chromosome mosaicism, ring chromosome, isochromosome, deletion, or duplication. Unlike patients who have Down syndrome, in which the dysmorphic features are fairly consistent, women who have Turner syndrome display a great variety of appearances. The phenotype varies with age. The stillborn fetus may be hydropic and have a massive cystic hygroma; newborns will have neck webbing and edema of the hands and feet. A young girl is likely to manifest short stature and minor anomalies that include low hairline, epicanthal folds, dysplastic and truly low-set ears, downslanting palpebral fissures, brittle nails, cubitus valgus, and short fourth metacarpal (manifested as a depressed metacarpal-phalangeal joint when the hand is fisted). The syndrome may be diagnosed for the first time in a teenager who is seen because of delayed secondary sexual development. Definitive diagnosis of Turner syndrome requires karyotype analysis.

An additional diagnostic pearl is to consider Noonan syndrome in a patient who is suspected of having Turner syndrome but has a normal karyotype, particularly if cardiac lesions are present in the right side of the heart (especially pulmonic stenosis). The phenotype of these two disorders is not identical, but similarities exist.

Cardiovascular malformations (CVMs) are a well-known feature of Turner syndrome, occurring in approximately 20% to 30% of patients. Typically they involve the left side of the heart. Although coarctation of the aorta is mentioned most often in connection with Turner syndrome, it occurs less frequently than bicuspid aortic valve (15% versus 30% incidence). Less common CVMs include aortic stenosis (with or without bicuspid aortic valve), mitral valve anomalies, and hypoplastic left heart syndrome (rare). In addition to left ventricular outflow tract obstructive lesions, ventricular and atrial septal defects, partial anomalous pulmonary venous return, and mitral valve prolapse may occur.

Although aortic root dilation occurs in only a few women who have Turner syndrome (approximately 9% in one study), it is an important cause of morbidity and mortality, especially in the older patient. This patient had chest pain, dyspnea, hypotension with wide pulse pressure, tachycardia, bounding pulses, a systolic click, a systolic murmur, and a diastolic murmur. She was suspected of having bicuspid aortic valve with aortic stenosis and regurgitation. Aortic dilation alone is asymptomatic and likely was present for many years prior to dissection. Her bicuspid aortic valve may have produced an innocent-sounding murmur initially, but over time it became stenotic and eventually regurgitant. This patient's chest pain was caused by her aortic dissection and provided a clue to the presence of that condition.

Coarctation of the aorta is a risk factor for aortic dilation, dissection, and rupture. The precise role played by the bicuspid valve in aortic dilation is unknown, although it also is acknowledged as a risk factor. As in the general population, systemic hypertension increases the risk of aortic disease and is more common in Turner syndrome. At present, exogenous estrogen administration and growth hormone are not thought to increase this risk.

Even when Turner syndrome is identified, aortic dissection often is not included in the differential diagnosis of chest pain and may be misinterpreted as anxiety or as a viral syndrome causing costochondritis or pleurisy. In some instances, only aortic valve disease is recognized.

Because some patients who have Turner syndrome with aortic dilation have been found to have cystic medial necrosis, an inherited connective tissue abnormality has been postulated. The hypothesis of a mesenchymal tissue defect is supported by the common association of Turner syndrome with abnormalities of the lymphatic vessels (lymphedema, cystic hygroma) and bone (broad chest, narrow palate, tibial exostoses, cubitus valgus, short fourth metacarpal, hip dysplasia, kyphoscoliosis).

Follow-up

Superior imaging of the aorta is obtained with MRI, which should be performed on patients in whom the findings on echocardiography are equivocal and on individuals who have an inadequate echocardiographic window because of chest wall configuration or obesity. MRI also can be valuable in assessing the possibility of aortic dissection.

In addition to general medical, genetic, renal, endocrinologic, orthopedic, and educational recommendations for patients who have Turner syndrome, the Committee on Genetics of the American Academy of Pediatrics advises prospective cardiologic supervision. All children should have blood pressure and peripheral pulse assessed routinely. An echocardiogram should be obtained in infancy, preferably as part of a cardiology consultation, with appropriate medical and surgical care dictated by results of the evaluation. Some patients will require antibiotic prophylaxis to prevent subacute bacterial endocarditis. Periodic echocardiograms or MRI scans should be performed to look for aortic root dilation, which usually is asymptomatic. It should be suspected, especially in patients who have coexisting risk factors such as hypertension, bicuspid aortic valve, or coarctation. Older adolescents leaving pediatric care must be reminded to continue cardiologic supervision, including echocardiography.

Lesson for the Clinician

This case illustrates a dilemma encountered by older adolescents and young adults who have genetic syndromes as they leave the care of pediatricians. It will become increasingly important for internists and other practitioners who deal with such patients to become familiar with their special medical needs. Women who have Turner syndrome often are healthy and may fail to seek medical care except for specific problems, neglecting health maintenance visits. During childhood, their routine care usually is supplemented with visits to the pediatric cardiologist and endocrinologist. After adolescence, a gynecologist often is the primary physician who cares for a woman who has Turner syndrome, addressing the issues of estrogen therapy, fertility, and reproductive options.

Angela E. Lin, MD, Westwood, MA

Constipation and Pain Upon Defecation

PRESENTATION

A 15-year-old Hispanic boy comes to the emergency department after passing a large, black, tarry stool. A similar problem occurred 5 years ago, when he was diagnosed as having "ulcer disease." After antacid treatment for 1 year, he was free of symptoms. The patient often is constipated and experiences pain upon defecation. He denies abdominal pain, diarrhea, emesis, fever, weight loss, night sweats, easy bruiseability, skin rashes, jaundice, passing red rectal blood, drug use, or any other systemic complaints, including problems with bleeding. He has had no surgery.

On physical examination, the patient is anxious and has both tachycardia and orthostatic hypotension. There is no blood in his nose and throat, but gastric lavage is positive for coffee ground material. His abdomen is soft and nontender; no organomegaly is noted. Rectal examination yields guaiac-positive stool, but no gross blood, fissures, or hemorrhoids are present.

Laboratory findings include: hematocrit, 0.44 (44%); platelet count, 283 x 10⁹/L $(283 \times 10^3/mcL)$; blood urea nitrogen, 4.28 mmol urea/L (12 mg/dL); bilirubin, 13.6 mcmol.L (0.8 mg/dL); aspartate aminotransferase, 36 U/L; alanine aminotransferase, 73 U/L; prothrombin time, 13 seconds (normal, 9.3 to 11.1 sec); partial thromboplastin time, 53 seconds (normal, 22.1 to 34.0 sec); and reticulocyte count, 10% of erythrocytes. His bleeding time is normal. Shortly after arrival, the patient begins to vomit blood, and his hematocrit drops to 0.21 (21%).

What is your differential diagnosis at this point?
Are there any elements of history or physical examination that would help you?
What additional diagnostic studies would you like performed?

DISCUSSION

Stabilization

For any patient who has hematemesis and hypotension, the immediate concern is stabilization. A logical series of steps involves obtaining central venous or adequate peripheral access with large-bore intravenous catheters, providing volume support with crystalloid fluids, and inserting a nasogastric tube for suctioning. A histamine₂ (H_2) receptor antagonist can decrease gastric acidity, packed erythrocytes can replace lost blood, and clotting factors may be infused if there is evidence of a coagulopathy. When the patient is stable, it is necessary to arrange for a diagnostic and possibly therapeutic endoscopic procedure.

Evaluation and Diagnosis

After stabilization with the previously mentioned measures, this patient underwent endoscopy, which revealed nodular antritis and superficial erosions in the body and fundus of the stomach. A large duodenal ulcer with a fresh adherent clot also was present and required injection therapy with saline and epinephrine.

This evaluation involved more than a simple reinvestigation of the patient's past problem with dyspepsia. Further examination revealed two additional findings: biopsy specimens were positive for *Helicobacter pylori*, and investigation into the etiology of the prolonged partial thromboplastin time revealed a factor VIII level of only 7%. This boy had two processes contributing to his hematemesis: *H pylori* gastritis with a duodenal ulcer and hemophilia A.

Treatment

Peptic ulcer disease is a relatively rare condition in childhood. Although recent research has established compelling evidence linking *H pylori* infection with duodenal ulcers and gastritis, it is unclear why some patients who harbor this organism develop ulcer disease and others experience only recurrent dyspepsia or are asymptomatic. In any case, it has been established that the recurrence rate of ulcers is reduced markedly by eradication of the bacterium. This patient was treated with 14 days of triple therapy (amoxicillin, metronidazole, and bismuth subsalicylate) to eradicate *H pylori*, then continued on an H_2 antagonist for an additional 6 weeks to manage his underlying gastritis and duodenal ulcer.

Additional Findings

Confounding this patient's upper gastrointestinal bleeding was the presence of an unsuspected coagulopathy, hemophilia A. Although severe cases of hemophilia frequently are diagnosed during infancy in association with a positive family history, easy bruiseability, or prolonged bleeding following trauma, it is not uncommon for mild cases to present later in life or never be diagnosed. In all cases, it is unusual for the initial presentation to be upper gastrointestinal bleeding, but because gastrointestinal bleeding is not common in children, screening tests for coagulopathy are worth considering in patients who have such bleeding.

Conversely, when faced with significant gastrointestinal bleeding in a patient who has or is suspected of having a coagulopathy, the clinician is wise to seek a specific lesion in the intestinal tract. This point is reinforced by recent experience with a 4-year-old boy who was known to have mild hemophilia A (factor VIII level of 12%) and who presented to the emergency department with a 4-day history of passing bright red blood with bowel movements. He also complained of intermittent, postprandial periumbilical pain and vomited twice on the day of admission. There was no history of diarrhea, fever, or medication use. Physical findings were normal except for a resting tachycardia, a grade III/VI systolic ejection murmur, generalized pallor, and abdominal tenderness. Blood test results were: hemoglobin, 0.81 mmol/L (5.2 g/dL); hematocrit, 0.16 (16%); prothrombin time, 11.3 seconds; and partial thromboplastin time, 56.2 seconds.

When the child's stools remained bloody after factor replacement, additional evaluation was undertaken. A Meckel scan was negative, and stool cultures were negative for *Salmonella*, *Shigella*, and *Escherichia coli* 0157. No ova or parasites were detected. The child underwent esophagogastroduodenoscopy and colonoscopy. He was found to have a discrete ulceration at the ileocecal valve, and his colonic stool aspirate was positive for *Campylobacter jejuni*.

Lessons for the Clinician

These cases remind clinicians of the importance of considering more than one etiology for a clinical presentation, particularly when a patient has serious problems. There is no relationship between hemophilia and peptic ulcer disease; they are independent entities. Yet, both of the patients discussed had both conditions. Clinicians often strive to unite all relevant information into one tidy diagnosis, but a patient is entitled to have more than one disease. In these cases, a fresh perspective yielded surprising additions to previously known diagnoses.

Joseph Colli, MD, Danny Thomas, MD, Leila Dane, MD, Childrens Hospital of Los Angeles, University of Southern California, Los Angeles, CA

Progressively Worsening Shortness of Breath With Sudden Drop in Oxygen Saturation

PRESENTATION

A 3-year-old girl is brought to the emergency department because of 24 hours of fever, nonproductive cough, and shortness of breath that has worsened progressively. She has no history of significant illness. She has been taking amoxicillin for 1 week to treat otitis media and pharyngitis.

On physical examination, the child appears in obvious respiratory distress. She has a temperature of 101°F (38.3°C), pulse of 150 beats/min, respiratory rate of 46 breaths/min, and blood pressure of 137/72 mm Hg. She is breathing with subcostal and intercostal retractions and nasal flaring. Her breath sounds are diminished in the area of the right upper lobe, and generalized inspiratory and expiratory wheezing is heard. Both tympanic membranes are red and distorted. Her pharynx is reddened but free of exudate. Other findings on the examination are normal.

Breathing 100% oxygen, the child has an arterial pH of 7.40, a P_{O_2} of 54 torr, and a P_{CO_2} of 28 torr. Radiography of her chest reveals collapse of the right upper lobe and a right apical pneumothorax. She is admitted to the intensive care unit and treated aggressively with beta-agonists and corticosteroids. While she is breathing 100% oxygen, her oxygen saturation suddenly drops to 80%. Her breath sounds now are diminished on both sides, and a radiograph reveals worsening of the right pneumothorax as well as a left pneumothorax with complete collapse of the left lung.

What is your differential diagnosis at this point?
Are there any elements of history or physical examination that would help you?
What additional diagnostic studies would you like performed?

DISCUSSION

Diagnosis

The child was taken to the operating room immediately, where her pneumothoraces were evacuated through chest tubes and she underwent rigid bronchoscopy. Pieces of a gelatinous foreign body, most consistent with a hot dog, were retrieved from her right upper and left mainstem bronchi. In less than 1 week she was extubated successfully, weaned to room air, and discharged home in stable condition.

Foreign body aspiration (FBA) into the tracheobronchial tree is a common pediatric problem that can result in chronic illness and even death if not recognized. The majority of children who aspirate foreign bodies are younger than 4 years.

Presentation

The clinical manifestations of FBA vary, depending on the location of the foreign body and the degree of obstruction that it causes. A large object may block larger airways, resulting in acute respiratory distress. Small objects aspirated into a peripheral location may cause local irritation and pneumonia, although the only sign might be a mild cough. They need to be removed, but are not life-threatening, as larger objects can be.

In most cases, the initial episode of FBA involves the immediate onset of choking, followed by recurrent spasmodic coughing and gagging. If this initial episode is not witnessed, a child may present with occasional coughing and mild wheezing without a history of aspiration. The lack of a positive history may be the greatest impediment to early diagnosis. The diagnosis of FBA should be entertained in all patients who have persistent wheezing unresponsive to bronchodilator therapy, persistent cough, atelectasis, or pneumonia.

Physical findings early in the course of an FBA may consist only of decreased aeration of the affected lung. Other signs seen in this condition are tracheal shift, wheezing, stridor, and bloody sputum.

Evaluation

Radiographic studies may reveal hyperinflation of the ipsilateral lung with shifting of the mediastinum to the contralateral side. Expiratory views may facilitate the diagnosis if the foreign body is radiolucent. Early in the course of this condition, however, it is not unusual for patients to have normal findings on chest radiography. If FBA is strongly suspected, rigid bronchoscopy is the recommended procedure.

Prognosis

FBA may be fatal if not diagnosed early. Most patients who are diagnosed recover rapidly and fully after the object is removed. If diagnosis is delayed, however, serious complications may develop, including tracheal trauma from inflammation, subglottic edema, infection manifested by fever and purulent sputum, lung abscess, and bronchiectasis.

Foreign bodies large enough to lodge in a central bronchus (usually a mainstem bronchus) can be remarkably silent from a clinical point of view, even for several days, unless they cause pneumonia. If a foreign body of this size moves, it may lodge beneath the vocal cords, causing immediate asphyxia. If such a foreign body shifts and obstructs the other mainstem bronchus, the lung that was blocked originally may be unable to support respiration because of a concomitant pneumonia and because it has little, if any, blood flow. With the originally healthy lung obstructed, the child cannot breathe.

Treatment

Because of the potential for these life-threatening events, any child suspected of having a foreign body in a central airway should be taken to the operating room immediately. Any intervention that might dislodge the object in the meantime should be avoided, including postural drainage, cupping, and bronchodilator therapy.

Early recognition of FBA is essential for the patient and a diagnostic challenge for the physician.

Martha Toledo-Valido, MD, University of Miami, Jackson Memorial Hospital, Miami, FL

Swollen Toes

PRESENTATION

As the pediatric consultant for a community hospital's emergency department, you are called in the early morning by the emergency physician on call. He describes a 5-month-old boy who was brought in because of swelling of his left third and fourth toes. His mother noticed the swollen toes when she removed him from his sleeper, which covers his feet loosely and which he had worn all night. She is sure his foot was normal the night before. The child seems irritable but otherwise normal to his mother. Nothing of this nature has happened to him before.

The physician describes the affected toes as being moderately swollen, especially distally. Both toes have a narrow, deep groove visible proximally, with surrounding erythema and swelling. The toes clearly are tender, as the infant vigorously resists their close examination. The remainder of the physical examination is normal, including the other toes and the rest of the foot.

The emergency physician has obtained radiographs of the toes, which are interpreted as normal. You offer suggestions that enable the diagnosis and treatment of the baby's condition.

What is your differential diagnosis at this point?
Are there any elements of history or physical examination that would help you?
What additional diagnostic studies would you like performed?

DISCUSSION

At your suggestion, the physician anesthetizes the toes with a digital lidocaine block, allowing him to examine them more closely. Using an otoscope for magnification, he discovers tightly wound hairs in both grooves, but is unable to remove them without damaging the toes further. He follows your advice and sends a family member to a nearby pharmacy to obtain a bottle of Nair™ hair remover. Several minutes after the product is applied, the hair becomes fragile enough to pick out with a fine forceps. The swelling and erythema resolve gradually.

Diagnosis

This condition, known as hair tourniquet syndrome, hair-thread tourniquet, hair wrapping, and toe tourniquet, is seen most commonly in infants. Because the tightly wound hair causes extensive local swelling, the hair itself may no longer be visible. Thus, inflammation due to trauma, insect sting, infection, or allergic reaction may be suspected. Left untreated, the constriction may lead to gangrene and eventual amputation. Recognition and early treatment are important to prevent permanent damage.

Although toes are afflicted most commonly, hair tourniquet syndrome may affect any extremity. Hair tourniquet of the fingers and penis are seen fairly commonly. Hair tourniquet of the clitoris, the labia majora, and even the uvula have been described. Interestingly, an affected great toe never has been reported. As in this case, several adjacent toes or fingers may be affected simultaneously. Because hair tourniquet syndrome may be the cause of otherwise unexplained irritability, it is important to examine the extremities of all irritable infants.

Many cases involve human hair, but the syndrome also may be caused by fine threads, usually from clothing. This circumstance occurs most commonly when the infant has been wearing a garment that covers the feet and has been washed repeatedly, leading to accumulation of loose threads and fibers near the toes. Mittens with loose threads have been implicated, as has a tight rubber band.

Etiology

The etiology of this condition often is mysterious. The question of child abuse may be raised. Indeed, the intentional malicious application of a penile hair tourniquet was described as long ago as 1832. Wrapping hairs about body parts also has been used in primitive societies to ward off evil spirits. Most contemporary cases seem to be accidental. It is postulated that repeated flexion and extension of the fingers or toes in the presence of loose threads or hairs gradually causes them to encircle the digits. Movement of the hips in the diapers may lead to similar involvement of the genitals. If the hairs are wet, they will constrict gradually as they dry, forming a tight band.

Treatment

The obvious treatment is timely removal of the encircling fibers. If one end can be grasped, the fibers simply may be unwound. If a fine forceps with teeth can be passed beneath the fibers, the strands can be isolated from the underlying skin and cut with a scalpel, fine scissors, or hollow needle. Application of hair remover is an elegant method of treatment, but it may not work with synthetic fibers and is not advisable on deeply cut skin. Because it may be difficult to judge the degree of involvement, hair remover should not be used if the tissue is markedly swollen or inflamed.

Surgical consultation may be required for hair tourniquet. Several operative techniques for cutting the encircling fibers without endangering the underlying nerves, tendons, or vessels have been described. Whatever the method, the clinician must be certain that all of the encircling fibers have been removed. Once the hairs or threads are removed, even severely affected extremities usually recover. Elective amputation should be delayed until the tissue clearly is not viable.

Gregory P. Conners, MD, University of Rochester School of Medicine
and Dentistry, Rochester, NY

Progressive Difficulty Walking and Headaches

PRESENTATION

A 6-year-old boy was first seen in the emergency department 6 days ago with complaints of generalized weakness, pain in the calves, and difficulty walking for 2 days. He also had vomiting and colicky abdominal pain at that time. His past medical history was unremarkable except for having had chickenpox 3 weeks prior to presentation. On physical examination, the boy was afebrile, had normal vital signs, and had normal physical findings except for a mildly unsteady gait. Results of a complete blood count, electrolyte levels, liver function tests, serum amylase, and serum lipase were normal, and he was sent home with the diagnosis of viral syndrome.

Five days later, he has returned because of worsening symptoms of weakness, pain in his legs, and difficulty walking. He also has developed global headaches of mild-to-moderate intensity and continues to experience abdominal pain and vomiting, but less intensely than before. On physical examination, his muscle strength is diminished (4/5 in upper extremities and 3/5 in lower extremities), and deep tendon reflexes are difficult to elicit. No ataxia, dysmetria, or tremor is noted. Further studies clarify the diagnosis.

What is your differential diagnosis at this point?
Are there any elements of history or physical examination that would help you?
What additional diagnostic studies would you like performed?

DISCUSSION

Diagnosis

A lumbar puncture yielded cerebrospinal fluid (CSF) that showed a protein level of 2,150 mg/L (215 mg/dL), white blood cell count of only 3/mcL (all mononuclear), and red blood cell count of 3/mcL. This pattern of elevated protein and normal white blood cell count suggested Guillain-Barré syndrome (GBS). The certainty of the diagnosis was strengthened when nerve conduction studies showed evidence of a sensory/motor demyelinating peripheral neuropathy compatible with GBS.

GBS is an acute demyelinating disease of the peripheral nervous system. The pathogenesis is autoimmune, and both cell-mediated and humoral immunity have been found to be altered. It usually presents a few days or weeks after the patient has had an upper respiratory tract or gastrointestinal infection. GBS has been reported to follow many infections. Among the associated viral infections are cytomegalovirus, Epstein-Barr virus, varicella, rubella, mumps, hepatitis, human immunodeficiency virus, and herpesvirus. Nonviral agents, such as *Campylobacter* sp (especially *Campylobacter jejuni*), *Mycoplasma* sp, and *Chlamydia* sp, also have been implicated. Less frequently, vaccines, neoplasms, surgery, epidural anesthesia, trauma, and drugs have been reported prior to the development of GBS.

Presentation

The clinical picture of GBS is characterized by progressive muscle weakness, usually more distal than proximal, and diminished or absent deep tendon reflexes in a generally symmetric distribution. Pain or paresthesia usually precedes the weakness. Most patients have an ascending progression of weakness, starting in the legs—like putting pants on—and progressing to the arms. For this reason, gait disturbance is the most common presenting symptom.

Respiratory weakness occurs in 12% to 20% of patients, causing some individuals to require mechanical ventilation. Therefore, vital capacity and sometimes arterial blood gases should be monitored frequently, especially at the beginning of the disease. The cranial nerves also can be involved. The seventh cranial nerve is involved most commonly, causing facial paresis. The third, sixth, ninth, and tenth cranial nerves also can be affected. Involvement of the ninth and the tenth cranial nerves manifests with difficulty swallowing.

Autonomic dysfunction sometimes is present and can range from diaphoresis to more serious manifestations, such as hypertension, postural hypotension, and cardiac arrhythmias. Bowel and bladder dysfunction have been reported but are extremely rare.

The disease progresses over a matter of weeks, with 90% of patients reaching their maximum deficits by 3 to 4 weeks. The majority of deaths are related to respiratory failure, pulmonary embolism, and autonomic dysfunction.

Many clinical variants of GBS have been described, the most common being Miller Fisher syndrome, which is characterized by ophthalmoplegia, ataxia, and areflexia with little weakness.

Laboratory Findings
The CSF characteristically demonstrates an elevated protein level with a normal cell count. This pattern is called albuminocytologic dissociation and can be absent early in the disease process, especially during the first week. Results of electrodiagnostic studies are abnormal in most patients and are manifested by a reduction in nerve conduction velocity. Multiple nerves should be studied because GBS is a patchy disease, and abnormalities may be missed in a limited study or when tested early, usually during the first week.

Differential Diagnosis
The differential diagnosis includes many disorders. Among the most important are spinal cord compression, transverse myelitis, acute cerebellar ataxia, myasthenia gravis, poliomyelitis, botulism, diphtheritic neuropathy, lead neuropathy, hexacarbon neuropathy, porphyria, metabolic myopathies, and tick paralysis.

Polio presents with myalgia, areflexia, and fever at the beginning of the paralysis, which is asymmetric and causes muscle atrophy later. Both the CSF cell count and protein levels are elevated. Children whose spinal cords are compressed due to tumors or epidural abscess have back pain, sensory deficit at a specific level, and bowel and bladder disturbances. Acute cerebellar ataxia presents with gait disturbance and hypotonia mimicking GBS, but the CSF usually shows pleocytosis with a normal protein level.

Treatment

Supportive care is a critical part of the treatment of patients who have GBS. Patients who experience declining vital capacities or oropharyngeal weakness require endotracheal intubation. Pneumonias and urinary tract infections can occur and require appropriate therapy. Specific therapy for GBS involves plasmapheresis or administration of intravenous immune globulin (IVIG). Both treatments are effective in shortening and improving the outcome of the disease, but they need to be started early, especially during the first 2 weeks of illness. Corticosteroids no longer are considered useful therapy for GBS. This boy was treated with IVIG and recovered completely.

Prognosis

The prognosis for patients who contract GBS is good; 70% to 80% recover completely within 1 year, and the majority recover during the first 6 months. Ten percent of patients will have permanent deficits, an outcome associated with a prolonged period of hospitalization. About 3% of patients will not survive the disease.

Carlos E. Sabogal, MD, University of Miami School of Medicine, Miami, FL

Persistent High Fever, Headache, and Sore Throat

PRESENTATION

A 5½-year-old boy is seen in the office because he has had 4 days of high fever, headache, and sore throat. For 2 days he has had "pink eye" and a rash, and for 1 day he has experienced vomiting, diarrhea, and general malaise. He has complained of pain in the left side of his neck, and his urine has been deep yellow. Two days ago he was seen at a clinic and was given amoxicillin for presumed streptococcal pharyngitis, but his condition has worsened since then.

On physical examination, the child is irritable and uncooperative and looks ill. His temperature is 38.8°C (101.9°F); other vital signs are normal. Bilateral, nonpurulent conjunctival inflammation is noted as well as a tinge of scleral icterus. His lips and tongue are erythematous, and his tonsils are moderately enlarged and appear inflamed. One 2.0 cm, somewhat tender lymph node is palpable on the left side of his neck. A maculopapular rash is present, most pronounced on his posterior trunk, and his palms and soles are reddened without desquamation. The remainder of the examination yields normal findings.

His white blood cell count is 11×10^9/L (11×10^3/mcL) with 53% segmented neutrophils and 31% band forms, platelet count is 336×10^9/L (336×10^3/mcL), and erythrocyte sedimentation rate (ESR) is 41 mm/h. Blood chemistry results include aspartate aminotransferase of 66 U/L (normal, 5 to 40 U/L), alanine aminotransferase of 152 U/L (normal, 7 to 56 U/L), and total bilirubin of 102 mcmol/L (6 mg/dL). His urine is deep yellow and is positive for bilirubin, blood, and nitrates; microscopic findings include 5 to 10 leukocytes per high-power field. A rapid streptococcal test and spot test for infectious mononucleosis are read as negative. Ultrasonography of the liver shows no abnormalities. Throat, blood, and urine cultures are obtained.

What is your differential diagnosis at this point?
Are there any elements of history or physical examination that would help you?
What additional diagnostic studies would you like performed?

DISCUSSION

Diagnosis

The child was admitted to the hospital and started empirically on parenteral antibiotics, but he continued to spike high fevers. All cultures yielded negative results, as did Epstein-Barr serology, hepatitis serology, and an antistreptolysin titer. Because of a clinical suspicion of Kawasaki disease, echocardiography was performed and revealed mild dilatation of the left ventricle, with a slight decrease in function and coronary artery diameters that were at the upper limits of normal.

The boy was given intravenous immune globulin (IVIG) on the second hospital day as well as high-dose aspirin. He also was given digoxin on the advice of the cardiologist. His fever subsided rapidly, and he was sent home after 4 days in the hospital. One week later, the skin on his fingers began to peel. Follow-up echocardiography was normal. The complete clinical picture was consistent with Kawasaki disease.

Kawasaki disease most often affects children younger than 5 years of age, with a peak age of occurrence at 18 to 24 months. The etiology of the disorder is unknown, although infectious and autoimmune mechanisms are suspected. The diagnosis is made primarily on clinical grounds, and the process involves exclusion of a wide range of diseases that have similar presentations.

Presentation

Diagnosis of Kawasaki disease requires the presence of fever for at least 5 days and any four of the following findings: bilateral nonpurulent conjunctivitis, oropharyngeal mucosal changes (inflamed pharynx; strawberry tongue; dry, fissured, erythematous lips), changes in the peripheral extremities (edema and erythema of the hands and feet, desquamation of the digits), rash (primarily truncal), and cervical lymphadenopathy. Affected children often manifest a striking irritability.

Atypical Kawasaki disease is diagnosed when fewer than four of the findings are present and usually occurs in infants younger than 1 year of age. The diagnosis often is missed in this group, resulting in higher morbidity. Therapy can be started even when all criteria have not been met fully if the clinical picture is strongly suggestive, as in the patient who has not yet had 5 full days of fever.

Complications

This disorder is multisystemic. The most serious complication is coronary artery dilatation and aneurysm formation, which can lead to myocardial infarction if not treated. When death occurs, it usually is due to this mechanism. Coronary artery complications usually develop 1 to 2 weeks after onset of the disease. Patients at higher risk for coronary artery disease are those whose fever persists longer than 10 days, those who have low concentrations of serum albumin or hemoglobin, males, infants younger than 12 months of age, and those who have signs of cardiac involvement (arrhythmias, pericardial effusion).

Pericarditis, myocarditis (with congestive heart failure), and endocarditis may occur, as can aneurysms of other arteries. Aneurysms may not regress completely, and the coronary artery disease can progress to stenosis or atherosclerosis. Involvement of other systems includes urethritis with sterile pyuria, hepatic dysfunction (as in this patient), arthritis or arthralgias, aseptic meningitis, and hydrops of the gallbladder.

Differential Diagnosis

The differential diagnosis of Kawasaki disease includes measles, other viral exanthems, scarlet fever, rickettsial infections, drug reactions, toxic shock syndrome, juvenile rheumatoid arthritis, leptospirosis, and mercury poisoning. Although no diagnostic test specific for Kawasaki disease exists, echocardiography is an essential procedure when this disorder is suspected. An experienced cardiologist must be involved early in the patient's course, and follow-up echocardiograms must be obtained. Depending on the type of cardiac involvement the patient has experienced, echocardiography may have to be repeated for years. Acute phase reactants, such as the ESR, C-reactive protein level, and platelet count, are elevated, the latter usually after the tenth day of illness. Liver enzymes may be elevated, as in this case, and ultrasonography may reveal hydrops of the gallbladder. Pyuria may be present, but cultures will be negative.

Treatment

The specific treatment of Kawasaki disease is administration of IVIG, which has been shown to decrease the prevalence of coronary artery disease and to hasten the resolution of other acute inflammatory processes, such as fever. It is administered as a single dose of 2 g/kg. Retreatment may be necessary if symptoms persist for more than 72 hours, the fever is recrudescent, and the clinical picture remains consistent with Kawasaki disease. High-dose aspirin (100 mg/kg per day in four divided doses) is used for its anti-inflammatory effect and reduced to a lower dose (3 to 5 mg/kg per day in one dose) when the patient becomes afebrile. The lower doses of aspirin are administered to take advantage of the drug's effect on platelet function. Components of the acute disease, such as congestive heart failure, require additional therapy.

Patients who do not have coronary artery disease can be continued on low-dose aspirin therapy for 6 to 8 weeks or until the platelet count and ESR return to normal. Those who have coronary artery disease should continue aspirin therapy indefinitely. Persistent or large aneurysms may require dipyridamole therapy and anticoagulation.

Lesson for the Clinician

Because the outcome of Kawasaki disease can be influenced significantly by early treatment and because damage from this disorder can be severe, clinicians should be quick to think of this disease when evaluating young children who have had fever for several days.

Michael K. Agyepong, MD, Malvern, AR

Labored Breathing, Lethargy, Lack of Appetite

PRESENTATION

A 16-month-old boy is brought to your urgent care center in mid-January because of a 3-day illness characterized by fever, cough, rhinorrhea, and wheezing. He has been ill several times in the past month, most recently with otitis media, which seemed to have resolved after a course of amoxicillin. His 2-month-old sister had been hospitalized 3 weeks earlier for bronchiolitis caused by respiratory syncytial virus. His mother says that his breathing is more labored, he is becoming lethargic, and he is not eating.

On physical examination the child appears lethargic and is breathing with difficulty. Wheezes are audible throughout his chest. His oxygen saturation by pulse oximetry is 82% in room air, and chest radiography demonstrates hyperinflation. He does not respond to two treatments of nebulized albuterol and is admitted to the hospital.

The child is given intravenous fluids and frequent albuterol treatments overnight; by morning, his oxygen saturation has improved and the wheezing has diminished. He is more lethargic, however, and his breathing is markedly more labored, with deep sternal retractions. His peripheral circulation has worsened. Arterial blood gas determinations are: pH, 7.04; Po_2, 192 torr; Pco_2, 9.2 torr; and HCO_3, 2.5 mEq/L. Another common laboratory test performed at the same time reveals the surprising cause of this child's distress.

What is your differential diagnosis at this point?
Are there any elements of history or physical examination that would help you?
What additional diagnostic studies would you like performed?

DISCUSSION

Diagnosis
This child initially was believed to be in septic shock. He was transferred to the intensive care unit, intubated, and given aggressive fluid resuscitation. Shortly after admission to the unit, his blood chemistry panel yielded the following results: sodium, 151 mmol/L (151 mEq/L); chloride, 119 mmol/L (119 mEq/L); bicarbonate, 5 mmol/L (5 mEq/L); blood urea nitrogen, 4.28 mmol urea/L (12 mg/dL); creatinine, 26.57 mcmol/L (0.3 mg/dL); and glucose, 25.31 mmol/L (456 mg/dL). In addition to having bronchiolitis, this child had diabetic ketoacidosis (DKA). He was started on an insulin drip and rehydrated. Gradually, the acidosis resolved and electrolyte status normalized. He was extubated and transferred to the pediatric ward, where his insulin regimen was adjusted. His improvement was steady, and he was discharged several days later. During his hospital stay, the wheezing persisted but responded to nebulized albuterol.

Presentation
The incidence of type 1 diabetes increases with age and peaks during early to mid-puberty. The classic presenting signs are polyuria, polydipsia, polyphagia, and weight loss. Patients also may be lethargic. Symptoms usually are present for more

than 1 month before the diagnosis is made. Mild-to-moderate symptoms may be present for several months. In infants and young children, the signs and symptoms often are difficult to recognize, sometimes mimicking more common childhood illnesses such as gastroenteritis. Type 1 diabetes commonly is not diagnosed in its early stages, allowing the patient to progress to DKA.

DKA can be defined by the following parameters: blood glucose greater than 13.88 mmol/L (250 mg/dL), pH less than 7.2 to 7.3, and HCO_3 less than 15 mEq/L. DKA often is the initial clinical presentation of type 1 diabetes. Usually there is a preceding history of polyuria, polydipsia, and weight loss that often is recalled in retrospect. DKA can be precipitated by an acute infection. In this case it is likely that the child was developing type 1 diabetes and that a respiratory syncytial virus infection precipitated the DKA.

The clinical pattern of DKA can vary. Patients may have nausea and vomiting. The level of consciousness may vary from alertness to lethargy to coma. Dehydration can result from vomiting and osmotic diuresis. Many children are seen by the pediatrician because of vomiting and dehydration. Type 1 diabetes should be suspected in those who appear clinically dehydrated yet are urinating regularly. Patients may have a fruity breath odor caused by ketosis. Respirations may be rapid and deep (Kussmaul respirations), as the body attempts to blow off carbon dioxide. Some patients may experience severe abdominal pain and have an elevated white blood cell count, leading the clinician to suspect problems such as appendicitis. Suspicion and a simple laboratory test can lead to early diagnosis and prevention of metabolic decompensation.

Evaluation

The clinician must inquire specifically about signs and symptoms of type 1 diabetes when evaluating patients who have unexplained illnesses that fall into one of the patterns consistent with that disorder. Polydipsia and polyphagia usually are evident to parents. Polyuria might be revealed by asking questions about the number of diaper changes, bedwetting, or frequent trips to the rest room during school. One can screen for type 1 diabetes easily by using urinary dipsticks for glucose and ketones.

In this case, the physicians were fooled by the patient's young age and by the presence of a respiratory infection, which halted further thought about the etiology of his condition. His dehydration and lethargy were attributed to the viral illness, and even the classic Kussmaul breathing was believed to be caused by the bronchiolitis.

It is likely that this child's bronchiolitis precipitated the clinical manifestation of his diabetes. Other disorders associated with metabolic acidosis that might be recognized initially during an intercurrent illness include later-onset forms of inborn errors of metabolism, such as maple syrup urine disease and methylmalonic, propionic, and isovaleric acidemias.

Lesson for the Clinician

Although cogent arguments are made against routine laboratory testing that might be costly and yield irrelevant data, it is reasonable to survey a range of physiologic parameters when evaluating a seriously ill patient. Sometimes, as in this case, the results may reveal an unsuspected condition, perhaps one obscured by a concomitant disorder.

Neil Russakoff, MD, Cigna Health Care of Arizona, Tucson, AZ

Sudden Refusal to Crawl

PRESENTATION

An 8-month-old boy is brought to your extended care facility because he has refused to crawl for the past 3 hours. The baby has had no fever, upper respiratory tract symptoms, rash, or joint swelling. He is accompanied by both parents, who appear to be loving and attentive to their child. The parents deny a history of trauma, but do recall an episode of crying while the infant was in his jumping device.

On physical examination, the child sits comfortably on his mother's lap and appears healthy and well. There are no obvious signs of trauma, but he refuses to bear weight on his right leg. The gluteal folds and leg lengths are symmetric. There is no warmth, erythema, induration, or swelling apparent in either leg. He responds with slight irritability to palpation along the proximal tibia. He has full range of motion without pain in his hips, knees, ankles, and subtalar joints. His abdomen is soft and nontender, with no palpable masses and normal bowel sounds.

What is your differential diagnosis at this point?
Are there any elements of history or physical examination that would help you?
What additional diagnostic studies would you like performed?

DISCUSSION

Presentation
Acute onset of a limp or inability to bear weight in a small child is a common clinical problem that can be difficult to diagnose. When seeking the cause of a painful limb in a child who has no definite history of trauma, infection or joint inflammation must be considered and ruled out first; occult trauma then would come to mind. In many cases of fracture, there will be no clear recollection of any traumatic event. Usual physical signs of traumatic injury, such as swelling or tenderness, may be absent. One study of occult fractures categorized the injuries by location (Oudjihane K, et al. Occult fractures in preschool children. *J Trauma.* 1988;28:858-860). Of 107 occult fractures of the lower extremity, 56 were in the tibia or fibula, 30 in the femur, and 11 in the metatarsals. The authors concluded that radiographic examination of the pelvis and all parts of both lower extremities should be performed if occult trauma is suspected and the exact site of injury cannot be located clinically. In the child presented, the subtle area of tenderness allowed radiographic examination to be localized to the area in question. This study revealed a hairline fracture of the proximal aspect of the medial tibia.

Etiology
Although some subtle fractures may have resulted from trauma, many are believed to be stress fractures, which are mechanical disturbances of trabeculae that occur in normal bone subjected to repeated episodes of minor stress. Such stress fractures are unlikely to occur in an 8-month-old infant; this patient's fracture is much more likely to have resulted from unrecognized or unacknowledged trauma. Remember that trauma can occur spontaneously and without witness, or it can result from abuse.

A third possibility is that a conscientious parent might observe a traumatic episode that has occurred from a lapse in watchfulness and is embarrassed to tell the clinician. An active 3- or 4-year-old child, however, could incur a real stress fracture.

In general, stress fractures usually are linear and transverse. A buckle or spiral fracture most likely results from one significant traumatic episode. The term "toddler's fracture" seems to be used in a variety of situations, particularly in reference to tibial or fibular fractures without apparent cause. Pediatric orthopedists do not use the term often, preferring to describe the specific fracture.

Normal findings on abdominal examination in this patient is important. Occasionally, a child will refuse to bear weight on one leg and have pain with motion of that leg because of a psoas abscess or retropsoas irritation from a ruptured appendicocele.

Evaluation

Diagnosis of occult fracture can be elusive and may require an experienced eye, multiple radiographic views, and in some cases, ^{99}Tc-polyphosphate bone scans. In this case, careful clinical examination allowed the physician to pinpoint the location of the fracture. Otherwise, radiologic examination of the entire lower extremity, including hips and pelvic area, would have been warranted. A technetium scan will show physiologic alteration in bone within hours of an occult fracture. If the child is healthy and happy, there is no fever or other systemic signs, findings on the physical examination are completely benign, the radiographs negative, and infection or tumor is not suspected, there is no need to perform a scan immediately. As long as the child is monitored carefully and improves gradually over the next 1 to 2 weeks, the presumptive diagnosis of a minor lower extremity fracture can be made. If the condition worsens, if new signs or symptoms appear, or if the child fails to improve over 5 to 7 days, further evaluation, including a bone scan, is warranted.

Treatment

Avoidance of weight bearing is the principal treatment of these minor fractures, with selected casting in some cases.

Harry S. Miller, MD, The Children's Hospital at Albany Medical Center,
Albany, NY

Sudden Seizure and Respiratory Arrest

PRESENTATION

An 11-month-old boy is brought to the emergency department in the midst of a seizure. He had been cared for by his grandparents and was eating and playful this morning. During breakfast, he developed tonic-clonic seizure activity, and while being rushed to the hospital, he suffered respiratory arrest in the car. His grandmother gave rescue breaths, and spontaneous respirations returned. On arrival, still seizing, he is intubated and treated with phenobarbital and diazepam. His grandparents state that he has always been healthy and takes no medication. There is no family history of seizures.

His seizure activity ceases, but soon he becomes hypotensive (blood pressure, 42 mm Hg by palpation), and premature ventricular contractions are noted on electrocardiographic rhythm strip. An irregular rhythm with a QRS complex of 0.16 seconds alternates with a sinus tachycardia of 180 beats/min. His temperature is 37°C (98°F), his blood pressure is 68/37 mm Hg, and he is receiving bag ventilation.

The child's sensorium is dull, but he shows no posturing or focal neurologic findings. There are no signs of head trauma. His pupils react sluggishly from 4 to 2 mm bilaterally; his fundi are normal with sharp discs. His neck is supple with no adenopathy. Irregular rate and rhythm are noted on cardiac examination, but no murmurs are heard. His perfusion is poor, and no femoral or radial pulses are palpable. Findings on the remainder of the physical examination are normal.

Laboratory findings include: venous pH, 7.24; Po_2, 35 torr; Pco_2, 29 torr; hematocrit, 0.31 (31%); white blood cell count, $9 \times 10^9/L$ ($9 \times 10^3/mcL$) with 55% neutrophils, 5% bands, and 30% lymphocytes; platelet count, $185 \times 10^9/L$ ($185 \times 10^3/mcL$); sodium, 140 mmol/L (140 mEq/L); potassium, 3.6 mmol/L (3.6 mEq/L); chloride, 102 mmol/L (102 mEq/L); and bicarbonate, 23 mmol/L (23 mEq/L). Chest radiography shows normal lung fields and cardiac silhouette.

The clinical pattern, an additional piece of history, and a laboratory finding establish the diagnosis.

What is your differential diagnosis at this point?
Are there any elements of history or physical examination that would help you?
What additional diagnostic studies would you like performed?

DISCUSSION

Diagnosis

The boy was stabilized in the pediatric intensive care unit, receiving sodium bicarbonate, antiarrhythmic drugs, and eventually cardioversion for wide complex arrhythmias. While he was being treated, the family returned home to search the house. They found a spilled purse; the strewn contents included several opened medications, including imipramine, which was reported the next day to be present in the patient's urine. Over the next several days, he stabilized without further seizures or abnormal cardiac activity. He was discharged with normal neurologic and cardiac status.

Although the causes of either seizures or sudden cardiac dysrhythmia in a toddler are extensive, the combination of both disorders in a previously healthy child is highly suggestive of tricyclic antidepressant (TCA) overdose. TCAs are commonly prescribed antidepressant medications for adults and antienuretic drugs for children. Although quite effective within their therapeutic ranges, they are extremely toxic in overdose. They are among the more commonly ingested toxic substances in the United States and are the most common cause of death in the database of the American Association of Poison Control Centers.

Because these drugs are absorbed rapidly, toxic effects usually occur within 2 hours of ingestion. TCAs are highly lipophilic and have an enormous apparent volume of distribution. Roughly 30% of an ingested dose is secreted into the bile and stomach and participates in enterohepatic and enterogastric circulation. Their toxic effects can persist for days. Acidemia leads to an increase in free serum concentration of the drug, enhancing toxicity.

Evaluation

Measuring serum levels of the drug is not helpful in the management of these patients. In addition to their high volumes of distribution, TCAs have variable free serum fractions; thus, the serum value may not reflect the total body load. It is difficult to predict the severity of outcome based on the amount of drug ingested or serum levels. However, toxicity may be predicted by measurement of the maximal limb-lead QRS duration from the electrocardiogram. A QRS duration of less than 0.10 seconds indicates minimal or no risk; a duration of 0.16 seconds or longer is highly predictive of seizures or ventricular arrhythmias. A duration of 0.10 to 0.16 seconds indicates a moderate risk for toxic effects.

Presentation

Classically, severe TCA toxicity causes a triad of cardiovascular, central nervous system (CNS), and anticholinergic effects. The cardiovascular complications of arrhythmias and hypotension account for the mortality associated with TCA overdose. Early in the clinical course, TCAs are concentrated in the myocardium and cause a quinidine-like effect that results in myocardial depression. They inhibit the fast sodium channel in the conduction pathways, which slows conduction through the heart and causes the dysrhythmia. However, sinus tachycardia, which occurs prior to ventricular dysrhythmias, is thought to result from the drug's anticholinergic effect and may be the only subtle clue to underlying cardiac involvement. TCAs also cause alpha-adrenergic blockage, which may contribute to systemic hypotension.

Simultaneously, a wide spectrum of CNS effects can occur. Patients who take an overdose of TCA often present with confusion, hallucination, lethargy, or seizures and coma, as in this patient. In the first 60 to 90 minutes after ingestion, patients may appear normal neurologically. However, their mental status can deteriorate abruptly. The neurologic effects of TCA drugs result either from their anticholinergic effect or by way of central norepinephrine depletion. TCAs cause a surge of central norepinephrine release. In an overdose, this effect may lead to depletion of the neurotransmitter. For example, a patient may present initially with hallucinations, then progress quickly to coma.

TCAs also manifest peripheral anticholinergic properties. The anticholinergic effects initially may be the sole indicator of toxicity or they may be overshadowed completely by the other effects of TCAs. The mnemonic mad as a hatter, red as a beet, dry as a bone, blind as a bat, hot as a hare helps the clinician recall some of the most common anticholinergic effects: confusion, hallucinations, flushing, dry mouth, mydriasis, and fever. This patient had mydriasis, which in combination with his CNS and cardiac signs, was a clue to his ingestion of a drug having anticholinergic effects.

Treatment

Treatment of TCA overdose is directed first at the ABCs. Because these patients may experience sudden changes in mental status, caretakers must be ready to protect the patients' airways. Correction of hypotension is of paramount importance, not only to improve oxygen delivery to tissues, but to reduce subsequent lactic acidosis, which can lead to increased free drug concentration in serum. Intravenous fluid boluses may not be adequate to correct hypotension quickly. Inotropic agents and placement of intravascular monitoring devices such as central venous catheters or a pulmonary (Swan-Ganz) catheter may be required.

Because dopamine, a commonly used inotropic agent, relies partly on release of central norepinephrine for its effect, some argue that this drug may be ineffective in treating a patient who has ingested an overdose of TCA and whose stores of norepinephrine may be exhausted. Adherents to this theory believe that direct-acting alpha-adrenergic agents, such as norepinephrine or phenylephrine, should be used to maintain blood pressure.

Seizures caused by TCA overdose usually are self-limited. However, because they potentiate acidosis, which leads to increased serum levels of free drug, seizures should be treated aggressively, even to the point of inducing paralysis. Phenytoin should be used with caution because of its cardiac depressing effects. Benzodiazepines (midazolam, lorazepam) and phenobarbital are the drugs of choice in managing seizures due to TCA overdose.

Therapy for tachycardia and cardiac dysrhythmia is administration of sodium bicarbonate (1 to 3 mEq/kg) with or without hyperventilation to increase the blood pH to a level greater than 7.45. The subsequent change in pH leads to dissociation of the drug from the sodium channels in the myocardial conduction pathways. For refractory abnormal rhythms, other antiarrhythmic medications such as lidocaine may be required. Quinidine, procainamide, and disopyramide are contraindicated in TCA-induced ventricular arrhythmias.

Because of the combination of a wide volume of distribution and tight protein binding, hemodialysis is not helpful in TCA overdose. Currently, no antidote exists for this poisoning, although the use of Fab fragment antibodies is being explored, with mixed results. Gastric decontamination should be undertaken as soon as the patient is stable. Syrup of ipecac is relatively contraindicated because seizure activity and depressed consciousness may occur rapidly. Gastric lavage with charcoal should be performed; the enterohepatic and enterogastric circulation of TCAs and their anticholinergic effect of slowing gut motility provide the rationale for this procedure. It is an important treatment, even late in the disease process.

In general, patients should be observed carefully for at least 6 hours in an emergency department or clinic. The electrocardiogram should be monitored and the limb-lead QRS duration measured. Asymptomatic patients may be discharged after a final dose of charcoal is administered and following any necessary psychiatric or social work consultation. Overtly symptomatic patients must be admitted for monitoring and supportive therapy until symptoms resolve.

TCAs are divided into generations. First-generation tricyclics are more likely to have toxic side effects; second-generation drugs were developed in the hope of decreasing the incidence of these effects. These newer drugs, including fluoxetine, trazodone, and sertraline, seem promising; they are less likely to have CNS or cardiovascular side effects when used as single agents.

Lesson for the Clinician

TCA overdoses are relatively common and can cause cardiac, CNS, and anticholinergic signs and symptoms. Recognition and supportive treatment can be lifesaving in this potentially fatal situation. It is important for clinicians to remember that TCA overdoses occur not only in depressed patients who take their own medication, but also in young children who have access to the drugs prescribed for other individuals, especially siblings and other family members.

Jeanette R. White, MD, University of Washington School of Medicine,
Seattle, WA

Update: Current treatment of patients who have been poisoned de-emphasizes lavage, while the role of activated charcoal alone has expanded. Gastric lavage, which is a hazardous procedure, confers little added benefit over the administration of activated charcoal alone. Proper treatment of this patient might include the use of activated charcoal, even later in the course, although such therapy might not interrupt the enterohepatic circulation of the drug sufficiently to alter the clinical outcome.

Two Days of Fever and Aching

PRESENTATION

A 9-year-old Hispanic boy is brought to the emergency department because of fever, headache, muscle aches, and abdominal pain for 2 days. He says that he has had no cough, vomiting, diarrhea, constipation, or urinary symptoms. There is no history of skin rash, trauma, or distant traveling. The other family members have been healthy. Two weeks prior to this episode the patient had been evaluated for fever and severe abdominal pain. He was observed for 8 hours, acute appendicitis was ruled out, and his symptoms resolved within 48 hours.

Physical examination reveals a temperature of 38.8°C (102°F), heart rate of 146 beats/min, diffuse abdominal tenderness without signs of peritoneal irritation, pain on palpation of the calves of both legs, and pain in the right ankle with passive movement (but no erythema, heat, or swelling). His pharynx is free of erythema and exudate. There are no skin lesions. The neurologic examination reveals generalized weakness of the muscles of all extremities, but deep tendon reflexes are normal.

The following laboratory data become available: white blood cell count, 10.5 x 10⁹/L (10.5 x 10³/mcL); hemoglobin, 2.17 mmol/L (14 g/dL); platelet count, 665 x 10⁹/L (665 x 10³/mcL); erythrocyte sedimentation rate (ESR), 100 mm/h; and creatine phosphokinase (CPK) level, 70 U/L. Results of a rapid streptococcal antigen detection test are negative, and an abdominal radiograph is read as normal.

The patient is kept in the emergency department and re-evaluated periodically. Twelve hours later, results of his cardiac examination have changed. The pulse rate is 160 beats/min and the apical impulse is hyperdynamic, felt best in the sixth intercostal space, on the left anterior axillary line. A holosystolic, high-pitched, blowing murmur is heard at the apex. The murmur is 3/6 in intensity, transmitted to the left axilla, and loudest when the patient assumes the left decubitus position. The second sound is widely split and fixed, and an accentuated third heart sound is audible.

What is your differential diagnosis at this point?
Are there any elements of history or physical examination that would help you?
What additional diagnostic studies would you like performed?

DISCUSSION

Diagnosis

The changing results of the cardiac examination suggest that this child probably had acute rheumatic fever (ARF). His murmur was typical of regurgitant blood flow through an incompetent mitral valve. A chest radiograph showed an enlarged cardiac silhouette and prominent pulmonary vascular markings. Electrocardiography (ECG) revealed left ventricular hypertrophy and prolongation of the PR interval. Two-dimensional echocardiography documented dilated left cardiac chambers and a small amount of pericardial fluid. A Doppler study demonstrated mitral insufficiency. All of these data were consistent with acute rheumatic carditis and congestive heart failure.

The elevated ESR, prolonged PR interval on the ECG, and presence of arthralgia on physical examination added to the likelihood that ARF was the underlying disorder. A serum antistreptolysin O level was 810 Todd units, providing evidence of preceding group A beta-hemolytic streptococcal infection and adding the critical element needed to make the diagnosis.

The patient received intramuscular benzathine penicillin and was hospitalized for further management. Bed rest, a low-sodium diet, diuretics, and corticosteroids brought about significant improvement. Aspirin was introduced during the last week of treatment with steroids. After 20 days, the patient was discharged home on aspirin and antibiotic prophylaxis, with ambulatory follow-up scheduled.

It is important to realize that abdominal pain is frequently nonspecific and that streptococcal pharyngitis may mimic appendicitis, presumably as with this boy. This case also shows that the diagnosis of ARF presenting without classic arthritis is challenging and requires a high degree of suspicion.

Although ARF is not encountered commonly by practitioners in this country, occasional clusters of patients have revived interest in this condition. ARF is a diffuse inflammatory process that involves the connective tissue and appears in approximately 3% of untreated patients who have group A beta-hemolytic streptococcal upper respiratory tract infections. Its epidemiology parallels that of the infection, with the greatest incidence occurring in children 5 to 15 years old. The pathogenic mechanism is uncertain.

Presentation
Clinical manifestations are protean. The diagnostic features are summarized by the

TABLE. Jones Criteria, 1992 Update*

MAJOR	MINOR	PLUS
Carditis	Arthralgia	Evidence of antecedent group A streptococcal infection
Polyarthritis	Fever	
Chorea	Elevated acute-phase reactants	
Erythema marginatum	Prolonged PR interval	
Subcutaneous nodules		

*Adapted from the Special Writing Group of the Committee on Rheumatic Fever, Endocarditis, and Kawasaki Disease of the Council of Cardiovascular Diseases in the Young of the American Heart Association. Guidelines for the diagnosis of rheumatic fever: Jones criteria, 1992. Update. *JAMA.* 1992;268:2069-2073.

A high probability of acute rheumatic fever exists if the patient has two major criteria OR one major and two minor criteria and if there is evidence of preceding group A streptococcal infection.

modified Jones criteria (Table). The manifestations encountered most commonly are arthralgias and polyarthritis. The polyarthritis, characterized by swelling, heat, redness, severe pain, tenderness to touch, and limitation of motion, almost always is migratory, involving large joints, particularly knees, ankles, elbows, and wrists, but it is benign, never resulting in chronic disease. It may recur.

By contrast, cardiac involvement is associated with long-term morbidity and can be life-threatening. Laseque's description remains true: "Rheumatic fever is a disease that licks the joints and bites the heart." For this reason, a thorough cardiac evaluation should be performed for all patients who have rheumatic fever, even in the absence of a cardiac murmur. ARF is one of the leading causes of acquired heart disease in the United States, with a 40% to 80% rate of cardiac involvement. This process often is a pancarditis, generating severe hemodynamic disturbances with or without evidence of congestive heart failure. Pericardial effusions and first-degree atrioventricular block are common.

Mitral insufficiency is the most common valvulopathy during the acute phase and may be followed by scarring and calcifications that can lead to stenosis. Concomitant involvement of the aortic valve is frequent. The tricuspid valve is affected occasionally, whereas involvement of the pulmonary valve is unusual.

Sydenham chorea, a delayed manifestation, is more common in young female patients. It is never present in conjunction with arthritis, although it sometimes coexists with carditis. Erythema marginatum, a distinctive, migratory, evanescent rash, occurs infrequently. The erythematous areas appear on the trunk and proximal extremities, never on the face; they vary in size and are nonpruritic and nonindurated, with pale centers and serpiginous margins. Subcutaneous nodules may be seen in some cases and present as firm, painless, freely movable lesions. They are located over the extensor surfaces of the elbows, knees, and wrists; in the occipital region; or over the thoracolumbar vertebral spinous processes, usually concomitant with severe carditis.

Differential Diagnosis
Several conditions other than ARF can affect the extremities acutely. Acute infectious myositis, a disorder entertained early in this patient's course, has a prodromal upper respiratory tract infection and is characterized by symmetric muscle pains and weakness, with normal deep tendon reflexes. However, the CPK is increased to levels more than 10 times normal. Infectious neuronitis causes muscle weakness, but patients become areflexic. Juvenile rheumatoid arthritis and other connective tissue disorders can mimic ARF, although the distinctive cardiac findings in rheumatic carditis allow differentiation.

Abdominal pain was a prominent aspect of this patient's early course. It is important to realize that abdominal pain often is nonspecific and triggered by a wide spectrum of disorders. Also, streptococcal pharyngitis may be accompanied by severe abdominal pain, which probably was what happened in this case.

Treatment
The treatment of ARF consists of antistreptococcal therapy at the time the diagnosis is made, anti-inflammatory medication, supportive management of congestive heart failure if present, benzodiazepines or haloperidol for chorea, and antibiotic

prophylaxis to prevent recurrent attacks. Aspirin can be strikingly efficacious for fever and joint symptoms. There is evidence supporting the use of corticosteroids in short courses for severe carditis, especially in the presence of congestive heart failure. In rare cases, valvuloplasty or surgical valve replacement is necessary.

Lesson for the Clinician
This case illustrates that repeated examination of a patient whose clinical picture is unclear may be the most important diagnostic procedure a clinician can perform.

Gheorghe R. Ganea, MD, Bronx-Lebanon Hospital Center, Bronx, NY

Fussiness and Infrequent Urination

PRESENTATION

A previously healthy 6-month-old girl is seen at the office for evaluation of fussiness and infrequent urination. The child has not voided in the past 9 hours despite her usual fluid intake. She is afebrile, with no focus of infection found on careful physical examination. A palpable mass is felt in the suprapubic area. Her external genitalia are normal.

Renal and pelvic ultrasonography reveal an echo-free area superior to a normal lower renal ureteral segment on the left side, with a circular echo-free area at the lower end of the ureter extending into and taking up about 25% of the space within a distended bladder.

What is your differential diagnosis at this point?
Are there any elements of history or physical examination that would help you?
What additional diagnostic studies would you like performed?

DISCUSSION

Diagnosis

A ureterocele is an uncommon congenital cystic dilatation of the distal ureter that protrudes into the bladder and usually has only a pinpoint stenotic ureteral orifice. Ureteroceles are more common in females than in males. Their embryogenesis is believed to be a failure of normal separation of the ureter from the wolffian duct as it migrates and is absorbed into the base of the bladder. If this expected separation fails to occur, the ureteral orifice potentially can end up in an ectopic location, most commonly the distal trigone of the bladder, the bladder neck, or the urethra itself.

Presentation

The child who has a ureterocele that is not detected antenatally usually presents with a urinary tract infection in early infancy, as did this child, whose urine culture grew greater than 100,000 colonies/mL of *Escherichia coli*. Although not always present, a palpable mass may be the first sign of a ureterocele and can result from either an obstructed, dilated upper segment of ureter or a distended, obstructed bladder.

Approximately 70% to 80% of ureteroceles are associated with duplicated draining systems and arise from the terminal intravesical position of the upper pole ureter. The ureteral orifice of the upper collecting system always is caudal to that of the lower collecting system. Bilateral ureteroceles occur in about 10% of cases. This child's findings on ultrasonography were typical and due to the dilated upper ureter, part of a double collecting system, with the ureterocele itself extending into the bladder.

Evaluation

With widespread obstetric use of ultrasonography, more cases of ureterocele are being detected before birth. Renal and bladder ultrasonography accompanying a voiding cystourethrogram now is recommended for children who have urinary tract infections, and ectopic ureteroceles may be diagnosed during this routine imaging. Once a ureterocele is diagnosed, prophylactic antimicrobial therapy should be maintained to prevent infection.

Differential Diagnosis

Occasionally a large ureterocele may prolapse through the female uretheral meatus and be visible on examination of the external genitalia. Confusion then may occur in deciding whether the child has a prolapsing ureterocele, a urethral prolapse, or sarcoma botryoides. Ultrasonography and radiologic dye studies with delayed imaging generally will resolve the issue and establish the correct diagnosis. The dilated cystic ureter can be visualized and identified on ultrasonography, and the ureterocele itself usually can be identified within the bladder. If uncertainty persists, excretory urography will identify the ureterocele as a round filling defect.

Ureteroceles can cause urinary retention, as in this child. However, retention also can result from neurogenic conditions of the bladder, such as occult spina bifida and, rarely, even from a urinary tract infection that causes the child to hold his or her urine to avoid the pain of urination.

Ectopic ureters also may exit outside the usual bladder sphincter mechanism. In females, this situation may cause continuous urinary dribbling or vaginal discharge and must be considered in evaluating a child whose diaper is constantly wet. A high degree of suspicion is necessary, and radiologic and endoscopic studies will lead to the correct diagnosis.

Treatment

Surgical treatment of ureteroceles often is quite difficult and complex and should be undertaken only by experienced pediatric urologists. In the asymptomatic neonate, endoscopic intervention prior to the development of infection should lead to improved long-term function of the obstructed segments, and subsequent operative intervention then can be deferred electively to a later date when reconstruction may be easier and performed more successfully.

John L. Green, MD, University of Rochester School of Medicine and Dentistry, Rochester, NY

Fever and Rash on Arms and Legs

PRESENTATION

You are asked to see a 13-year-old boy who has been ill for 2 days with fever, headache, and a rash on his arms and legs. Previously in good health, he has had no exposure to others with such symptoms. On physical examination, he does not appear sick. His temperature is 38.3 °C (101 °F), but there are no other abnormal findings except for the rash, which consists of distinct erythematous macules on the distal arms and legs and the dorsa of both feet.

A test for streptococci is negative, and antipyretics are prescribed.

The fevers continue to occur daily, often to 39.4 to 40 °C (103 to 104 °F), sometimes with chills and sometimes with headache. By the ninth day of illness he has lost 2.25 kg. The rash remains much as it was, with a few lesions suggestive of petechiae on his legs; new spots appear as older lesions fade. Results of urinalysis and white blood cell count are normal; erythrocyte sedimentation rate (ESR) is 26 mm/h, and blood culture results are negative.

On the fifteenth day, although he is feeling better, he develops a similar rash on his chest. On the sixteenth day he seems weaker and complains of multiple joint pains. His white blood cell count remains normal, although the ESR is 40 mm/h; another blood culture is drawn and grows nothing.

On the twenty-second day of his illness, he is hospitalized. No other new findings are noted. A number of cultures are taken, as are antibody studies for rickettsiae.

What is your differential diagnosis at this point?
Are there any elements of history or physical examination that would help you?
What additional diagnostic studies would you like performed?

DISCUSSION

Diagnosis

Fever is a regular occurrence in children, but an accompanying rash frequently is helpful and often diagnostic. Distress, confusion, lethargy, or signs of shock raise the suspicion of meningococcemia with or without meningitis. In contrast, patients who have chronic meningococcemia present more often as remarkably well. Paradoxically they may have almost daily fever spikes, often with chills, in the latter part of the day, at which time there may be some headache, weakness, and arthralgia.

Evaluation

Diagnosis of this infection requires bacteriologic confirmation. Blood cultures, if initially negative, should be repeated. A blood culture taken at the time of a fever spike may be more helpful. The only blood cultures that were positive in this case were performed in the hospital when the fever was high. Throat or nasopharyngeal cultures are only occasionally positive; they must be performed with proper technique and are of little help if negative. Another diagnostic technique, antigen testing of blood and urine samples, is less likely to yield a positive result in chronic rather than acute meningococcemia, so a negative result does not rule out the infection. Bacteria have been found in skin lesions on biopsy.

Differential Diagnosis

The rash of chronic meningococcemia tends to be scanty, occurring primarily on the extremities and appearing rather scattered. This pattern contrasts with the more localized and polymorphous rash of Henoch-Schönlein purpura, which is confined to the legs, buttocks, and extensor surfaces of the arms. Rickettsial infections, such as Rocky Mountain spotted fever, cause a more widespread and progressive rash that usually starts on the extremities. Patients who have typhoid fever at times have a rash (rose spots) on the trunk and frequently experience abdominal pain. Gonococcal disease may cause a similar rash and characteristically causes septic arthritis. The clinician should consider an enteroviral etiology in similar cases, especially where there is a low or normal white blood cell count, but the duration of the rash is far shorter than 3 weeks. Rheumatoid arthritis in its pauciarticular form may have a lengthy febrile course before much joint involvement appears, but seldom do chills occur with the fever, and there tends to be a high white blood cell count.

Treatment

This patient recovered uneventfully with treatment. High-dose intravenous penicillin G is the drug of choice, with chloramphenicol, cefotaxime, and ceftriaxone as alternatives. The penicillin-resistant strains of meningococci found in other parts of the world have not emerged in the United States, so sensitivity testing is not performed routinely. Meningococci were not recovered from family members or contacts in this case, but nasopharyngeal cultures are not always accurate. Recommendations for chemoprophylaxis of household members and other close contacts are delineated clearly for cases of acute meningococcal disease, but they are not as well-defined for situations such as this one, in which the illness persisted for weeks before diagnosis. In any case of chronic meningococcemia, proper management of contacts must be individualized and should be determined by the primary physician in consultation with infectious disease and public health specialists.

James W. Sayre, MD, Rochester, NY

Irritability, Lethargy, Peripheral Ecchymoses

PRESENTATION

It is 9:15 PM and a 2-year-old boy is brought to your office by his father, 45 minutes later than his scheduled appointment time. The boy had appeared well during the day except for slight yellow nasal discharge and perhaps mild pallor. His father knows of no change in the child's symptoms other than the sudden onset of fever, and no accident was reported to the boy's mother, who had picked him up at 5:00 PM. You note what smells like the odor of alcohol on the father's breath.

On physical examination, the child appears acutely ill and pale. His rectal temperature is 40.1°C (104.2°F). He is both irritable and lethargic, constantly attempting to lie down and preferring the examination table to his father's lap. There is no evidence of meningismus. There are 8 to 10 reddish-blue ecchymoses on his arms, chest, back, and lower legs. In addition, you note 10 to 12 sharply defined, flat, 0.5- to 1.0-cm purplish areas on the neck, the tips of two fingers of the right hand, the ankles, and the plantar surface of the right foot. His pulse is 170 beats/min, respiratory rate is 32 breaths/min, breathing is unlabored, and capillary refill time is 3 to 4 seconds. The systolic blood pressure is approximately 70 mm Hg. Findings on the remainder of the physical examination are normal.

A complete blood count shows a hematocrit of 0.28 (28%), hemoglobin of 1.49 mmol/L (9.6 g/dL), and white blood cell count of 5.3 x 10⁹/L (5.3 x 10³/mcL) with 85% polymorphonuclear leukocytes, 6% bands, 4% lymphocytes, and 4% monocytes. Platelets appear decreased on smear, but there are no clumps.

What is your differential diagnosis at this point?
Are there any elements of history or physical examination that would help you?
What additional diagnostic studies would you like performed?

DISCUSSION

Diagnosis

The peripheral distribution of the purpuric lesions in an acutely ill child, particularly when combined with evidence of poor perfusion, portends a catastrophic course for the patient unless prompt treatment of presumptive systemic bacterial infection ensues.

Treatment

This patient was thrombocytopenic and hypotensive. A consumption coagulopathy appeared to be in progress, which should prompt vigorous supportive therapy and treatment of the triggering infection as soon as possible. Group A *Streptococcus pyogenes*, *Branhamella catarrhalis*, and *Haemophilus influenzae* infections have been associated with purpura fulminans — the formal name for this rapidly progressive purpura — but the chief offender is *Neisseria meningitidis*, which was the case in this patient, as revealed in a positive culture for meningococcemia. Thus, broad-spectrum antibiotic coverage with penicillin or ampicillin and chloramphenicol should be initiated as soon as reliable vascular access is obtained. Fresh frozen plasma and platelet infusions may be needed to address clotting abnormalities. Heparin infusion, while controversial, also is employed to block further consumption of clotting factors.

Evaluation

Diagnostic studies should be performed simultaneously with initiation of therapy and should include blood culture and clotting studies (platelet count, prothrombin time, partial thromboplastin time, and possibly fibrin split products and fibrinogen assays). Meningitis should be ruled out with lumbar puncture when the patient's condition allows the procedure to be done safely. Treatment should not be delayed by time-consuming diagnostic maneuvers.

Differential Diagnosis

Some consideration should be given to the diagnosis of idiopathic purpura fulminans, a rare disorder of dermal vasculature seen in children, usually in the setting of an antecedent skin exanthem. Although this disorder may be devastating to skin, it usually is not associated with thrombosis or hemorrhage of other organs, and most patients do not present with the circulatory collapse characteristic of septic shock.

In this patient, purpura due to abuse might be suspected. Although it is appropriate for clinicians to be sensitive to the possibility of abuse, such concerns should not be allowed to become a distraction in a situation such as the one presented here, where the possibility of a life-threatening infection takes precedence in dictating management.

Thomas C. Bisett, MD, Manchester, NH

Update: The organism formerly termed *Branhamella catarrhalis* now goes by the name of *Moraxella catarrhalis.*

Sudden Fever and Generalized Rash

Presentation

A 2½-year-old girl living in the south central United States is seen in mid-July because of a temperature of 39.5 °C (103 °F) and a painless but itchy generalized rash of sudden onset. She has no other signs or symptoms. On physical examination, the child looks well, without signs of toxicity. A maculopapular rash covers all parts of her body, including her palms and soles. In addition, her tonsils appear to be mildly inflamed. She is diagnosed as having a throat infection, and oral cephalexin is prescribed.

One week later, the girl continues to run high fevers, and the rash is noted to be petechial in some areas. A complete blood count, measurement of serum electrolytes, and urinalysis all yield normal results, but an erythrocyte sedimentation rate is elevated at 27 mm/h. Further history is obtained from her mother, leading to the performance of a specific test that reveals the diagnosis.

What is your differential diagnosis at this point?
Are there any elements of history or physical examination that would help you?
What additional diagnostic studies would you like performed?

DISCUSSION

Diagnosis

On direct questioning, the patient's mother stated that she had removed an engorged tick from the child's body several days before she became ill. The girl's indirect fluorescent antibody titer for Rocky Mountain spotted fever (RMSF) was 1:1,024, establishing the cause of her illness.

RMSF is an infection caused by *Rickettsia rickettsii*, which is carried by ticks. The ticks acquire the organism from infected animal hosts such as dogs and rodents and by transovarian passage. Human infection occurs through the bite of an infected tick and usually is seen during the summer months, when tick counts are highest. Most cases are contracted in the south Atlantic, southeastern, and south central United States, although the disease is spread widely throughout the entire country.

Presentation

The incubation period of RMSF varies from 2 to 14 days and probably is influenced by the dose of the inoculum. Usually there is a prodrome of headache, high fever, anorexia, restlessness, general malaise, vomiting, and diarrhea. Myalgia is a symptom that is suggestive of this infection. Often a careful examination will reveal the area of the tick bite as an indurated, inflamed papule. A history of tick bite is invaluable in making the diagnosis, as in this case. Engorgement of the tick, which is a result of the feeding process, usually is a prerequisite to infection. Unfortunately, this history may not be given unless specifically requested.

After about 5 days, a maculopapular exanthem starts peripherally on the wrists and ankles and spreads rapidly to the entire body, including the palms and soles. If the patient is not treated, the rash becomes purpuric and ecchymotic. Thrombosis of large vessels may occur, leading to gangrene of distal parts of the body, such as the limbs, digits, scrotum, and ear lobes. Facial edema may be present as well as hepatosplenomegaly. Myocarditis, renal failure, pneumonia, and shock may result from the infection. Mortality is highest in those who develop disseminated intravascular coagulation. Patients who have coagulation inhibitors and glucose-6-phosphate dehydrogenase deficiency tend to have an accelerated form of the infection that is associated with a profound coagulopathy and high mortality.

In about 10% of patients who have RMSF, no rash develops, and the diagnosis is delayed, leading to higher morbidity and mortality in this group.

Evaluation

The diagnosis usually is confirmed by serology. Antibodies are detected about 7 to 14 days after the onset of illness. Thrombocytopenia and hyponatremia are present in about 50% of patients and are diagnostically useful findings early in the disease process. Because of the fever, blood cultures usually are obtained and typically are negative.

Differential Diagnosis

Infection with *Ehrlichia canis*, which is a canine tick-borne disease, can present similarly to RMSF, although the incidence of rash is only 40% to 50%. When evaluating a patient for RMSF, serologic testing for *Ehrlichia* infection should be included.

Many other conditions bear some resemblance to RMSF, although usually there are specific characteristics that enable differentiation. In the initial evaluation, meningococcemia must be the first entity considered in a febrile child who has a widespread rash. Enterovirus is another agent that can produce a clinical picture similar to that of RMSF. In this case, the presence of a rash that involved the palms and soles and the persistence of the rash were the major clues to the diagnosis of RMSF.

Treatment

Therapy may be started on clinical and epidemiologic grounds to ensure the likelihood of successful treatment. Drugs of choice include doxycycline, tetracycline, and chloramphenicol. Treatment may be given intravenously or orally and is continued for 3 to 5 days after the patient becomes afebrile for a total of 7 to 10 days. Chloramphenicol generally is preferred for children younger than 8 years of age, although doxycycline can be used if the patient has not been exposed previously to the tetracycline family. Doxycycline is potentially less destructive to tooth enamel than tetracycline. Other antibiotics are not effective, and sulfonamides actually may worsen the disease by augmenting rickettsial replication. Supportive measures such as parenteral fluids, platelet infusions, or blood transfusion may be necessary. This patient was admitted, started on intravenous doxycycline, and switched later to oral doxycycline. She responded well and was discharged from the hospital after 2 days.

Lesson for the Clinician

This case reminds clinicians to think of RMSF in febrile children who live in or have visited areas where the infection is likely to be present. A history of tick bite is helpful. The specific bite reported by the parent may not be the one that spread the infection, but it can lead the investigation in the right direction. RMSF and other less common infections should be considered for children whose disease course is thought to be viral and does not resolve or is thought to be bacterial and does not respond to antibiotic therapy.

Michael K. Agyepong, MD, Malvern, AR

Persistent Pain in the Ear

PRESENTATION

A 6-year-old boy is seen in the office because of persistent pain in his left ear. There is no history of rhinorrhea, cough, or elevated temperature. He was exposed to a child who had streptococcal pharyngitis 1 week ago. Results of physical examination are completely normal, including tympanic membranes, external auditory canals, and teeth. No cervical adenopathy is noted. A throat culture is negative for Streptococcus. You treat him with a decongestant for possible eustachian tube dysfunction and acetaminophen for pain.

One week later, the boy returns because of persistent pain. Again, results of the physical examination are normal. He is referred to an otolaryngologist, who finds no cause for the pain. Results of tympanography and audiography are normal.

Because of persistent pain, he is referred to a pediatric dentist, who makes the diagnosis.

What is your differential diagnosis at this point?
Are there any elements of history or physical examination that would help you?
What additional diagnostic studies would you like performed?

DISCUSSION

Diagnosis

Although most ear pain in children is caused by processes within the ear, experienced clinicians know that disease processes in other structures can be responsible for pain that is referred to the ear. Pharyngitis commonly causes this phenomenon, and dental problems also can be responsible for ear pain.

In this case, the dentist noted tenderness over the child's left temporomandibular joint (TMJ). When the boy opened his mouth, his mandible deviated to the left. A panoramic radiograph showed a density in the area of the left condyle. The lesion was excised and revealed to be a benign fibro-osseous tumor comprised of collagen, fibroblasts, and varying amounts of osteoid tissue. The joint was reconstructed, and his recovery was uneventful, with return of full range of motion.

Presentation

TMJ dysfunction is well known in adults, but it may not be a common consideration among children. The condition is characterized by TMJ pain and tenderness, decreased motion, and joint noise. The prevalence appears to increase with age. TMJ dysfunction may present as headache, facial pain, earache, sore throat, or toothache as well as pain localized to the joint.

The term temporomandibular dysfunction actually may be more precise in many cases because most problems in this anatomic area are extracapsular (myofascial) rather than intracapsular (inflammation or derangement of the joint itself). This discussion will use the commonly applied term TMJ dysfunction, but the reader should keep in mind that other elements of the masticatory apparatus may be responsible for the pain, rather than the joint itself.

Disease Classification

TMJ dysfunction can be classified into two categories. One group consists of true somatic disorders in which patients have recognizable diseases or anatomic abnormalities causing their pain. The most common etiologies in this category include juvenile rheumatoid arthritis (JRA), trauma, primary bone tumor, and congenital developmental defects such as hemifacial microsomia. In JRA, the joint may be swollen, erythematous, warm, and tender, and the erythrocyte sedimentation rate and antinuclear antibody test may be abnormal.

Hemifacial microsomia and trauma may produce asymmetry, resulting in joint pain. Tumors will cause pain and occasionally present as a palpable mass. Panoramic radiographs, tomograms, and computed tomographic scans are helpful in diagnosing these conditions. Correction of the anatomic pathology usually relieves symptoms.

The second category of TMJ dysfunctional pain includes a diverse group of patients who have what can be termed psychophysiologic disorders. There may be a physical tendency toward jaw joint dysfunction, which can combine with psychosocial factors to cause the TMJ disorder. Malocclusion or hyperlaxity may be predisposing physical factors. Aggravating habits include bruxism, jaw clenching, nail biting, pencil chewing, wide yawning, vocal straining, self-induced clicking maneuvers, and excessive gum chewing. These children usually are tense and anxious. They have increased muscle activity and hypertrophy, sometimes leading to degenerative changes in the TMJ. Most children in this category respond to counseling, physiotherapy, biofeedback, behavior modification, analgesics, or splint therapy. Even when the joint actually is involved, conservative therapy usually suffices. Surgery rarely is necessary, and when it is, endoscopic techniques are available that may obviate the need for open-joint operations.

Some patients have no objective signs of disease or anatomic joint changes, and their TMJ symptoms resolve when their underlying psychiatric disorder is treated. In these cases, the primary condition may be anxiety disorder, depression, anorexia nervosa, encopresis, or similar emotionally based disorders. Patients also may have a family history of psychiatric illness. In this group of individuals, subjective symptoms are out of proportion to physical findings.

Lesson for the Clinician

The clinician managing a child who has otalgia and no detectable abnormalities of the ear should consider conditions involving other areas, including dysfunction of the masticatory system.

Vincent J. Menna, MD, University of Pennsylvania Health System,
Doylestown, PA

Blood in the Urine

PRESENTATION

An 18-year-old boy consults you because of "blood in the urine." Over the past 6 months he has experienced nine episodes of painless passing of bright red urine for 1 day. There has been no trauma, and he has no family history of renal disease. Dipstick examination of the urine shows a small amount of blood, 1+ protein, and a positive test for leukocyte esterase. Microscopy reveals 5 to 9 leukocytes and 0 to 2 erythrocytes per high-power field; no casts are seen. A urine culture is negative, and testing for the following parameters reveals normal or negative results: complete blood count, antistreptolysin O titer, C3 and C4 complement, prothrombin time, partial thromboplastin time, and erythrocyte sedimentation rate. His blood urea nitrogen (BUN) and creatinine levels are 7.85 mmol urea/L (22 mg/dL) and 97.43 mcmol/L (1.1 mg/dL), respectively. No definitive diagnosis is established.

Five months later, the boy is hospitalized because of gross hematuria and pain over both flanks. Except for the discomfort, his physical examination yields normal findings. His urine is bright red, with a positive dipstick test for blood, but only a rare red blood cell (RBC) is seen on microscopy. His BUN level is 7.85 mmol urea/L (22 mg/dL), creatinine is 221.43 mcmol/L (2.5 mg/dL), and creatine phosphokinase (CPK) is 317 U/L (normal, 24 to 195 U/L). Plain radiographs and computed tomography of the abdomen show normal findings.

A review of the boy's recent activities suggests the diagnosis, which is confirmed by a laboratory test.

What is your differential diagnosis at this point?
Are there any elements of history or physical examination that would help you?
What additional diagnostic studies would you like performed?

DISCUSSION

Diagnosis

This patient's diagnosis was suggested by the disparity between finding a large amount of blood on dipstick analysis and seeing few RBCs on microscopy. Not all positive dipstick results are caused by the presence of RBCs in the urine. These highly sensitive chemical sticks are capable of detecting small numbers of RBCs (3 to 4 per high-power field), but they also react to the presence of free hemoglobin (as in hemolytic disorders or when very dilute urine causes RBCs to lyse) or myoglobin. Thus, a microscopic examination is the necessary next step when the dipstick is positive for blood. The differentiation of hemoglobin from myoglobin can be confirmed by specific biochemical assays.

A detailed history revealed that this boy's episodes of red urine occurred on the days after he played the bongo drums with his band for 1 to 2 hours. His urine was sent for quantitative analysis and was reported to contain large amounts of myoglobin. Although it also contained a few erythrocytes, RBCs commonly are found in small-to-moderate numbers in the sediment of patients who have rhabdomyolysis. Hence, their presence does not mean that myoglobin should not be sought if there is reason to suspect it is present. The relationship between playing the bongo drums and the presence of hematuria and myoglobinuria has been described with the term "bongo drum hematuria" since 1973, and it is highly probable that this boy's myoglobinuria was caused by exertional rhabdomyolysis.

The patient was treated with intravenous fluids containing added bicarbonate to alkalinize his urine. Analgesics were administered for pain. His urine cleared, and his pain subsided over 4 days. His BUN level dropped to 4.64 mmol urea/L (13 mg/dL), creatinine to 124 mcmol/L (1.4 mg/dL), and CPK to 57 U/L. A modified activity and exercise plan was devised, and he has been free of symptoms for 1 year after the hospitalization.

Etiology

Rhabdomyolysis with myoglobinuria has a host of potential etiologies. The most common probably is strenuous exercise, especially when performed by untrained individuals. Electric shock, crush injury, ingestion of drugs and toxins, viral and bacterial infections, and metabolic defects also are frequent causes. More frequently involved drugs are alcohol and cocaine; nonsteroidal anti-inflammatory agents may initiate or perpetuate injury. Infectious etiologies include coxsackievirus, infectious hepatitis, and influenza.

Metabolic defects include muscle phosphorylase deficiency, muscle type lactic acid dehydrogenase deficiency, phosphofructokinase deficiency, phosphoglycerate mutase deficiency, and carnitine palmitoyl transferase deficiency. The disorders related to enzyme defects all share essentially the same presentation: fatigue, muscle pain, and myoglobinuria after strenuous exercise. Other characteristics of muscle metabolic disorders are onset in childhood, a positive family history, recurrent presentations, and the development of overt muscle necrosis after mild exercise or even in the absence of an obvious precipitating event. These defects usually are differentiated by muscle biopsy. Because these studies were not undertaken in this case, it cannot be said with absolute certainty that this patient did not have a metabolic defect, but the total clinical picture is much more consistent with exertional rhabdomyolysis.

Myoglobinuria due to rhabdomyolysis frequently results in renal failure (9% of all cases of acute renal failure). Clinicians should keep this mechanism in mind when a patient presents having acute renal failure, even if signs and symptoms of muscle involvement are not obvious, as in a comatose person. The elevated creatinine level in this boy is a sign that his kidney function was affected. The mechanism of renal injury could be direct nephrotoxicity of myoglobin, although other mechanisms have been suggested. Predisposing factors include dehydration, hypovolemia, acidosis, high ambient temperatures, high humidity, and subclinical enzyme defects.

Treatment

It has been demonstrated that tubular elimination of myoglobin is pH-dependent. Thus, treatment includes aggressive intravenous fluid therapy and alkalinization of urine, which is accomplished by adding sodium bicarbonate to the fluids. Acetazolamide has been used for the same purpose. Early use of cation exchange resins and phosphate binders, while avoiding the administration of exogenous calcium, is required, as is prompt institution of dialysis in patients who have refractory electrolyte disturbances. Nonsteroidal anti-inflammatory agents should be avoided. Fasciotomy is an option that might preserve a limb when compartment syndrome is associated with the muscle damage. Acute renal failure due to rhabdomyolysis has an excellent prognosis if appropriate management is provided.

Shoeb Amin, MD, Haverstraw, NY

Agitation and Confusion Leading to Seizure

PRESENTATION

A 19-year-old male college student is brought to the emergency department by his roommate because he has been agitated and confused since late morning. On arrival, the student has a 2-minute generalized tonic-clonic seizure. Intravenous lorazepam is administered as prophylactic therapy. There is no significant past medical history and no known history of seizure disorder.

Physical examination reveals a tremulous adolescent who appears to comprehend commands but has difficulty putting together complete sentences or recalling the day's events. His heart rate is 120 beats/min, respiratory rate is 14 breaths/min, blood pressure is 150/90 mm Hg, and oral temperature is 38.1°C (100.6°F). His mucous membranes are slightly dry, but the rest of his physical findings are normal.

Laboratory tests, including measurement of serum sodium, potassium, chloride, bicarbonate, and glucose, yield normal findings. His white blood cell count is 10 x 10^9/L (10 x 10^3/mcL). Computed tomography (CT) of the head reveals no acute hemorrhage or other abnormalities. A urine sample is sent for drug screening, and a blood alcohol level is drawn.

On further questioning of the roommate, an element of history is revealed that leads to the diagnosis.

What is your differential diagnosis at this point?
Are there any elements of history or physical examination that would help you?
What additional diagnostic studies would you like performed?

DISCUSSION

Diagnosis

The roommate revealed that the patient had a history of heavy ethanol use. Reportedly he was known by all his friends as someone who "liked to party." His serum ethanol level was found to be 50 mg/dL. No other drugs were detected on screening.

The patient was admitted to the hospital and treated for a presumptive diagnosis of alcohol withdrawal seizures. His agitation and tremor responded to lorazepam. While in the hospital, he disclosed that he had been drinking on a frequent basis since his early teenage years. He denied using recreational drugs. In the past, he had experienced tremors when abstaining from alcohol, but never to this extent, nor had he ever suffered a seizure. Over the subsequent 24 hours, all symptoms resolved gradually. He was discharged the following day and was referred to the university health services for follow-up and enrollment in a rehabilitation program.

Differential Diagnosis

The differential diagnosis of agitation and seizures in the young adult is extensive. Traumatic head injury must be ruled out either by careful, accurate history or by CT. Infectious processes, both viral and bacterial, should be considered. If meningitis or encephalitis is suggested by clinical findings, a lumbar puncture should be performed. A first presentation of metabolic disease would be unusual at this age. Toxic ingestion is another important category in the differential diagnosis.

The number of drugs and other substances associated with generalized seizures is extensive (Table). Many of these agents, including ethanol, produce seizures as part of an abstinence syndrome rather than as a manifestation of acute intoxication. Regardless of the age of the patient, chronic heavy ethanol intake can lead to alcohol withdrawal seizures. Although clinicians are asking their adolescent patients more often about the use of alcohol, questions about the extent of alcohol abuse often go unasked, including inquiry about previous alcohol-related trauma, withdrawal symptoms, and seizures.

Alcohol withdrawal and alcohol-related seizures reflect a complex interaction between the neuropharmacology of alcohol and the characteristics of the individual patient. Alcohol withdrawal may mimic several disease processes that could be considered in the differential diagnosis of this patient, including benzodiazepine withdrawal, amphetamine or cocaine intoxication, encephalitis, anticholinergic poisoning, and hypoglycemia. (It should be noted that acute alcohol poisoning in the young child can lead directly to hypoglycemia, often associated with hypothermia and coma and sometimes with seizures.)

Epidemiology and Etiology
Ethanol abuse among adolescents is widespread. According to recent surveys, there has been a consistent increase in the use of all drugs, including ethanol. Binge drinking, defined as the consumption of five or more drinks in a row, is distressingly prevalent, with 16% of 8th graders, 25% of 10th graders, and 30% of 12th graders reporting such intake within the previous 2 weeks. Use of ethanol by adolescents is associated strongly with other risk-taking behaviors, and alcohol ingestion is a significant factor in motor vehicle fatalities, sexual assaults, and other serious injuries.

Withdrawal symptoms from alcohol can begin within 24 hours of discontinuing or decreasing alcohol intake in the patient who is habituated to alcohol. Most of these seizures occur within 24 hours of elimination or reduction of alcohol intake. Alcohol has many neurotransmitter effects, one of which is an increase in the amount of gamma-aminobutyric acid (GABA), an inhibitory neurotransmitter. Removing alcohol from this and other neuronal systems promotes an unchecked excitatory process, demonstrated as central nervous system hyperactivity. Removal of alcohol's effect on GABA also is postulated to be the etiology of alcohol withdrawal seizures.

Treatment
Treatment of alcohol withdrawal seizures as well as other features of the alcohol withdrawal syndrome focuses on the substitution of another GABA agonist to replace alcohol. Benzodiazepines will interact with similar chloride-ion channels on the GABA site and are effective both in reducing the symptoms of alcohol withdrawal and in treating alcohol withdrawal seizures. Phenytoin is ineffective in treating this type of seizure. Benzodiazepines have been shown to be more effective in reducing further seizure activity and are the agents of choice. A typical regimen consists of 2 mg of lorazepam administered intravenously at the appearance of withdrawal signs (piloerection, agitation, tachycardia, and diaphoresis).

TABLE. Agents Associated With Seizures*

Drugs of Abuse

- Amphetamines
- Cocaine
- Benzodiazepine (withdrawal)
- Barbiturate (withdrawal)
- Ethanol (withdrawal)
- Inhalants
- Ma huang
- Lysergic acid diethylamide (LSD)
- Phencyclidine (PCP)
- Jimson weed

Medicinal Agents

- Baclofen
- Bupropion
- Caffeine
- Camphor
- Carbamazepine
- Chlorpromazine
- Colchicine
- Diphenhydramine
- Ergotamine
- Fluvoxamine
- Haloperidol
- Isocarboxazid
- Isoniazid
- Lidocaine
- Lithium
- Meperidine
- Nicotine
- Orphendrine
- Phenylpropanoloamine
- Propoxyphene
- Salicylate
- Sulfonylurea antidiabetic agents
- Theophylline
- Tricyclic antidepressants
- Tramadol

Nonmedicinal Agents

- Aniline
- Arsenic
- Arsine
- Bromates
- Carbon monoxide
- Chlordane
- Chlorpyrifos
- Cyanide
- Dicholorodiphenyltrichloroethane (DDT)
- Diazinon
- Diquat dibromide
- Hydrogen sulfide
- Lead
- Malathion
- Mercury
- Naphthalene
- Pesticides
- Strychnine
- Thallium
- Toluene
- Water hemlock

*This is a partial listing compiled from *Lexi-Comp® Clinical Reference Version 99.1.* Hudson, Ohio: Lexi Comp, Inc; 1999.

Adolescents who have a significant history of substance abuse require prompt intervention, beginning with referral to a mental health or substance-abuse counselor. For those adolescents who have the most serious problems, admission to an inpatient rehabilitation program may be necessary. If there are psychiatric comorbidities, inpatient psychiatric care is likely to be required.

Lesson for the Clinician

This case demonstrates the importance of considering alcohol and drug use in the young adult presenting with new-onset seizures. A directed history and laboratory investigation for chemical evidence of alcohol and drugs are necessary. Recreational drug use typically is included in the differential diagnosis of such a patient, but a complete alcohol history should be sought as well and should include age of onset of consumption, amount and frequency of alcohol use, and the previous occurrence of withdrawal symptoms.

K. Sophia Dyer, MD, Michael Shannon, MD, MPH, Children's Hospital, Harvard Medical School, Boston, MA

Bruising on the Face

PRESENTATION

A 2-year-old girl is brought to the office by her anxious mother because of bruises that have appeared on the child's face over the past 2 weeks. She spends all day in a child care center, whose director called the mother expressing concerns about child abuse and stating that she had called child protective services.

The child has been healthy and has no history of bruising or prolonged bleeding. There has been no witnessed trauma to the face. She has occasional episodes of asthma, and 10 days ago she received two albuterol treatments in which a mask was held against her face. She is taking no medications now. The mother and stepfather deny abusing her. Family history reveals that the mother bruised easily as a young child but now has no bleeding tendency and has normal menstrual periods.

On physical examination, the child appears well-developed, healthy, and happy. Her growth parameters and vital signs all are normal. There are several bruises on her face, with some resembling marks made by fingers. There are no bruises on her neck or any other parts of her body. Palpation of her head reveals neither tenderness nor bumps. The remainder of her examination is normal.

The following laboratory results are obtained: white blood cell count, 5.2 x 10⁹/L (5.2 x 10³/mcL); hemoglobin, 1.83 mmol/L (11.8 g/dL); platelet count, 184 x 10⁹/L (184 x 10³/mcL); prothrombin time, 11.6 seconds (normal, 11.5 to 14 sec); and activated partial prothrombin time (APPT), 30.5 seconds (normal, 25 to 39 sec). A urinalysis yields normal findings.

Additional laboratory findings clarify the situation.

What is your differential diagnosis at this point?
Are there any elements of history or physical examination that would help you?
What additional diagnostic studies would you like performed?

DISCUSSION

Diagnosis

A more extensive evaluation was necessary to pursue further the possibility of a bleeding disorder. The child's bleeding time was prolonged at 14 minutes (normal, 2.5 to 10 min). Her von Willebrand factor (vWf) antigen level was normal at 1.13 (113% of normal) (normal, 0.60 to 1.30 [60% to 130%]), as were the factor VIII (FVIII) activity level at 1.27 (127%) (normal, 0.50 to 1.50 [50% to 150%]) and quantitative fibrinogen level at 6.87 mcmol/L (233 mg/dL) (normal, 5.46 to 12.42 mcmol/L [185 to 421 mg/dL]). The level of her ristocetin cofactor (a test for vWf activity), however, was low at 0.27 U/mL (normal, 0.45 to 1.25 U/mL), indicating that she had von Willebrand disease (vWd).

vWd is the most common of the inherited bleeding disorders, affecting about 1% of the population. It is caused by an abnormality of the protein vWf and a variable deficiency of factor VIII:C (FVIII:C). vWf is responsible for the adherence of platelets to damaged endothelium, and it functions as a carrier protein for plasma FVIII.

Eric von Willebrand described the disorder in 1925 in 24 of 66 members of a family from Åland, an island off the coast of Finland. Both genders are affected, and the condition is inherited in an autosomal dominant fashion. It is a heterogenous disorder that is due either to a congenital absence of vWf or to the formation of that protein with an abnormal molecular structure. The condition often is very mild, but children of two parents who have the mild form (autosomal trait) can develop severe vWd. The genes encoding vWf are located on band 21 of chromosome 12. This protein is a macromolecule synthesized in megakaryocytes and endothelial cells. Deficiency of vWf is associated with a variable deficiency of FVIII:C and impaired platelet adhesion.

Disease Classification

vWd is classified into four main types. Type 1 is characterized by mild-to-moderate quantitative deficiencies of vWf and FVIII:C, with normal multimeric protein; 70% of patients who have vWd have type 1. Type 2 is caused by qualitative abnormalities of vWf.

Type 3 involves a severe quantitative deficiency of vWf to less than 3%. The FVIII level also is low (0.1 to 1.0 [1% to 10%]). These patients experience hemarthrosis and muscle hematomas. Although both parents have contributed genetically, one or both usually are asymptomatic.

Type 4 vWd is called pseudo-vWd or platelet vWd and may be associated with a decreased platelet count. Acquired forms of vWd can be seen in association with myeloproliferative disease, systemic lupus erythematosus, cardiovascular defects, Wilms tumor, adrenal cortical carcinoma, and valproic acid therapy.

Ristocetin cofactor activity is absent in those who have vWd, and they exhibit prolonged bleeding time and possibly prolonged APTT.

Presentation

The clinical manifestations of vWd are variable, as would be expected from the spectrum of defects. Many patients have no bleeding symptoms, 60% of individuals experience epistaxis, 40% have ecchymoses, 20% suffer postoperative bleeding, 35% experience gingival bleeding, 50% bleed after dental extraction, and 35% demonstrate menorrhagia (heavy menstrual bleeding can be the first manifestation in a girl who has vWd). Those who have the severe type (type 3) experience atraumatic hemarthrosis and can develop petechiae, especially after taking aspirin. Almost all of the clinical manifestations in patients who are mildly or moderately affected ameliorate by the second or third decade of life.

Evaluation

Patients who have vWd may exhibit a normal APTT and even a normal bleeding time, although most have prolonged bleeding times. Also, test results in the same patient may vary at different times. Definitive evaluation requires both quantitative and qualitative study. vWf activity is measured in vitro by quantifying ristocetin cofactor. The vWf multimer protein can be visualized by autoradiography. Prenatal diagnosis is possible in selected families by polymerase chain reaction assays, using amniotic fluid samples or chorionic villus biopsy specimens.

The reduced ristocetin cofactor activity and prolonged bleeding time in association with normal levels of vWf antigen and FVIII suggest that this child has either type 1 or type 2 vWd. A test for the multimeric protein pattern is needed; if it is normal, she has type 1, but if it is abnormal, she would have one of the type 2 variants. FVIII levels in type 1 and the type 2A variant may respond to desmopressin (DDAVP) administered by the intravenous, subcutaneous, or nasal routes. The platelets of patients who have type 2B and pseudo-vWd (the platelet type) are hyperresponsive to DDAVP, which can result in thrombocytopenia. (DDAVP has been found to be effective in raising the FVIII level in patients who have mild hemophilia A as well.) In those patients in whom DDAVP is contraindicated (type 2B, pseudo-vWd, and type 3) or in whom it is ineffective, appropriate treatment is administration of a plasma-derived vWf.

Lesson for the Clinician

The possibility of a bleeding disorder must be considered when evaluating bruised children for child abuse. One study showed that 16% of children evaluated for bruising had a bleeding disorder. The usual time in life for a bleeding disorder to become manifest is when children begin to walk, which also is an age when child abuse occurs frequently.

The bruises of abused children are found predominantly in areas that are injured infrequently by accident, such as the back. Facial petechiae occur either naturally, from such circumstances as severe cough or upper airway obstruction, or as a result of intentional injury, such as strangulation. Although it is tragic to miss recognizing that a child has been abused, it also is tragic to accuse a parent falsely of abuse, especially when the child is ill and the signs and symptoms are due to undiagnosed illness. Holding a nebulizer mask on the face of an uncooperative, crying child could create bruises if that child has a bleeding disorder. Clinicians should measure the bleeding time in a child who is being evaluated for bruising.

Najla N. Falaki, MD, Prince Georges Medical Center, Hyattsville, MD

Dilated Pupils and Difficulty Focusing

PRESENTATION

A 10-year-old boy comes to you complaining that his pupils have been dilated for 24 hours and that he is having a difficult time focusing. He has a slight headache and noted some mucoid discharge in his eyes that morning, but has no other ophthalmologic complaints. He has allergies and has taken pseudoephedrine periodically, but not for more than 1 week. He also uses eye drops containing lodoxamide tromethamine, a mast cell stabilizer. A review of systems reveals no neurologic or anticholinergic symptoms.

On physical examination, the boy is alert, cooperative, and friendly. His blood pressure is 92/60 mm Hg, heart rate is 80 beats/min, and temperature is 36.1°C (97.0°F). Visual acuity is 20/50 bilaterally. His pupils are symmetrically fixed and dilated at 6 mm. Neither pupil reacts to light, directly or consensually. Extraocular movements are normal. On funduscopy, his optic disks are sharp. Testing of cranial nerve function, motor abilities, and sensation yields normal findings. Deep tendon reflexes are symmetric and 2+. His toes are down-going bilaterally on plantar reflex testing.

Findings on the remainder of the examination are normal. Pilocarpine eye drops at concentrations of 1/8% and at 1% cause no pupillary constriction.

Three days later, his pupils are normal and he can see well. After you obtained an additional piece of history, wearing dark glasses was the only intervention prescribed.

What is your differential diagnosis at this point?
Are there any elements of history or physical examination that would help you?
What additional diagnostic studies would you like performed?

DISCUSSION

Diagnosis

This young boy's fixed and dilated pupils resulted from a pharmacologic blockade, the most common reason for that condition. Further history from the child's mother revealed that his father had instilled the grandmother's atropine sulfate 1% eye drops that she used for iritis in the boy's eyes instead of the lodoxamide tromethamine drops intended for his allergic conjunctivitis. The history was negative for ingestion of sympathomimetic drugs (amphetamines, cocaine, pseudoephedrine), parasympatholytic drugs (tricyclic antidepressants, phenothiazines, gastrointestinal or genitourinary antispasmodics, antihistamines), or anticholingergic plants or foods (panther mushrooms, jimson weed, wild sage, nutmeg, wild tomato). A urine screen for toxins was negative, and magnetic resonance imaging of his head yielded normal findings.

Differential Diagnosis

The differential diagnosis of a fixed and dilated pupil can be understood best by examining the neuroanatomy of the visual system. Light comes in through the afferent system (retina and optic nerve) to the Edinger-Westphal nucleus in the midbrain. At the midbrain level, a vascular accident, a demyelination process, or a tumor can damage the Edinger-Westphal nucleus and theoretically could result in bilateral mydriasis. Optic nerve and retinal disease can result in the Marcus Gunn pupil. In this condition, the affected pupil does not react to light directly, and the contralateral pupil does not react consensually. However, when light is flashed on the normal eye, both pupils react appropriately.

The efferent pathway to the ciliary ganglion in the oculomotor nerve (the "preganglionic" portion) may be damaged by meningitis, compression of the nerve by displacement of the brain stem, uncal herniation, aneurysm, or parasellar tumor. These are problems with which we are more familiar in a pediatric intensive care unit. Adie tonic pupil may result from inflammation, injury, or tumor of the oculomotor nerve at the "postganglionic" level. After the injury, imperfect reinnervation occurs, causing the pupil to react poorly to light and then to redilate in a slow, tonic manner.

As the efferent pathway moves into the orbit, the suprachoroidal path or ciliary plexus may be damaged by blunt trauma to the globe, resulting in a traumatic iridoplegia. Finally, at the muscle level, the iris sphincter may be damaged by traumatic iridoplegia, acute glaucoma, or iris disease.

It is at the muscle level that the most common cause of a fixed, dilated, and unreactive pupil—pharmcologic blockade—occurs. Purposeful or accidental instillation of a cycloplegic substance (typically atropine-like) blocks the cholinergic receptor, thus allowing the iris sphincter to relax. Instillation of pilocarpine (pilocarpine test) helps differentiate a neurologic mydriasis from a pharmacologic blockade. One or two drops of 1% pilocarpine (a cholinergic agent) will constrict the affected dilated pupil when neurologic iridoplegia is present, but will not do so when the pupil is dilated because of pharmacologic blockade.

Lesson for the Clinician

Although residency training sensitizes clinicians to the relationship between fixed and dilated pupils and intracranial mass effects, which suggests a worrisome prognosis, poisoning is the more likely culprit causing this problem. When the patient has otherwise normal findings on neurologic examination, the poisoning is likely to be caused by an agent acting directly in the eye.

John J. Spitzer, MD, Kalamazoo, MI

Apparent Limb Paralysis in an Infant

PRESENTATION

A mother brings her 2-month-old son to the emergency department because she is concerned over his lack of movement. There is no history of trauma or illness. The baby always has been placid, but otherwise has been healthy and has fed and grown well. His sleeping, voiding, and stool patterns have been normal.

The family is from a rural area. No prenatal care was sought, and the baby has had no immunizations. The pregnancy was full term and uncomplicated, as was the delivery.

On physical examination the baby appears alert and calm, and he smiles at the examiner. He does not move his arms or legs spontaneously and cries when they are palpated. No deformities or edema are present. His weight and length are at the 40th percentile; his head circumference is at the 20th percentile. Except for a liver edge palpable 3 cm below the right costal margin, the remainder of his examination is normal, including his eyes, anterior fontanelle, head control, muscle tone, and suck.

Laboratory findings include an erythrocyte sedimentation rate of 59 mm/h, a white blood cell count of 14×10^9/L (14×10^3/mcL) with 8% bands and 14% eosinophils, and a hematocrit of 0.40 (40%). His cerebrospinal fluid contains no cells and normal levels of glucose and protein. Radiographs and additional chemistry values clarify the diagnosis.

What is your differential diagnosis at this point?
Are there any elements of history or physical examination that would help you?
What additional diagnostic studies would you like performed?

DISCUSSION

Diagnosis

A radiographic skeletal survey revealed generalized, bilateral, symmetric periosteal reaction of the humerus, radius, and femur as well as metaphysitis of the distal humerus and femur. A rapid plasma reagin (RPR) test was positive at a titer of 1:64, and a fluorescent treponemal antibody absorption test (FTA-ABS) also was positive. Maternal RPR testing was positive at a titer of 1:8. An RPR test of the baby's cerebrospinal fluid (CSF) was negative. This infant had pseudoparalysis of Parrot caused by congenital syphilis (CS).

Presentation

Although bone involvement occurs in as many as 90% of patients who have CS, it is rare for musculoskeletal manifestations to be the principal signs and symptoms of this infection. The inflammation is painful and often results in refusal to move the extremities. The clinician should suspect CS when an infant who has had poor prenatal care appears to have limb paralysis and pain upon motion. The radiologic evaluation is critical. Typical findings include diffuse involvement of the shaft and metaphysis of the long bones (most often humerus and femur) in a bilateral, symmetric pattern.

Much more commonly, CS is asymptomatic in its early stages or will cause generalized signs such as fever, growth failure, restlessness, and irritability. Highly infectious, mucocutaneous wart-like lesions of the mouth, anus, or genitalia can develop as well as maculopapular, erythematous, or vesicular rashes that can involve palms and soles. Nasal congestion known as snuffles is caused by extensive involvement of nasal mucosa. Hepatosplenomegaly almost always is present, and lymphadenopathy often is found. Renal involvement manifesting as glomerulonephritis or nephrotic syndrome occurs rarely. Other less common disorders that can be part of the CS clinical spectrum include gastroenteritis, peritonitis, pancreatitis, pneumonia, eye problems (glaucoma, chorioretinitis), nonimmune anemia with hydrops, and testicular masses. The differential diagnosis of CS includes sepsis, blood group incompatibility, child abuse, neonatal hepatitis, osteomyelitis, and the TORCH disorders (toxoplasmosis, rubella, cytomegalovirus, herpes simplex).

Evaluation

Evaluation for central nervous system (CNS) involvement is mandatory, although the significance of positive laboratory results in the CSF remains controversial. As many as 25% of patients who have neurosyphilis will have a normal CSF cell count and protein level, and the FTA-ABS test does not identify CNS involvement reliably.

Nontreponemal serologic quantitative tests (RPR, Venereal Disease Research Laboratory [VDRL] test) are very sensitive and inexpensive. The FTA-ABS test is a more specific, nonquantitative treponemal indirect antigen detection test that costs more. Higher serum serologic titers in the infant than in the mother are very unusual, but when present, they are most helpful in documenting active infection. Declining titers can document the response to treatment but are unnecessary.

Treatment

Bone lesions are self-limited, healing in the first 6 months of life, but a symptomatic infant warrants prompt treatment. Patients who have proven disease or who have a high probability of having CS should receive penicillin therapy, the most common regimen being aqueous crystalline penicillin G, 100,000 to 150,000 U/kg per day intravenously for 10 to 14 days. Clinical response is rapid, and radiologic follow-up in 6 weeks should reveal nearly complete resolution. Patients who have CS should be reported to the health department. Their parents should be evaluated, not only for syphilis, but also for human immunodeficiency virus infection and other sexually transmitted diseases.

Nora Riani-Llano, MD, University of Rochester School of Medicine and Dentistry, Rochester, NY

Progressive Sore Throat and Difficulty Swallowing

PRESENTATION

A 19-year-old girl comes to the university health service with complaints of difficulty swallowing and fever. The illness began 2 days ago with a minor sore throat. Although she has been able to take in sufficient fluids, she has had progressively more difficulty swallowing and has became febrile. There has been no known exposure to other illnesses, nor does she have any specific complaints of a chronic nature. Her last menstrual period was 3 weeks ago; she denies sexual activity.

Physical examination reveals a febrile young woman in no acute distress but complaining of throat discomfort. Pertinent findings include a markedly swollen oropharynx, with erythema of the uvula and marked cervical adenopathy.

Findings on the remainder of the examination are normal.

What is your differential diagnosis at this point?
Are there any elements of history or physical examination that would help you?
What additional diagnostic studies would you like performed?

DISCUSSION

Diagnosis

Acute epiglottitis, as we traditionally view it in pediatrics, involves an acutely toxic, febrile child who suddenly begins drooling and has difficulty swallowing and impaired breathing. Traditional intervention consists of a controlled examination of the epiglottis, securing of a patent airway, and administration of appropriate antimicrobial drugs, preferably a second-generation cephalosporin or, alternatively, ampicillin and chloramphenicol to cover *Haemophilus influenzae* type b, the likely pathogen in the preschool child.

This patient illustrates the phenomenon of acute epiglottitis in the young adult population. Although usually thought of as an infection of preschool or early school-age children, acute epiglottitis has been described regularly in the adult population. The signs and symptoms seen in the traditional pediatric patient may be missing in the adolescent, in whom the toxicity and so-called "febrile dysphagia" often can be absent.

This young woman was examined by an otolaryngologist in a controlled environment and was found to have a swollen and inflamed epiglottis. A culture of the epiglottal area grew *H influenzae* of a nontypeable variety. She was hospitalized and treated conservatively, without airway intervention, with intravenous antibiotics and fluids. After 48 hours, the swelling of her epiglottis had diminished markedly, and she was discharged on oral antibiotics.

Evaluation

The management of epiglottitis in the young patient clearly includes the critical element of establishing a patent airway, a task best accomplished by trained personnel working in a team led by physicians skilled in anesthesiology and otolaryngology. Traditional pediatric wisdom has stated that the use of a tongue blade by an unskilled individual to examine the epiglottis can be dangerous and should be avoided. In addition, the young patient who may have epiglottitis should be kept as quiet and unagitated as possible.

Visualization is the critical procedure in diagnosing epiglottitis, with blood culture, culture of the epiglottis, and white blood cell count of secondary importance. The predominant organism causing epiglottitis in young children is *H influenzae* type b. Most series in the adult and older adolescent population have indicated that 50% of cases are caused by *H influenzae* type b, with the other 50% due to group C *Streptococcus* and a variety of other bacterial pathogens.

Lesson for the Clinician
This case illustrates how important it is for the pediatric practitioner who is caring for adolescents and young adults to be aware of the possibility of acute epiglottitis when these individuals present with sore throat and fever. Although viral and streptococcal pharyngitis, infectious mononucleosis, and even peritonsillar cellulitis and abscess are more common, epiglottitis, with its potential for serious consequences, should be kept in mind. Epiglottitis in children presents a true respiratory emergency. In the young adult population, conservative management with close observation may be possible, but each case needs to be evaluated on its own merits and carefully monitored, and the physician must be ready to intervene more aggressively.

Bradley J. Bradford, MD, The Mercy Hospital of Pittsburgh, Pittsburgh, PA

Update: Immunization against *H influenzae* has diminished considerably the incidence of epiglottitis caused by this organism and, thus, the occurrence of epiglottitis in general. Other pathogens, however, are capable of causing this infection, including pneumococci, streptococci, staphylococci, and *Klebsiella pneumoniae*, and antibiotic coverage should be adjusted accordingly. Herpes simplex type 1 also has been described as a cause of epiglottitis. Finally, clinicians must be aware that epiglottitis is more likely to affect immunocompromised individuals and can be caused by *Candida* sp.

Unexplained Fever

PRESENTATION

A 2-year-old boy is referred for a second opinion because of abnormal laboratory results and maternal anxiety. His past history includes two hospital admissions for fever. On both occasions, findings on all investigations were unremarkable, and he was treated with antibiotics. The first hospitalization occurred 1 year ago, soon after the unexpected death of his 2-year-old sibling. The brother had been evaluated at the emergency department of a local hospital for fever and was discharged on antibiotics. He returned within hours and died. The autopsy reported bronchospasm and congestive heart failure as causes of death. Another sibling, who is 8 years old, suffers from epilepsy and had undergone a lobotomy. The child's father had a brain aneurysm that was operated on recently.

The patient is a well-appearing Caucasian boy running around in the office. His physical examination yields only normal findings. Laboratory findings include platelet count, 567 x 10^9/L (567 x 10^3/mcL); hemoglobin, 1.78 mmol/L (11.5 g/dL); and white blood cell count, 7 x 10^9/L (7 x 10^3/mcL) with a normal differential count. The peripheral blood smear reveals anisocytosis and the presence of schistocytes, poikilocytes, target cells, and occasional erythrocytes that contain Howell-Jolly (HJ) bodies. Because this child is nearly the same age as his sibling was at his death, his mother is extremely frightened that this child might die soon. To reassure the mother, a repeat blood count is obtained, which is similar to the first one. Further history leads to a broadening of the evaluation.

What is your differential diagnosis at this point?
Are there any elements of history or physical examination that would help you?
What additional diagnostic studies would you like performed?

DISCUSSION

Diagnosis

Although the family history was impressive, the absence of abnormal physical findings and the lack of dramatic laboratory findings made it appear at first glance that the child's mother was overreacting. However, when she called back later with more details of the sibling's death, the clinical picture became clearer. The postmortem blood culture taken from the boy's brother had grown *Streptococcus pneumoniae*. The presence of HJ bodies, target cells, and thrombocytosis in this child suggested the absence of a functional spleen. Abdominal ultrasonography failed to demonstrate the presence of a spleen. Asplenia was confirmed by a technetium-99 radionuclide scan.

Because the mother wanted to know if her deceased son also had asplenia, an autopsy report was obtained. Although the presence of a spleen was documented, it weighed only 10 g; a normal spleen in a 2-year-old child weighs between 38 and 47 g.

The presence of HJ bodies in the peripheral smear raises the suspicion of asplenia, hyposplenia, or the lack of a functional spleen. HJ bodies are small, round, densely stained nuclear remnants formed during erythropoiesis. Normally, they are removed from the interior of red blood cells by the spleen; the cells then continue to circulate. HJ bodies often are seen in the newborn period and are found in patients who have certain anemias (megaloblastic, dyserythropoietic, and thalassemia). The presence of HJ bodies beyond the first week of life should raise the suspicion of splenic dysfunction.

HJ bodies also appear after surgical removal of the spleen for trauma, malignancy, or hematologic conditions such as hereditary spherocytosis. Asplenia may develop when "autosplenectomy" has occurred, as in sickle cell anemia and related conditions in which repeated vaso-occlusive episodes occur, followed by infarction and progressive fibrosis of the spleen.

Asplenia is diagnosed most often in association with significant abnormalities of the cardiovascular, pulmonary, and gastrointestinal systems, as in the Ivemark syndrome. In contrast, isolated asplenia or hyposplenia is far less common and often missed, as in the case of the sibling described previously. Although no genetic defect has been recognized, the presence of asplenia or hyposplenia in multiple members of the family suggests that genetic factors play an important role in this condition. The three surviving siblings of this patient were screened and found to be normal.

Because the spleen plays a critical role in phagocytosis, production of antibodies and complement, and the clearance of bacteria from the bloodstream, asplenic patients are at significantly increased risk of fulminant sepsis, especially in the first 2 years of life. Gram-negative enteric organisms (*Klebsiella* and *Escherichia coli*) are the most common pathogens in children younger than 6 months; encapsulated organisms such as *Streptococcus pneumoniae* and *Haemophilus influenzae* type b are more common in older children. Patients who undergo splenectomy due to trauma become immunocompromised to a much lesser degree than those who have congenital asplenia. Whenever possible, elective splenectomy should be deferred until after the age of 5 years.

Evaluation
Routine peripheral blood smear examination may reveal several abnormalities due to the derangement of the normal clearing function of the spleen. These include the presence of HJ bodies and target cells, thrombocytosis, and leukocytosis. The presence of increased numbers of "pocked" erythrocytes (pit count) is a helpful finding, but that determination requires special equipment. Ultrasonography can be used to determine the presence of a spleen, but it does not provide information regarding its function. Technetium-99 radionuclide scan is extremely helpful in confirming the absence of a functional spleen.

Treatment
Aggressive management is mandatory and includes parent education, early and appropriate management of suspected infections, antibiotic prophylaxis with oral penicillin, and appropriate immunizations, including pneumococcal, *Haemophilus*, and meningococcal vaccines.

Lesson for the Clinician
Because isolated absence or hypoplasia of the spleen often is unrecognized, the true incidence of these conditions may be underestimated. There may be virtually no clues to the presence of underlying asplenia, and the patient may present with an overwhelming infection, often fatal, as happened to the sibling of this child. Increased awareness of the existence of asplenia or hyposplenia without coexisting abnormalities is critically important and may lead to prompt and early diagnosis of these potentially fatal conditions.

Mudra Kohli-Kumar, MD, Fran Gross, MD, All Children's Hospital,
St. Petersburg, FL

Repeated Right Upper Quadrant Abdominal Pain

PRESENTATION

A 13-year-old girl is brought to your office because she has experienced three episodes of right upper quadrant abdominal pain over the past several weeks. The first episode began suddenly while she was eating. The pain initially is dull but becomes sharp spasmodically. It radiates to her back and is associated with nausea but not vomiting. In between attacks she is totally free of pain, although she has had intermittent diarrhea. Her appetite is diminished, but the pain is not associated with specific foods. She experienced menarche 1 year ago and has regular periods; she denies sexual activity.

On physical examination, the girl is afebrile. She weighs 75.9 kg (95th percentile for age). Her abdomen is diffusely tender, with exquisite tenderness in the right upper quadrant associated with localized guarding but no rebound tenderness. Her bowel sounds are normoactive, and no hepatomegaly or splenomegaly is noted.

Blood chemistry findings include: alanine aminotransferase, 11 U/L; aspartate aminotransferase, 17 U/L; gamma glutamyl transferase, 8 U/L; and total bilirubin, 10.2 mcmol/L (0.6 mg/dL). Her white blood cell count is 6.8×10^9/L (6.8×10^3/mcL) with 68% segmented neutrophils and 26% lymphocytes. Serum amylase level and urinalysis results are normal, and a urine culture is negative. Abdominal ultrasonography reveals normal kidneys, liver, and spleen. The gall bladder is unremarkable. No stones are seen, and the common bile duct is not distended. One additional study reveals the diagnosis.

What is your differential diagnosis at this point?
Are there any elements of history or physical examination that would help you?
What additional diagnostic studies would you like performed?

DISCUSSION

Differential Diagnosis

This adolescent presented with right upper quadrant abdominal pain and right upper quadrant tenderness on physical examination but normal laboratory study and abdominal ultrasonographic findings. The differential diagnosis of right upper quadrant abdominal pain in the adolescent patient is extensive and includes viral illnesses such as infectious hepatitis and acute mononucleosis, gallbladder disease, peptic ulcer disease, pyelonephritis or nephrolithiasis, pneumonia or pleuritis, pancreatitis, pelvic inflammatory disease with perihepatitis (Fitz-Hugh—Curtis syndrome), and even appendicitis or ectopic pregnancy with radiation of pain to the right upper quadrant.

In this patient, viral illnesses seemed unlikely in the absence of systemic symptoms and the presence of a normal complete blood count and liver function tests. In addition, an infectious mononucleosis spot test, Epstein-Barr virus titers, and urine culture for cytomegalovirus were negative. Peptic ulcer disease also was unlikely given the colicky rather than burning nature of the patient's pain and her striking abdominal tenderness, which is unusual in peptic disease. As further negative evidence, a *Helicobacter pylori* titer was negative.

Kidney disease seemed improbable in a patient who had normal results on urinalysis and renal ultrasonography and a negative urine culture. The absence of respiratory symptoms rendered pneumonia and pleuritis unlikely diagnoses, and the normal amylase level ruled out pancreatitis. The patient's negative sexual history made sexually transmitted disease and ectopic pregnancy unlikely (but not impossible); a serum human chorionic gonadotropin level was negative. Finally, the patient reported having had an appendectomy 2 years ago, which ruled out the possibility of appendicitis.

Diagnosis

The colicky nature of this patient's pain, in association with nausea, exquisite tenderness to palpation and guarding of her right upper quadrant, and her relative obesity, led to further investigation for gallbladder disease, despite the normal results of ultrasonography of her biliary tract. A provocative 99mTc-dimethyliminodiacetic acid scan with cholecystokinin stimulation was performed and revealed delayed filling of the gallbladder at 2 hours (normal filling time, 10 to 40 min) and a reduced gallbladder ejection fraction of 11% at 30 minutes (normal, 50%). Chronic acalculous cholecystitis was diagnosed. She underwent laparoscopic cholecystectomy and recovered uneventfully, with complete resolution of her symptoms.

Gallstone and gallbladder disease are uncommon in children and adolescents. Gallstone disease indicates the presence of either gallstones or sludge in the biliary tract, usually the gallbladder. Gallbladder disease indicates defective function or morphologic changes (inflammation, fibrosis) in the gallbladder. Usually gallbladder and gallstone disease are found together. The one exception to this association is acalculous cholecystitis, which is more common among children than adults. Conditions that lead to an increased risk of gallstone and gallbladder disease in children and adolescents include obesity, pregnancy, chronic hemolytic disease (such as sickle cell anemia), cystic fibrosis, and prolonged parenteral nutrition. Cholecystitis may be found in association with viral, bacterial, and parasitic infections, but the causal link between infection and gallbladder inflammation has not been proven. Cholecystitis also may accompany metabolic, vascular, traumatic, malignant, or congenital diseases. A family history of gallbladder disease is another risk factor; this girl had an aunt who had had gallbladder disease. Individuals who belong to some ethnic groups—people of Hispanic heritage, for example—have an increased incidence of gallbladder disease.

Presentation

The most common presentation of cholecystitis and cholelithiasis is recurrent abdominal pain, which often is colicky and localized to the right upper quadrant. The pain may radiate to the back or the right scapula, down the arm, or into the neck. The symptoms may be exacerbated by ingestion of fatty foods. The pain may be associated with nausea and vomiting. Typically, patients who have attacks of biliary colic are asymptomatic between episodes, as this girl was.

Physical examination may reveal right upper abdominal tenderness, often with guarding. Occasionally jaundice is present. There are no overt peritoneal signs, and often the examination is completely normal. Results of laboratory studies may be normal or may include elevations of serum alkaline phosphatase, direct bilirubin, aminotransferase, or gamma glutamyl transferase. Although ultrasonography usually will reveal thickening of the gallbladder wall, biliary sludge, or stones, occasionally the scanning yields normal results, as in this case. If gallbladder disease still is suspected, a test of gallbladder function, such as hepatobiliary scintigraphy, may be useful.

Evaluation

Since the introduction of 99mTc-iminodiacetic acid compounds in 1975, the role of these agents in imaging pediatric biliary tract disorders has become well established. The radiopharmaceutical is administered intravenously, and sequential images of the liver, biliary system, and bowel are obtained. In healthy children, the liver, intrahepatic and extrahepatic ducts, gallbladder, and bowel are visible within 1 hour after injection. Concentration of the material within the liver usually is maximal 5 to 20 minutes after injection, visualization of the gallbladder occurs at 10 to 40 minutes, and activity reaches the small bowel at 20 to 40 minutes. Delayed visualization of the gallbladder, as seen in this patient, suggests the diagnosis of chronic cholecystitis. Corroborating evidence may be obtained by infusion of cholecystokinetic agents following hepatobiliary scintigraphy. Failure of the gallbladder to contract by more than 50% of its volume also suggests chronic cholecystitis.

Treatment

At this time, cholecystectomy generally is considered to be the definitive treatment for patients who have cholecystitis. Treatment of gallstones (particularly asymptomatic ones) is more controversial; new therapies such as medical dissolution and lithotripsy may provide alternatives to cholecystectomy.

Lesson to the Clinician

This child's history reinforces the need to consider gallbladder disease when the clinical picture is suggestive of that disorder, even when ultrasonography fails to yield conclusive results, and to use more specific diagnostic techniques.

Mary Ann P. Rigas, MD, Coudersport, PA

Weekly Paroxysms of Diffuse Abdominal Pain

PRESENTATION

A 7-year-old girl comes to your office because of a 5-year history of paroxysms of diffuse abdominal pain. Her mother states that the events occur about once a week and are not related to any particular circumstance or time of day, although the child has missed several days of school during some of the episodes.

Just before the attacks of pain, the girl becomes nauseated, then feels a very sharp, diffuse pain in her stomach. The pain lasts for several minutes and is followed by vomiting and sleep. After sleeping for an hour, the child resumes her usual activities without sequelae. There has been no weight loss, diarrhea, or headaches. The child has always had a good appetite.

Previous evaluation of these pain attacks has involved performance of blood chemistry panels that included liver function tests, complete blood count, erythrocyte sedimentation rate, urinalysis, plain abdominal radiographs, an upper gastrointestinal radiographic series, and abdominal ultrasonography. Results of all tests have been normal.

Physical examination reveals a well-developed, well-nourished, friendly young girl. Her vital signs are normal, as are the results of her entire examination, including abdominal and neurologic evaluations.

The diagnosis is revealed when more history is obtained.

What is your differential diagnosis at this point?
Are there any elements of history or physical examination that would help you?
What additional diagnostic studies would you like performed?

DISCUSSION

Diagnosis

Further history revealed that both parents suffer from severe migraine headaches. After learning this, the girl's physicians decided that her paroxysmal abdominal pains most likely were abdominal migraines, and she was started on prophylactic cyproheptadine. She has been symptom-free for several months.

Migraine headaches and their variants are the most common episodic disorders of childhood. It is estimated that 5% to 10% of children experience migraines in some form. Migraines are defined as recurrent episodes of pain (usually in the head) that often are accompanied by nausea, vomiting, and photophobia. The headache commonly is unilateral and throbbing or pulsatile in nature. The pain often is relieved by sleep. More than 90% of these children have a family history of migraines. Somnambulism and motion sickness are much more common among children who have migraines. Females suffer from migraine more than males after puberty, although the incidence is about equal in prepubertal children.

The etiology of migraines is unknown, but vasomotor instability seems to be an important factor. There appears to be an initial focal decrease in cerebral blood flow, which results in a spreading reduction in perfusion and concomitant cortical depression. A central dysautonomia actually may exist, with secondary vascular changes.

Increased levels of circulating serotonin and substance P may act directly on the intracranial and extracranial blood vessels. Hormonal changes (as during a menstrual cycle), stress, allergies, elements of diet, bright flashing lights, and excessive sound all have triggered migraine attacks.

Disease Classification

Migraines can be divided into four categories: classic, common, complicated, and variant. Classic migraines occur in 14% to 30% of children, and the attack is preceded by an aura. The aura can be visual and take the form of blurred vision, scotoma (an area of depressed vision within the visual field), photopsia (flashes of light), fortification spectra (brilliant white zigzag lines), spots, colors, or image distortions. The aura also can take the form of vertigo, numbness, or paresthesias. Headache follows the aura by several minutes.

Common migraines account for 60% to 85% of all migraines and are not preceded by an aura. The headache is characterized by throbbing pain in the bifrontal or temporal regions that often does not assume a unilateral pattern in children. The headache typically lasts for 1 to 3 hours, but the pain can persist for as long as 24 hours. Nausea, vomiting, a behavior prodrome that involves mood changes, and withdrawal from activity often are components of the clinical picture.

Complicated migraines are associated with transient neurologic signs or symptoms that occur before, during, or after the headache or in the absence of headache. Complicated migraines are divided into five types. Hemiplegic migraines are characterized by hemiparesis or numbness. Basilar migraines cause dizziness, weakness, ataxia, tinnitus, diplopia, and occipital headache. Opthalmoplegic migraines are associated with third, fourth, or sixth cranial nerve involvement and paralysis of eye muscles. In Alice in Wonderland syndrome, headache is not a prominent feature, but the patient experiences distortions of vision, space, or time together with sensory hallucinations. Confusional migraine is characterized by sensory impairment as well as agitation, lethargy, or stupor, but not headache.

Migraine variants include benign paroxysmal torticollis of infancy (recurrent episodes of head tilting), benign paroxysmal vertigo of childhood (recurrent episodes of vertigo and ataxia with nystagmus), and abdominal migraines. Abdominal migraine is characterized by episodes of abdominal pain accompanied by nausea or vomiting. The attacks can last several hours, and there is no associated headache. If the episodes are prolonged, dehydration can become a concern. After the event, there is a period of sleep followed by a symptom-free awakening. As these children grow older, they develop the more typical features of migraine headache. Individuals who have a course of cyclic vomiting as children develop migraine syndromes later in life, causing some clinicians to suggest that cyclic vomiting of childhood and abdominal migraine are the same entity.

Differential Diagnosis

Abdominal migraine is a diagnosis of exclusion, and other causes for vomiting must be considered, including increased intracranial pressure.

Another disorder that can cause a similar pattern is epilepsy. In certain forms of epilepsy, vomiting followed by sleep may be the only initial manifestation. Electroencephalography is indicated for children who have stereotyped histories of this kind of vomiting, even when there is a strong family history of migraine. The overlap of migraine and partial complex seizures is well-known.

Treatment

Drugs used to treat individual attacks of migraine include analgesics, such as acetaminophen, and nonsteroidal anti-inflammatory drugs, such as ibuprofen and naproxen, the latter of which currently is being used by some pediatric neurologists to treat migraine attacks in children who are at least 7 years old. Vasoconstrictors such as ergotamine are another class of drugs useful in treating some patients. The serotonin agonists, such as sumatriptin, comprise a newer group of agents. Sumatriptin is not recommended for children younger than 18 years of age, but it has been used successfully for pediatric patients and is available as an injection, tablet, and nasal spray. Some clinicians use combinations of drugs, such as ergotamine with caffeine; butalbitol with caffeine and aspirin or acetaminophen; and isometheptene (a vasoconstrictor), dichloralphenazone (a sedative), and acetaminophen. For the child who cannot retain oral medication, the route of administration of therapeutic agents as well as the nature of supportive treatment become critical.

Drugs used to prevent migraines include anticonvulsants, antidepressants such as amitriptyline and paroxetine, antihistamines such as cyproheptadine, and beta-blockers such as propranolol. Some clinicians employ a combination of ergotamine, phenobarbital, and belladonna. The serotonin antagonist sumatriptin in an oral form also has been advocated by some pediatric neurologists for prophylaxis.

Because treatment of migraine can be complex, primary care practitioners might want to consult a pediatric neurologist in some cases.

Scott A. Barron, MD, Southern Illinois University School of Medicine,
Springfield, IL

Lack of Menstruation at Nearly Age 15

PRESENTATION

As you finish examining a 14-year, 11-month-old girl for an upper respiratory tract infection, she asks when she might expect to stop growing. When told that most girls stop growing after menarche, she explains that she has never had a menstrual period.

On examination, her height is 69.5 cm (95th percentile) and her weight is 53.6 kg (50th percentile). Her breast development is at Sexual Maturity Rating (SMR) (Tanner) stage 4, and she says that her breasts have remained at their present state of development for at least 3 years. She lacks both pubic and axillary hair. Her external genitalia are normal, as is the remainder of her physical examination.

What is your differential diagnosis at this point?
Are there any elements of history or physical examination that would help you?
What additional diagnostic studies would you like performed?

DISCUSSION

Diagnosis

As is frequently the case, the presenting complaint is the passport for discussion of a patient's prime concern—in this teenager's case, her tall stature.

The androgen resistance (or insensitivity) syndrome, formerly known as the testicular feminization syndrome, is an X-linked disorder in which genotypic males present as phenotypic females. With a reported incidence of between 1 in 20,000 and 1 in 64,000 individuals, it is the third most common cause of primary amenorrhea, after Turner syndrome and congenital absence of the vagina. This X-linked disorder may come to mind if there is a sibling or maternal aunt similarly affected, but the diagnosis usually is delayed until puberty, when menarche fails to occur in a girl who has demonstrated normal linear growth and appropriate breast development. The absence of pubic and axillary hair is the clue to the diagnosis and is believed to be due either to an inadequate quantity of androgen receptors or to androgen receptors that are functionally defective. The diagnosis may be made in a prepubertal girl who undergoes inguinal herniorrhaphy and is found to have testicular tissue.

The average age for menarche in the United States is 12.5 years, with a range of 9 to 16 years. SMR staging of breast and pubic hair development serves as an important guideline for assessing adolescent maturation. Although breast and pubic hair development follow nearly parallel tracks, breast development usually precedes pubic hair maturation. Once initiated, however, pubic hair development proceeds to full maturation in an average of 2.7 years, contrasted with 4.2 years for breast maturation. Thus, the young woman who attains the latter stages of breast development without the inauguration of pubic hair growth presents a unique clinical picture. In response to this patient's question about her height, peak height velocity usually occurs at SMR stage 3 breast development, just prior to menarche, and height rarely increases more than 5.1 cm once menstrual periods have begun.

Despite adequate testosterone production by the testes during embryogenesis, the lack of satisfactory receptors in patients who have androgen resistance syndrome results in absence of differentiation of the wolffian duct into the vas deferens, epididymus, and prostate as well as failure of masculinization of the external genitalia. The müllerian-inhibiting factor produced by these testes, however, acts to repress the development of the müllerian structures (uterus, fallopian tubes, and upper vagina). Therefore, these patients have normal female external genitalia with an absent or blind vagina and no internal genitalia except for the male gonads.

Evaluation
Plasma testosterone levels in androgen resistance syndrome are in the normal-to-elevated range for an adolescent boy. Pelvic ultrasonography reveals the absence of the uterus. Diagnosis is confirmed by a 46 XY karyotype in a patient whose clinical findings are characteristic. Another diagnostic consideration in a 46 XY phenotypic female would be enzymatic testicular failure; however, plasma testosterone in this disorder is very low.

Differential Diagnosis
Primary amenorrhea is defined clinically as the lack of menses by the age of 16 years or by 2 years after sexual maturation. In the case presented here, the amenorrhea occurred despite the normal progression of breast development. Other causes of primary amenorrhea in the patient whose breast development is adequate include genital abnormalities such as congenital absence of the uterus, imperforate hymen, vaginal agenesis, and transverse vaginal septum. Hypothalamic-pituitary disorders, although less likely, should be considered and can be due to anorexia nervosa, emotional stress, and chronic illness.

Treatment
Therapy for this patient consists of genetic counseling; gonadectomy because of the high incidence of neoplasia in these testes; possible vaginoplasty for adequate sexual functioning; and sensitive discussion of the diagnosis with the patient and her family.

Dennis J. McCarthy, MD, Butte, MT

Progressive Respiratory Distress in an Infant

PRESENTATION

You admit a 4-month-old girl to the hospital in November because of respiratory distress. She has had nasal congestion for 4 days and a cough that has become progressively more severe; for the past day her temperature has fluctuated, with a high of 38.3 °C (101 °F). She has fed poorly and occasionally has gagged after feedings. On the evening prior to admission, her mother noted an episode of apnea. The child was born at 36 weeks' gestation and had mild respiratory distress syndrome and bronchopulmonary dysplasia, requiring oxygen until 6 weeks of age. Her mother has had a lingering cough.

On physical examination, her temperature is 37.6 °C (99.7 °F), pulse is 140 beats/min, and respiratory rate is 48 breaths/min. She is breathing with mild retractions; auscultation reveals scattered wheezes bilaterally and a prolonged expiratory phase. Culture for respiratory syncytial virus and swabs for pertussis detection are negative. Her initial white blood cell (WBC) count is 6.8 x 10^9/L (6.8 x 10^3/mcL), but it rises to 12.3 x 10^9/L (12.3 x 10^3/mcL) on hospital day 7; both counts show a predominance of lymphocytes. Cultures of urine, cerebrospinal fluid, and blood are negative.

On hospital day 5, her status worsens, with the development of respiratory failure and hypotension. Despite aggressive measures, she dies on day 7.

What is your differential diagnosis at this point?
Are there any elements of history or physical examination that would help you?
What additional diagnostic studies would you like performed?

DISCUSSION

Diagnosis

Pertussis often is diagnosed on clinical grounds based on a history of exposure or the findings of characteristic cough and posttussive vomiting. Supportive laboratory evaluation includes fluorescent antibody (FA) testing and isolation of the organism by culture on Bordet-Gengou media. Because these tests lack sensitivity, pertussis cannot be excluded when they are negative.

In this patient, an FA was repeated because of clinical suspicion, and this second test was positive. A leukemoid reaction to pertussis, which she also demonstrated, first was reported 90 years ago and has served as a marker for the disease ever since. The leukocytosis results from a toxin called leukocytosis-promoting factor. Although an elevated WBC count also can indicate secondary bacterial infection, this patient evidenced no such infection. The WBC count is useful in predicting outcome. Patients who have a count of more than 100 x 10^9/L (100 x 10^3/mcL) fare poorly.

Serology rarely is helpful in diagnosing pertussis. Present serologic tests lack specificity and sensitivity. Newer serologic methods are available in research laboratories and may become clinically useful in the future.

Pertussis is a highly contagious disease with secondary attack rates of 80% to 90%. Humans are the only known hosts of *Bordetella pertussis*, and transmission occurs via close contact with respiratory secretions. As in this case, there frequently is contact with an older individual who has had a prolonged cough; older children and adults provide a reservoir of infection. Pertussis should be considered as an etiology in a child or adult whose cough persists.

Despite immunization programs, which are now more than 3 decades old, increasing numbers of pertussis cases have been reported. The epidemic of 1993 was the most extensive since the early 1960s. Although some of the increase may be attributed to improved reporting, most cases occurred in inadequately immunized patients; in these children, proper immunization might have prevented the disease. Immunization rates of 50% to 60% in the United States attest to the need for improvement in this area.

This child had not received her first set of immunizations, underscoring the wisdom of immunizing preterm babies with diphtheria-tetanus toxoids with pertussis (DTP) and other vaccines at the appropriate postnatal age, regardless of gestational age at birth.

Disease Stages

The incubation period for pertussis is 1 to 3 weeks and is followed by the first, or cararrhal, stage, which is indistinguishable from a viral upper respiratory tract infection and lasts from a few days to 1 week. The diagnosis of pertussis is likely to be entertained during the second, or paroxysmal, stage, in which the characteristic inspiratory whoop follows paroxysms of coughing. This phase lasts from 2 to 4 weeks. The paroxysms are worse in the evening and are precipitated by external stimuli, such as the swallowing of dry food or the inhaling of polluted air. Older children appear relatively well between paroxysms. The paroxysmal stage is followed by the convalescent stage, in which the cough may last from weeks to months, giving rise to the name, "the 100-day cough."

The whoop rarely occurs in infants younger than 6 months of age. Unfortunately, the disease is most severe in the group that presents the most difficulty in diagnosis. Clues to detection of pertussis include contact with someone who has had a prolonged cough, posttussive vomiting, and the seasonal nature of this infection. Outbreaks tend to occur every 3 years in the early summer and late fall. Complications of pertussis include pneumonia (20%), seizures (2.6%), and encephalophathy (0.8%), as reported in one series.

Treatment

Treatment of pertussis is limited by the course not being altered at the paroxysmal stage when it is most likely to be discovered. Erythromycin is the drug of choice, and treatment does reduce the infectivity of the index patient as well as household contacts; if given in the catarrhal state, it can have a beneficial effect on the course of the disease. An alternate drug for the patient who cannot tolerate erythromycin is trimethoprim-sulfamethoxazole, the efficacy of which is unproven. This child was given erythromycin on the second hospital day, when coughing paroxysms were noted. Broad-spectrum antibiotics were given later. Her mother was not tested for pertussis, but was treated with erythromycin after the baby's diagnosis was confirmed by FA testing.

Lesson for the Clinician

Analysis of this child's clinical course revealed little that could have been done differently in her management and emphasizes the importance of prevention.

Harry S. Miller, MD, The Children's Hospital at Albany Medical Center, Albany, NY

Hematologic Abnormalities in Sickle Cell-Hemoglobin C Hemoglobinopathy

PRESENTATION

A 4-year-old boy who has SC (sickle cell-hemoglobin C) hemoglobinopathy comes to the Resident Practice Group Clinic for a preschool evaluation. At present he has no complaints, although he has had several hospital admissions related to febrile illnesses and painful crises from his sickle cell disease. He has been receiving penicillin prophylaxis and folic acid supplementation.

A complete blood count yields the following findings: white blood cell count, 27.9 x 10^9/L (27.9 x 10^3/mcL), with 1% band forms, 19% segmented neutrophils, 26% lymphocytes, 9% monocytes, and 45% eosinophils; hemoglobin, 1.69 mmol/L (10.9 g/dL); hematocrit, 0.318 (31.8%); and platelet count, 464 x 10^9/L (464 x 10^3/mcL).

Further evaluation is undertaken because of his abnormal hematologic picture, revealing two unsuspected conditions.

What is your differential diagnosis at this point?
Are there any elements of history or physical examination that would help you?
What additional diagnostic studies would you like performed?

DISCUSSION

Diagnosis

This child was discovered to have two separate conditions, both related to an acquired habit. The very high number of eosinophils in his peripheral blood smear prompted further evaluation. Causes of eosinophilia include parasitic infection, allergic conditions, dermatologic disorders, Hodgkin disease, and immunodeficiency. Because the degree of eosinophilia can provide an additional clue to the causative condition, reference to standard tables on eosinophilia might narrow the diagnostic search.

In this case, the possibility of parasitic infection prompted more detailed questioning that revealed a history of pica; the child's mother had witnessed him eating paint chips a few months earlier. Stool examination for ova and parasites was negative, but serology was positive for both *Toxocara canis* and *Ascaris*. Because of the history of pica, venous blood was drawn and showed a lead level of 2.93 mcmol/L (61 mcg/dL), which warrants chelation.

Helminthic infection in human beings can be caused by tissue nematodes such as *T canis* or intestinal nematodes such as *A lumbricoides*. Both of these infestations are acquired by ingesting the eggs of the parasite. *T canis* is distributed widely in dog and cat populations and can manifest viscerally and ocularly. Visceral larva migrans occurs most frequently in children younger than 10 years and is most common in children ages 1 to 4 years, especially in those who engage in pica. It is characterized by fever, hepatomegaly, pulmonary disease, and eosinophilia. Cough with wheezing, abdominal pain, seizures, and rash may be present. Ocular toxocariasis usually occurs in older children and presents most commonly with decreased visual acuity.

The diagnosis is based on clinical manifestations and serologic testing, although the demonstration of larvae in a biopsied tissue is the only sure method. Eosinophilia is common in patients who have the visceral syndrome but occurs less often in ocular disease. Treatment usually is not required, but several antiparasitic drugs, some experimental, are available.

Ascariasis is the most prevalent human helminthiasis in the world, producing an estimated 1 billion cases worldwide. Its clinical manifestations are variable. The infestation can cause a pulmonary symptom complex consisting of cough, blood-stained sputum, and eosinophilia, which may be difficult to differentiate from visceral larva migrans. Abdominal symptoms are rare in pulmonary ascariasis.

Involvement of the small intestine may produce vague abdominal pain or abdominal distention. Intestinal obstruction is rare but may result from a mass of worms in a heavily infected child. Fat or vitamin A malabsorption also may occur. Diagnosis is based on stool examination, clinical data, serologic testing, and high suspicion. Therapy employs mebendazole or pyrantel pamoate.

Screening

Had he been involved in a screening program, this child's lead poisoning might have been detected sooner. In 1991, the Centers for Disease Control and Prevention recommended universal screening for lead poisoning. Screening should focus on children younger than 72 months of age. The combination of hand-to-mouth activity and rapidly developing central nervous systems makes them more vulnerable to the effects of lead. Children who have developmental delay may have extensive hand-to-mouth activity and pica even when older.

Risk Factors

Lead-based paint is a major source of lead. Homes built before 1960 that undergo renovation are of greatest concern. Therefore, children at highest risk for lead poisoning are those 6 to 72 months old who live in or frequent old buildings, including child care centers. Children who have parents whose work or hobbies involve lead or those who live near industries that process lead may be at increased risk for lead intoxication, as are other children in the same environment as a child in whom poisoning has been proved.

The clinician should suspect lead poisoning in children who have unexplained seizures, neurologic symptoms, abdominal pain, growth failure, developmental delay, hyperactivity, behavioral disorders, hearing loss, and anemia. Venous blood lead levels are preferred, but finger stick collection is accurate if the skin is prepared very carefully to avoid contamination.

Lessons for the Clinician

The lessons learned from this case derive from the importance of following up any unusual findings. The laboratory result of eosinophilia that was discovered on testing for another reason led to a more extensive history, revealing the pica. Those two elements pointed toward a parasitic infection. The two parasites discovered share a similar life cycle and often are acquired together. As the child ingests parasite eggs, he also is likely to ingest lead; thus, the clinician should suspect lead poisoning. This case also emphasizes the patient's right to have more than one disorder.

John Kidd, MD, Donald L. Batisky, MD, University of Tennessee
College of Medicine, Memphis, TN

Brachial Palsy and Respiratory Distress in a Newborn

PRESENTATION

You are assisting in the care of a 3-day-old term infant who has brachial palsy and mild respiratory distress. Her birthweight was 3.25 kg, and the delivery was complicated by posterior asynclitism, an oblique presentation of the infant's head. Delivery of the infant from her exhausted mother was accomplished with "low" forceps. A cord wound tightly three times around the neck was reduced immediately. Because of a lack of respiratory effort, positive pressure ventilation was given for 2 minutes with bag and mask, producing a good response.

On physical examination, the baby is hypotonic and demonstrates a poor cry and suck. Her right arm is extended, internally rotated, and limp; only a slight grip is present. The Moro reflex is absent on that side. There is no movement at the shoulder or elbow. No swelling or crepitus is noted on examination of the arm and clavicle. Deep forceps marks are present on both sides of the face. Midway down the right side of the infant's neck is a small bruise underlying a tiny break in the skin. The baby demonstrates mild nasal flaring, intercostal retractions, and very little bulging of the abdomen upon inspiration. Auscultation reveals good air exchange bilaterally.

Ampicillin and cefotaxime have been administered since the baby was 18 hours old; at this point, a blood culture shows no growth. The required concentration of inspired oxygen has decreased from 32% to 28% over the past 24 hours. Chest radiographs performed on the first and second days of life appear normal. You order a procedure that clarifies the diagnosis.

What is your differential diagnosis at this point?
Are there any elements of history or physical examination that would help you?
What additional diagnostic studies would you like performed?

DISCUSSION

Diagnosis

Real-time fluoroscopy was performed to evaluate diaphragmatic motion. The left hemidiaphragm rose with expiration and fell with inspiration, but the right side showed no movement during the respiratory cycle, confirming the diagnosis of right hemidiaphragmatic paresis.

Presentation

Diaphragmatic paralysis should be suspected in newborns who have brachial palsy, irregular or labored respirations, and cyanosis. Signs may be present on the first day of life or may be delayed as long as 1 month. Breathing occurs in a thoracic pattern, with the abdomen remaining relatively scaphoid and not bulging with inspiration. Phrenic nerve injury is caused by overstretching of the anterior roots of cervical nerves 3, 4, and 5. This insult results from lateral hyperextension of the neck, usually during breech births or difficult forceps deliveries. Mild cases often are overlooked because signs and symptoms are minimal. Although most cases of phrenic nerve palsy are associated with an ipsilateral brachial palsy, as many as 25% of these infants may not have a concomitant brachial plexus injury.

Radiologic findings typically consist of elevation of the affected hemidiaphragm with perhaps some atelectasis in the lung above the paralyzed hemidiaphragm and a mediastinal shift to the opposite side of the chest. In some cases, chest radiographs may appear normal during the first few days of life, as they did for this baby. The right hemidiaphragm, which is affected more commonly, normally is slightly higher than the left, a phenomenon that can mask a paralysis. Phrenic nerve palsy is diagnosed definitively by ultrasonographic or fluoroscopic examination, in which the affected diaphragm is noted to be elevated and the two sides of the diaphragm move in a see-saw pattern during the respiratory cycle.

Brachial plexus injury occurs in 0.1% to 0.5% of deliveries. The most common type, Erb-Duchenne paralysis, results from injury to cervical nerves 5, 6, and in 50% of cases, 7. Associated obstetric factors include high birthweight, shoulder dystocia, and a parity of 1. Up to 50% of cases of Erb palsy occur without ostensible signs of birth trauma. On examination, the infant lacks the power to abduct the arm with the shoulder, rotate the arm externally, and supinate the forearm. The recurrence rate in subsequent deliveries approaches 30%.

Injury to cervical nerves 7 and 8 and the first thoracic nerve may result in the rarer Klumpke paralysis, a condition affecting the small muscles of the hand and wrist that produces paralysis of the hand, which lacks the ability to grip. Up to one third of affected infants have Horner syndrome, which consists of ipsilateral ptosis and miosis resulting from damage to the sympathetic fibers of the first thoracic nerve.

Treatment

Treatment of these injuries usually is supportive. The majority of cases are mild, and the patients recover by 1 to 3 months of age. Most infants who have phrenic nerve injury maintain sufficient lung volume by employing those respiratory muscles that still function. It is recommended that the infant be placed on the affected side and be given oxygen as needed. Continuous positive-pressure breathing by nasal cannula has been effective in the management of some patients. Paralysis may persist with more severe damage. Rarely, surgical plication of the diaphragm is indicated if phrenic nerve function does not return in an appropriate time, especially if the infant is affected severely. Microsurgical intervention should be considered if there is no brachial biceps muscle function by 3 to 5 months or sooner in very severe cases.

For the first 7 to 10 days, light binding of the palsied arm to the chest has been suggested, although there is no firm evidence showing that this modality will prevent further injury to the phrenic nerve. After this period, passive range-of-motion exercises of the shoulder, elbow, wrist, and hand of the palsied arm are begun to prevent contractures. Wrist splints to stabilize the fingers also are helpful in preventing contractures. Consultation with a physical therapist is recommended.

A pediatric neurologist should be involved as soon as possible to delineate the extent of neurologic damage and assist in planning rehabilitation. The consultant in this case found slight ptosis of the right eye and miosis, with the right pupil 0.5 mm smaller than the left, confirming the presence of Horner syndrome at 2 weeks of age. By 3 weeks of age, the infant had almost normal movement of her right arm. She was weaned successfully from oxygen by 5 weeks of age. This period of supplemental oxygen was unusually long; most affected infants require oxygen only for several days.

John C. Leopold, MD, Ehrling Bergquist Hospital,
Offutt Air Force Base, NE

Bilateral Hip Pain in a Teenager

PRESENTATION

A 17-year-old boy complains of bilateral hip pain that has bothered him for the past year. He participates in high school football and track, but the hip pain is worse in the off season. When pain occurs, he is able to "run it out." He denies other medical problems except for recurrent allergic conjunctivitis, for which he has been followed by another physician over the past 2 years.

On physical examination, his eyes are normal, as are his arm and leg joints. He is unable to bend over and touch his toes. Deep palpation of the back reveals some tenderness in the sacral region, but no hip tenderness or limitation of motion is noted. Deep tendon reflexes are normal, but his gait appears deliberate and stiff. A radiograph of the pelvis shows bilateral sacroiliitis.

What is your differential diagnosis at this point?
Are there any elements of history or physical examination that would help you?
What additional diagnostic studies would you like performed?

DISCUSSION

Diagnosis

Adolescent athletes frequently come to the pediatrician's office because of musculoskeletal pain. In addition to assessing patients for the more common sprains, strains, and overuse syndromes, the physician should examine joints thoroughly for evidence of rheumatologic disease.

Ankylosing spondylitis occurs in approximately 0.2% to 0.3% of the population; it should be remembered in the evaluation of low back pain and especially when evaluating hip pain, because sacroiliac pain is often felt as hip pain. Caucasians are affected more than African-Americans, and the occurrence of the disorder follows the racial distribution of human leukocyte antigen (HLA) B27. Ankylosing spondylitis usually is thought of as a disease affecting young men, but recent studies suggest a more equal gender distribution, although young women have milder disease.

Ankylosing spondylitis is the prototype of the seronegative spondyloarthropathies, a group of overlapping entities that includes Reiter syndrome, psoriatic arthropathy, the enteropathic spondylitis of Crohn disease and ulcerative colitis, and the reactive arthropathies. The seronegative arthropathies are characterized by negative findings on rheumatoid factor testing, sacroiliac joint involvement, and peripheral inflammatory arthropathy.

Pathologic changes occur around the enthesis, the site of ligamentous insertion into bone. The joints of the axial skeleton are involved most frequently.

Presentation

Five historical features suggest inflammatory spinal disease: 1) insidious onset of chronic low back pain or stiffness, 2) age less than 20 years, 3) persistence beyond 3 months, 4) morning stiffness, and 5) improvement with exercise.

Physical examination may show loss of normal lumbar spine lordosis, with local muscle spasm and restriction of forward flexion. Extra-articular manifestations include recurrent attacks of acute iridocyclitis, which is often symptomatic in the early stages, unlike that of rheumatoid arthritis in children. Iridocyclitis is best diagnosed by slitlamp examination rather than conventional ophthalmoscopy. Also seen in ankylosing spondylitis are pericarditis, aortic valve incompetence, and rarely, upper lobe pulmonary fibrosis with pleural thickening.

Evaluation
Laboratory testing may reveal a hypochromic anemia, an elevated erythrocyte sedimentation rate, and a negative rheumatoid factor. Radiographs are diagnostic and show involvement of the sacroiliac joint as sclerosis and erosions of the joint margins. HLA B27 testing is positive in about 95% of patients, but it is expensive and does not influence patient management.

Treatment
Management goals in this chronic condition include reduction of inflammation with medications and maintenance of good posture and function with strengthening exercises and other measures. Indomethacin is the drug of choice for treatment; if not tolerated, other nonsteroidal anti-inflammatory drugs may be tried. In general, the younger the patient at the onset of symptoms, the more severe the outcome. With early diagnosis and intervention, these teens should enjoy a normal life span with maximum function.

Summer Smith, MD, Medical College of Virginia, Richmond, VA

Update: Current therapy of ankylosing spondylitis is likely to start with naproxen, with a second choice being the combination of sulfasalazine and naproxen. This condition responds most consistently to indomethacin, but concerns about adverse gastrointestinal effects induce clinicians to reserve this agent for cases refractory to other medications. It is possible that Cox-2 inhibitors may prove useful in this inflammatory disorder.

Recurrent Abdominal Pain and Vomiting

PRESENTATION

A 4-year-old Indian boy is brought to the emergency department because he has suffered all day with abdominal pain. He has eaten nothing, has kept down very little liquid, and has vomited several times. Over the previous 3 months he has experienced a number of similar episodes for which he was seen by his pediatrician; each time he was felt to have viral gastroenteritis. A radiograph of his abdomen was obtained on one occasion and was normal. He has had no constipation, diarrhea, hematochezia, hematemesis, or fever. The abdominal pain is ameliorated by vomiting. His past medical history is significant only for repair of an incarcerated umbilical hernia at 3 years of age.

On physical examination, the boy is alert but subdued and appears to be 5% to 8% dehydrated. His height and weight are both at the 75th percentile, and his temperature is 37.4 °C (99.3 °F) rectally. His abdomen is soft and nontender, with hypoactive bowel sounds; no masses are palpated. Rectal examination reveals normal tone and soft stool that is free of blood. A radiographic abdominal series for free air is normal.

The child is rehydrated and admitted for observation. During the night he passes a grossly bloody stool. A specific test reveals the source of his illness.

What is your differential diagnosis at this point?
Are there any elements of history or physical examination that would help you?
What additional diagnostic studies would you like performed?

DISCUSSION

Diagnosis

A technetium-99 scan was strongly suggestive of a Meckel diverticulum. The child was taken to the operating room, and a significantly inflamed outpouching of the ileum was found with a diverticulum that was attached to the anterior abdominal wall. This diverticulum was in the typical location, 70 cm above the ileocecal valve. The affected bowel was resected and the child did well postoperatively.

Meckel diverticulum is the most common intestinal malformation, occurring in approximately 2% of the population. A Meckel diverticulum is the embryonic remnant of the vitellointestinal duct and usually is located within the terminal 100 cm of the ileum. As in this case, the diverticulum may be connected by a fibrous cord to the abdominal wall, and the cord can contain cystic structures. About 50% of Meckel diverticula contain ectopic mucosa, which is gastric in 65% to 85% of cases but can be pancreatic, derived from the small bowel, or colonic. The vast majority of Meckel diverticula that bleed will be found to have ectopic gastric mucosa.

Differential Diagnosis

In evaluating a 4-year-old child who has intermittent abdominal pain associated with vomiting, the clinician must be concerned about malrotation with intermittent midgut volvulus, a Meckel diverticulum with intermittent volvulus, and internal or inguinal hernias. When this child passed a grossly bloody stool, the likelihood of his having a Meckel diverticulum became greater.

Intussusception also should be considered in any young child who has intermittent pain with vomiting, but it is an unusual cause of recurring pain over a period of months. Most pediatric surgeons feel that recurring intussusception that resolves spontaneously is rare and that intussusception caused by invagination of a Meckel diverticulum never resolves spontaneously (and rarely can be reduced with contrast enemas). It is possible that the intermittent abdominal pain experienced by this boy over the previous months was caused by volvulus of the terminal ileum around the fibrinous band connecting the umbilicus to the diverticulum.

Intussusception, the most frequent cause of intestinal obstruction among infants beyond the immediate newborn period, is a telescoping of one portion of bowel into another segment, most commonly ileum into colon. Most cases of intussusception occur during the first year of life and have no identifiable cause. In children older than 2 years, intussusception usually is associated with a lead point; Meckel diverticulum is responsible for the majority of cases. Other etiologies include polyps, lymphoma, foreign bodies, and parasites.

Patients who have intussusception typically present with intermittent bouts of crampy abdominal pain, which tends to occur at 10- to 15-minute intervals. Vomiting, which usually follows the pain, may bring temporary pain relief. The abdomen usually is soft between episodes of pain; in approximately 85% of cases, a sausage-like mass can be palpated in the right upper or lower quadrant. Classic currant jelly stools are present early in the disorder in only 10% of cases but eventually are noted in about 90% of cases.

Presentation

Unlike this situation, Meckel diverticula usually are asymptomatic and discovered as an incidental finding during surgery or autopsy. Signs or symptoms of hemorrhage, intestinal obstruction, or diverticulitis occur in 25% to 30% of cases. The most common presentation is painless rectal bleeding, which occurs in 40% to 60% of symptomatic patients. Blood usually is passed without accompanying stool and commonly is dark red. Intestinal obstruction occurs in approximately 20% of patients who have Meckel diverticulum and are symptomatic. Obstruction can result from intussusception (with the diverticulum as lead point), volvulus around the fixed end of the diverticulum, internal herniation, or incarceration in an inguinal hernia. Diverticulitis and perforation occasionally occur, possibly secondary to peptic ulceration.

Evaluation

Meckel diverticulum is diagnosed by technetium-99 scan. This nuclide is taken up readily by the secretory cells of the thyroid and salivary glands as well as by those of the gastric mucosa. The ectopic tissue found in a Meckel diverticulum, most commonly gastric mucosa, will show up as a "hot spot" within the abdomen, usually in the right lower quadrant. The test is accurate and specific, with rare false-positive but a few false-negative results. In patients who have bleeding from the diverticulum, there is a 10% false-negative rate, presumably because the area of ectopic gastric mucosa is not large enough to concentrate enough technetium.

Treatment

Once the diagnosis is made by scan, the treatment is surgical excision of the diverticulum. If there is a peptic ulcer in the adjacent ileum, the involved ileal segment also should be resected.

Lesson for the Clinician

Both Meckel diverticulum and intussusception must be kept in mind when evaluating children who have abdominal pain or rectal bleeding.

Rubia Khalak, MD, Robert Gadawski, MD, University of Rochester School of Medicine and Dentistry, Rochester, NY

Fainting After Exercise

PRESENTATION

The mother of a 10-year-old girl brings her into the office because of a fainting spell that occurred earlier at school. After playing basketball, she was standing against the wall and suddenly slumped to the floor, apparently unconscious. The gym teacher estimated that she started to regain consciousness in "about a minute." One of her classmates described jerking of a leg, but the history is vague. The child recalls only awakening and seeing people surrounding her. By the time her mother arrived to take her home, she felt tired but otherwise "pretty good."

A fainting spell had occurred last summer on vacation after a vigorous lake swim. The youngster had recovered quickly with rest, and her parents ascribed the episode to overexertion. The mother is adopted and does not know her family history. There is a cousin with "epilepsy" on the father's side. You perform a complete examination, with particular attention to the neurologic appraisal. All findings are normal. An electroencephalogram is ordered.

What is your differential diagnosis at this point?
Are there any elements of history or physical examination that would help you?
What additional diagnostic studies would you like performed?

DISCUSSION

Differential Diagnosis

Pediatricians are used to thinking of seizures or vasovagal syncope when children have spells involving the sudden loss of consciousness. Cardiac disturbances in a young person who has no apparent heart disease are less likely to come to mind. Although they are rare, cardiac arrhythmias can cause syncope and even seizures in children and should be considered in the diagnostic process, even if no heart disease is evident. Other symptoms associated with arrhythmias include dizziness, discomfort in the chest, and decreased exercise tolerance.

The prolonged QT syndrome can occur in a child who has normal hearing or in conjunction with sensorineural hearing loss. Many cases have a familial basis, and a careful family history is warranted, looking especially for evidence of syncope, atypical seizures, and sudden death. Syncope or seizures are induced by a ventricular tachycardia, often of the dangerous "torsade de pointes" pattern, which can progress to ventricular fibrillation and sudden death. Arrhythmias also are associated with the Wolff-Parkinson-White syndrome and the sick sinus ("bradytachy") syndrome. Syncope also can result from cardiac conditions that obstruct blood flow, such as valvular stenoses, pulmonary hypertension, cardiac tamponade, and hypertrophic cardiomyopathy (previously called idiopathic hypertrophic subaortic stenosis) as well as aberrant left coronary artery and the rare intracardiac myxoma.

The occurrence of syncope during or immediately after exertion can be a clue to a cardiac cause. Emotional excitement can trigger arrhythmia, a point to remember especially when leaning toward a psychological diagnosis.

Evaluation
Prolonged QT syndrome can be identified on electrocardiography, as can Wolff-Parkinson-White syndrome and some of the other disorders that cause arrhythmias. This test is noninvasive and relatively inexpensive and always should be obtained in a youngster who has syncope if a noncardiac cause for the spells cannot be identified clearly. Some cardiac disorders that can cause loss of consciousness will not be detected by electrocardiography. If the clinician suspects a cardiac etiology despite normal findings on conventional electrocardiography, further testing can be undertaken, including Holter continuous rhythm monitoring, exercise testing, and more sophisticated electrophysiologic testing under the direction of a pediatric cardiologist.

Treatment
Treatment of the prolonged QT syndrome usually starts with the use of a beta-adrenergic blocker. Pacemakers also have been employed. Because this condition is believed to result from an imbalance between the left- and right-sided sympathetic innervation of the heart, surgery on the left stellate ganglion has been performed in some cases. However, surgery is employed only after medical attempts have failed and is not indicated in the usual situation.

Lesson for the Clinician
This child had normal findings on electroencephalography, but electrocardiography led to the correct diagnosis. The major lesson to be learned from this case is to think of cardiac causes, particularly arrhythmias, in children who have fainting spells or seizures that do not fall clearly into some other diagnostic category.

Lawrence F. Nazarian, MD, Penfield, NY

Update: There are many aspects of this unique condition that clinicians must know, including the relationship of arrhythmic episodes to emotional responses, especially those of the "fight, flight, or fright" variety, and to activity. Exertional syncope should be considered cardiac until proven otherwise and requires thorough cardiovascular evaluation. Many medications can prolong the QT interval, including such commen agents as erythromycin, trimethoprim-sulfamethoxazole, cisapride, terfenadine, ketoconazole, and fluconazole, as can hyponatremia and hypokalemia.

Physicians should calculate the corrected QT interval themselves, rather than rely on automated methods. Once the diagnosis of inherited long QT syndrome is established (about 50% of cases can be linked to gene mutations), relatives should be screened by history and electrocardiography. Current therapy includes the use of beta-adrenergic blockers, implantation of a pacemaker or defibrillator, and left cervicothoracic sympathetic ganglionectomy. Gene therapy may be of help to some of these patients in the future. Readers are referred to the excellent review by Ackerman in *Pediatrics in Review.* 1998;19:232-238.

Diffuse Rash Following Ampicillin Administration

PRESENTATION

A 10-month-old boy is brought to the emergency department because of fever, irritability, and rash. When the fever started 3 days ago, he was diagnosed as having pharyngitis and was given ampicillin. A rash developed 2 days later.

On physical examination, the child is pale, looks ill, and is very irritable. His temperature is 40 °C (104 °F), heart rate is 190 beats/min, respiratory rate is 45 breaths/min, and blood pressure is 84/45 mm Hg. Peripheral vascular perfusion appears to be poor. A rash is present that resembles a diffuse sunburn. His hands and feet are edematous, and there is mild peeling. Bilateral, nonpurulent conjunctival inflammation is present. Two small lymph nodes are palpable on each side of his neck.

The white blood cell (WBC) count is 3 x 10⁹/L (3 x 10³/mcL), with 70% neutrophils, 15% lymphocytes, 9% monocytes, and 6% eosinophils. The platelet count is 75 x 10⁹/L (75 x 10³/mcL). Blood chemistry testing reveals the following levels: total bilirubin, 24 mcmol/L (1.4 mg/dL); aspartate aminotransferase, 125 U/L (upper limit of normal, 41 U/L); alanine aminotransferase, 167 U/L (upper limit of normal, 45 U/L); creatine kinase, 628 U/L (upper limit of normal, 225 U/L); albumin, 25 g/L (2.5 g/dL); and calcium, 2.0 mmol/L (7.9 mg/dL). Urinalysis shows 30 to 40 WBCs per high-power field. Lumbar puncture yields clear spinal fluid that contains 650 mg/L (65 mg/dL) of protein. The clinical picture and results of a culture reveal the diagnosis.

What is your differential diagnosis at this point?
Are there any elements of history or physical examination that would help you?
What additional diagnostic studies would you like performed?

DISCUSSION

Diagnosis

Cultures of urine and cerebrospinal fluid grew no bacteria, but a throat culture grew both *Staphylococcus aureus* and group A *Streptococcus pyogenes*. Toxic shock syndrome (TSS) was diagnosed, and the infant was treated with antibiotics, intravenous immune globulin (IVIG), repeated infusions of colloid, and dopamine for inotropic support. He was discharged 1 week after admission and currently is thriving.

TSS results from infection somewhere in the body by *S aureus* or *S pyogenes*. The condition initially was described in 1978 by Todd as occurring in children and was reported as a disorder in menstruating young women in 1980. It was noticed later to be associated with a variety of clinical conditions. Since its initial description, and probably because of publicity about the danger of inappropriate tampon use, the incidence of TSS has decreased. In 1994, only 192 cases were reported to the Centers for Disease Control and Prevention (CDC), although this may represent an underestimate of the true incidence of this disorder.

At present, TSS occurs with equal or greater frequency outside the setting of menstruation and tampon use. The incidence of postoperative cases after all types of surgery has been estimated to be 3 per 100,000 population. For ear, nose, and throat surgery, the incidence is 16.5 per 100,000 population. Patients who are colonized in the anterior nares by *S aureus* are at risk for TSS when the respiratory mucosa is disrupted by surgery, trauma, or a respiratory infection, such as influenza. Menstruating women 16 to 30 years of age are at particular risk, especially 72 to 96 hours after beginning menstruation and when using high-absorbency tampons. Cases of TSS may result either from inapparent colonization of a mucous membrane or wound or from invasive disease caused by *S pyogenes* or *S aureus*.

Etiology

Both staphylococcal and streptococcal TSS are believed to be mediated by toxins known as superantigens, the most common of which are the staphylococcal TSST-1 exotoxin and the streptococcal pyrogenic exotoxins A, B, C, and F. The superantigens interact with the major histocompatibility class II proteins and activate the T cells. This T-cell stimulation leads to polyclonal activation, which results in massive release of cytokines such as tumor necrosis factor and interleukin-6. These substances are responsible for the shock and multiorgan dysfunction. Polyclonal activation generally results in reversible reduction in the number of circulating (CD4+) lymphocytes. Other infections also may be associated with superantigen activity.

A concomitant magnesium deficiency might increase the production of TSST-1. It should be noted that 40% to 50% of nonmenstrual TSS caused by *S aureus* and 5% to 10% of menstrual TSS isolates do not produce TSST-1; therefore, a role for other exotoxins and enterotoxins has been proposed.

Presentation

The criteria established by the CDC for staphylococcal TSS are listed in Table 1; those for streptococcal TSS are presented in Table 2. In children, there usually is a prodromal period of 1 to 6 days that is characterized by conjunctivitis, fever, diarrhea, and irritability. Hypotension usually is a very late symptom in children who have TSS. Streptococcal TSS has a slower onset (over several days), a lower incidence of vomiting, and a higher incidence of diarrhea and conjunctival injection. No specific test establishes the diagnosis, but the results of several nonspecific tests, as indicated by the criteria, can form a diagnostic pattern.

Differential Diagnosis

Infectious diseases that might simulate TSS include rash-associated viral syndromes, Rocky Mountain spotted fever, Kawasaki disease, streptococcal scarlet fever, sepsis, leptospirosis, tick typhus, and Legionnaire disease. Mention should be made of the distinction between the rashes of TSS and Kawasaki disease. The rash of TSS is diffuse and resembles sunburn. The eruption seen in Kawasaki disease can take many forms, but most frequently it is deeply erythematous, pruritic papules and plaques. Urticaria is another common skin manifestation, as is a macular-papular morbilliform eruption. The rash often is accompanied by reddish-purple erythema of the palms and soles and edema of the hands and feet. Kawasaki disease rarely may cause a sunburn-like rash, but the other visible features should help to differentiate it from TSS.

TABLE 1. Criteria for Staphylococcal Toxic Shock Syndrome

- Fever of 38.9°C (102°F)
- Presence of diffuse macular erythroderma ("sunburn" appearance)
- Desquamation 1 to 2 wk after onset of illness, particularly of the palms and soles
- Hypotension, defined as a systolic blood pressure of 90 mm Hg for adults and 5th percentile for children younger than 16 y; an orthostatic decrease in diastolic blood pressure of 15 mm Hg with a position change from lying to sitting; orthostatic syncope; or orthostatic dizziness
- Involvement of three or more of the following organ systems:
  - Gastrointestinal: history of vomiting or diarrhea at the onset of illness
  - Muscular: elevated creatine phosphokinase level or severe myalgia
  - Mucous membrane: nonpurulent conjunctivitis, oropharyngeal hyperemia, or vaginal hyperemia or discharge
  - Renal: abnormal results of renal function tests or urinalysis
  - Hepatic: elevated serum transaminase and bilirubin levels
  - Hematologic: thrombocytopenia
  - Central nervous system: disorientation or alteration in consciousness without focal neurologic signs and in the absence of hypotension or fever

In addition, normal results of the following tests, if performed: Blood, throat, cerebrospinal fluid cultures (blood culture may be positive for *Staphylococcus aureus*); antibody tests for Rocky Mountain spotted fever, ehrlichiosis, leptospirosis, and rubella.

Toxic shock syndrome is probable when at least four of the five criteria are fulfilled

Modified from American Academy of Pediatrics. Staphylococcal toxic shock syndrome. In: Peter G, ed. *1997 Red Book: Report of the Committee on Infectious Diseases.* 24th ed. Elk Grove Village, Ill: American Academy of Pediatrics; 1997:481.

Noninfectious processes such as acute rheumatic fever, hemolytic-uremic syndrome, systemic lupus erythematosus, and adverse drug reactions must be excluded.

Treatment

The course of TSS can be complicated by hypotension, oliguria from acute tubular necrosis, interstitial water leakage, and pulmonary edema. Severe rhabdomyolysis can occur, as can hypophosphatemia, metabolic acidosis, and adult respiratory distress syndrome. Therapy is supportive. Albumin infusion can correct hypovolemia and restore perfusion. Inotropic support, such as dopamine infusion, can be helpful if the response to fluid administration is sluggish. An elevated creatinine level, usually above 265 mcmol/L (3 mg/dL), is a predictor of prolonged hospitalization. Systemic administration of a beta-lactamase-resistant antistaphylococcal antibiotic such as nafcillin or vancomycin is recommended. Any potential focus of infection should be removed. Infected wounds should be explored and drained even when they do not show dramatic signs of inflammation.

Adjuvant therapy of TSS has included IVIG, steroids, plasmapheresis, and monoclonal antibodies. At present, these therapies should be considered experimental.

TABLE 2. Proposed Case Definition for the Streptococcal Toxic Shock Syndrome

1. Isolation of group A streptococci
   A. From a normally sterile site (eg, blood, cerebrospinal fluid, peritoneal fluid, tissue biopsy, surgical wound)
   B. From a nonsterile site (eg, throat, superficial skin lesion)
2. Clinical signs of severity
   A. Hypotension: systolic blood pressure 90 mm Hg in adults or 5th percentile for age in children, and
   B. Two or more of the following signs:
      - Renal impairment: creatinine 2 mg/dL for adults or at least twice the upper limit of normal for age
      - Coagulopathy: platelets 100,000/mm^3 or disseminated intravascular coagulation
      - Liver involvement: serum alanine aminotransferase (SGOT), asparate aminotransferase (SGPT), or total bilirubin concentrations at least twice the upper limit of normal for age
      - Adult respiratory distress syndrome
      - A generalized erythematous macular rash that may desquamate
      - Soft-tissue necrosis, including necrotizing fascitis or myositis, or gangrene

An illness fulfilling criteria 1A and 2 (A and B) can be defined as a definite case. An illness fulfilling criteria 1B and 2 (A and B) can be defined as a probable case if no other etiology for the illness is identified.

Modified from the Centers for Disease Control and Prevention. The Working Group on Severe Streptococcal Infection. Defining the group A streptococcal toxic shock syndrome: rationale and consensus definition. *JAMA.* 1993;269:390-391.

Table from American Academy of Pediatrics. Group A streptococcal infections. In: Peter G, ed. *1997 Red Book: Report of the Committee on Infectious Diseases.* 24th ed. Elk Grove Village, Ill: American Academy of Pediatrics; 1997:484.

Prolonged muscle weakness, fatigue, loss of fingers or toes, behavior changes, and reversible hair or nail loss have been reported as sequelae in patients who have TSS. There is a high rate of recurrence, which usually is associated with inadequate initial therapy.

Lesson for the Clinician

Clinicians should be aware of the constellation of symptoms caused by TSS and suspect this disorder, especially when faced with a febrile, hypotensive patient who has a diffuse erythematous rash.

Thomas Spentzas, MD, St. Mary's Medical Center, Evansville, IN

Two Days of Abdominal Pain, Nausea, and Vomiting

PRESENTATION

A 17-year-old girl is seen in the emergency department because of abdominal pain, nausea, and vomiting of 48 hours' duration while camping. She has had no fever. Although her intake has been poor, she did pass a normal stool the day before. She reports irregular menstrual cycles and claims not to be sexually active.

On physical examination, she appears uncomfortable and shows guarding when palpated in the right lower quadrant and suprapubic areas. She has a few widely intermittent bowel sounds. On rectal examination, there is fullness on the right side; the stool is guaiac-negative. On bimanual pelvic examination, the adnexa on the right are tender and seem to be enlarged, although her pain interferes with the examination.

Her white blood cell count is 22 x 10⁹/L (22 x 10³/mcL) with 88% segmented cells. Supine and upright radiographs of the abdomen demonstrate small bowel air-fluid levels in the right lower quadrant and no free air. No fecolith is seen. Urinalysis shows moderate ketone levels and 8 to 10 white blood cells per high-power field; no bacteria are noted. An additional diagnostic study is done and subsequently an operation is performed.

What is your differential diagnosis at this point?
Are there any elements of history or physical examination that would help you?
What additional diagnostic studies would you like performed?

DISCUSSION

Diagnosis

The symptoms and signs of torsion of an ovary are similar to those of an acute painful abdomen caused by appendicitis, volvulus, intussusception, and other causes of small bowel obstruction. Other important causes of acute abdominal pain are inflammatory bowel disease, mesenteric adenitis, and constipation.

Most often, torsion of the ovary is associated with an ovarian cyst. Benign follicle cysts are common, frequently bilateral cysts that appear on the surface of ovaries and are filled with clear fluid. They are found most commonly after the onset of puberty and after anovulatory cycles. Their size varies from microscopic to 4 cm in diameter (rarely larger). These cysts represent the failure of an incompletely developed follicle to resolve. A large cyst and ovary can twist, leading to lymphatic and venous obstruction. Hemorrhage and rupture can occur. Benign solid ovarian tumors, such as a dermoid or teratoma, also can lead to ovarian torsion. Malignant teratoma of the ovary and cystadenoma or carcinoma of the ovary also are known to occur in this age group.

Evaluation and Treatment

Female patients experiencing acute abdominal pain should have a rectal examination to assess the ovaries and adnexa. In some patients, a bimanual pelvic examination may be possible, but often it is deferred in lieu of pelvic ultrasonography, which will demonstrate a large ovary with an edematous wall. It also may show, as it did in this patient, an enlarged ovary with multiple ovarian cysts. Gynecologic consultation then would be indicated. Surgery always is indicated, but the degree of torsion and ischemia of the ovary will determine how much tissue can be salvaged.

Andrea C. Bracikowski, MD, Rochester, NY

Muffled Voice and Lymphadenopathy

PRESENTATION

A 4-year-old boy is seen in your office with a 4-day history of sore throat and low-grade fever. Two months earlier he was seen with a fever and sore throat and was felt to have a viral illness; he did not receive antibiotics, and he recovered. His mother reports that he is not eating well, and she believes he has a stomach ache.

On physical examination, the boy appears well but somewhat apprehensive. When he speaks, his voice sounds distorted and muffled. His temperature is 38°C (100.4°F). On both sides of his anterior neck you palpate several 2-cm nontender, freely moveable lymph nodes. You have difficulty getting the child to open his mouth wide and stick out his tongue, but you do catch one quick glimpse of his oropharynx, which is mildly erythematous but free of exudate. His right tonsillar region is swollen, and his uvula appears to deviate to the left.

What is your differential diagnosis at this point?
Are there any elements of history or physical examination that would help you?
What additional diagnostic studies would you like performed?

DISCUSSION

Diagnosis

Peritonsillitis is a term that includes both cellulitis and abscess of the tissues surrounding the tonsils. Peritonsillar abscess is the most common deep abscess in the head and neck and the most frequent complication of tonsillitis. The distinction between the two entities depends on whether pus can be obtained (abscess) by aspiration or by incision and drainage. Peritonsillar cellulitis and peritonsillar abscess appear to be different points on the spectrum of the same disease process.

Presentation

The more common presenting features of peritonsillitis include dysphagia, fever, trismus, voice change ("hot potato voice"), drooling, and otalgia; frequently there is a history of recent tonsillitis. Rancid breath and pain on lateral rotation of the neck also may be present.

Etiology

The organisms isolated from both peritonsillar cellulitis and peritonsillar abscesses essentially are the same. Group A and non-group A beta-hemolytic streptococci account for the majority of cases in which pathogens have been isolated by culture. Other relatively frequent etiologic organisms include group D streptococci, *S pneumoniae*, alpha streptococci, anaerobic diphtheroids, coagulase-negative staphylococci, and *S aureus*. Frequently, more than one pathogenic organism is identified from cultures of an abscess.

Evaluation

Several studies have attempted to determine distinguishing clinical features of peritonsillar cellulitis and abscess, with conflicting conclusions. Peritonsillitis in general is seen most commonly in adolescents, but patients who have peritonsillar cellulitis tend to be younger than those who have peritonsillar abscess, which is uncommon before age 10 years. The results of studies taken as a whole suggest that there are no reliable signs or symptoms to help differentiate a peritonsillar abscess from cellulitis in an individual patient and that aspiration is necessary for a definitive answer. Radiographs can provide an estimate of soft-tissue edema and are used by some clinicians in the management of this disorder.

Treatment

The standard of practice for treating peritonsillitis is not firmly established. Most current literature recommends aspirating the swollen peritonsillar region, usually with an 18-gauge needle, and sending any material obtained for culture. If pus is obtained, the abscess needs to be drained. Aspiration, however, may be difficult and dangerous in very young or uncooperative patients. The procedure also can cause the patient to aspirate abscess contents, and there is a risk of inserting the needle into the carotid artery. Furthermore, failure to yield pus does not rule out an abscess.

The importance of differentiating between peritonsillar abscess and cellulitis is unclear. Some studies suggest that culture results may make no difference in antibiotic selection or patient outcome, bringing into question the need to culture patients who have peritonsillitis. In light of the difficulties and risks of aspiration, clinical judgment must be exercised to decide which patients may be treated without attempting to drain the region. A nontoxic-appearing child may be treated empirically with antibiotics without the benefit of culture. The patient then can be observed for signs of worsening illness or complications of peritonsillitis.

Antibiotic treatment of patients who have peritonsillitis should not be delayed because of the risk of sudden airway obstruction, meningitis, or extension of the infection to the retropharyngeal or prevertebral spaces. Penicillin, almost always given parenterally, is the usual treatment of choice, but many use a penicillinase-resistant penicillin pending culture results. Clindamycin, erythromycin, metronidazole, and cephalosporins are good alternatives for patients who are allergic to penicillin. Because *S pneumoniae* is an occasional etiologic agent, and in some geographic areas penicillin resistance is high, a second- or third-generation cephalosporin may be an attractive alternative.

The decision for immediate or subsequent tonsillectomy for peritonsillitis remains controversial, with the pediatric literature presenting a more conservative approach to treatment than the otolaryngologic literature.

Differential Diagnosis

The differential diagnosis of peritonsillitis includes other infections of the region, such as tonsillar and retromolar abscesses and abscesses of the retropharyngeal and lateral pharyngeal spaces. Infectious mononucleosis, extensive cervical adenitis, and neoplasms also may mimic peritonsillitis.

Randy Cron, MD, PhD, University of Washington, Seattle, WA

Bruising Following Parental Discipline

PRESENTATION

A 4-year-old boy is brought to the office because of bruising that his mother had noticed while bathing him 2 days previously. He has not had nosebleeds or noticeable blood in his stool or urine, and he has been well except for a bout of gastroenteritis 2 weeks earlier. His parents are separated, and his mother states that the youngster's father spanked and kicked him and his brother during a visit last weekend. An 11-year-old sister is present and says that the father grabbed the boy's arm and "kicked his rear with his boot."

On physical examination, the child has multiple bruises—some appearing fresh, some apparently several days old—on his back, anterior torso, arms, and anterior thighs. Over his buttocks are linear areas composed of clusters of petechiae. There is a cluster of bruises over the right upper posterior thigh. The remainder of the examination is normal. You discuss a child protective referral with the mother, who says she will report the situation through her lawyer. You also draw a blood sample and send it to the laboratory.

What is your differential diagnosis at this point?
Are there any elements of history or physical examination that would help you?
What additional diagnostic studies would you like performed?

DISCUSSION

Diagnosis

The report of a complete blood count on this boy showed a platelet count of 5×10^9/L (5×10^3/mcL) and normal white blood cell count, differential count, and hemoglobin level, which was suggestive of idiopathic thrombocytopenic purpura (ITP). He was restricted in his activities and followed carefully. His platelet count rose spontaneously within days, and he went on to full recovery.

Because the child protective referral had been made, the pediatrician had to explain to the agency that the degree of trauma inflicted on the boy was difficult to ascertain, given the low platelet count. In fact, the physician felt that the child may have been subjected to inappropriate punishment, judging by history and some of the bruising patterns. However, the usual standards for evaluating the extent of abuse are difficult to apply when the bleeding status is impaired, as in this case.

Presentation

One should suspect thrombocytopenia when bruising, petechiae, and purpuric areas are widespread or involve the mucous membranes. The normal bruising that occurs in active children usually predominates over the anterior legs and other areas subject to the trauma of play. Petechiae are unusual in areas other than those that obviously have been scraped or traumatized, and diffuse petechiae are especially unusual in a normal child.

ITP is a relatively common cause of thrombocytopenia and is characterized by a low platelet count but otherwise normal findings in the peripheral blood. Often the patient reports a viral illness about 2 weeks prior to the skin changes, and the causative mechanism is felt to be immune in nature. Results of physical examination usually are normal except for the areas of bleeding. Lymphadenopathy and liver and spleen enlargement are not characteristic.

A platelet count below 150×10^9/L (150×10^3/mcL) is considered low. In ITP, platelet counts are frequently below 20×10^9/L (20×10^3/mcL). Although a rare complication, intracranial bleeding can occur in ITP, usually early in the course; mucous membrane bleeding, epistaxis, and gastrointestinal bleeding also can occur in patients who have thrombocytopenia or functional platelet disorders. Be aware, however, that deep muscle or joint bleeding rarely results from these conditions and should raise the suspicion of trauma or hemophilia.

Treatment
Children who have ITP and platelet counts more than 20×10^9/L (20×10^3/mcL) or minimal bleeding symptoms simply may be followed without specific therapy. Corticosteroids can cause a rapid rise in the platelet count, and intravenous gamma globulin has been shown in recent years to be an effective treatment in many cases. Most hematologists recommend a bone marrow study, if corticosteroids will be prescribed, to make sure the patient does not have leukemia.

Differential Diagnosis
Many other conditions can cause low platelet counts, including drug-induced thrombocytopenia, aplastic anemia, leukemia, microangiopathies, and inherited thrombocytopenias, such as the Wiskott-Aldrich syndrome, in which the patient also has eczema and immune deficiency. Patients who have systemic lupus erythematosus or lymphoma can have thrombocytopenia, although these disorders usually are seen in older children. Sepsis and disseminated intravascular coagulation states can cause low platelet counts, but these conditions have many other distinct characteristics.

Petechiae and purpura can occur in patients who have normal platelet counts. Some viral illnesses cause petechial eruptions, and disorders characterized by vasculitis can cause purpura and bruising in the face of a normal or increased platelet count. Anaphylactoid (Henoch-Schönlein) purpura is a relatively common example of such a condition. Most children bruised by abuse have normal platelet counts.

Lesson for the Clinician
The pediatrician evaluating a bruised child must keep an open mind, realizing that the bruises could be caused by abuse, an underlying medical condition (with or without hematologic abnormality), or even a combination of both.

Lawrence F. Nazarian, MD, Penfield, NY

Update: There is a new feature in therapy for ITP since this case was published. As stated in the discussion, corticosteroids can cause a rapid rise in the platelet count. Intravenous gamma globulin (IVIG) is even more effective in this regard; most children respond within 3 days and often the response lasts for weeks. There is a high incidence of headaches, vomiting, and fever after IVIG administration. Anti-D antibody is a new and effective agent that also causes a prompt rise in the platelet count, but it is effective only in Rh-positive patients. Most hematologists recommend obtaining a bone marrow study before using corticosteroids to be sure that the patient does not have leukemia. A bone marrow examination also is recommended for children who do not respond to IVIG or anti-D antibody therapy.

History of Fractures in a Toddler

PRESENTATION

A 3-year-old boy is brought to the emergency room because he tripped while wrestling with his brother and now will not bear weight on his right leg. The child was born with transposition of the great arteries, for which he has had a Mustard procedure. He is doing well on no medications, although he is described as being a "picky" eater. When he was 3 months old, his father turned him over and "heard a snap"; subsequently, he was found to have transverse fractures of the radius and ulna. At 8 months of age he sustained a spiral fracture of the left tibia after falling from a changing table.

On physical examination, the boy weighs 14.85 kg (50th percentile) and is 88.9 cm tall (10th percentile). He sits quietly in his mother's arms and looks pale but is in no distress. There is obvious swelling of his lower right leg, with bruising.

Radiographs reveal a spiral fracture of the midshaft of the right tibia and mild osteopenia. His leg is casted, and the emergency department social worker is contacted. You also arrange follow-up with a specialist.

What is your differential diagnosis at this point?
Are there any elements of history or physical examination that would help you?
What additional diagnostic studies would you like performed?

DISCUSSION

Diagnosis

This child had been seen twice before in the emergency department; both times child abuse had been suspected because the injuries appeared too severe for the explanation given. Although child abuse again was suspected on this visit, the examining resident wondered about an underlying bone disorder, and on careful re-examination of the child noted a subtle blue cast to his sclerae, leading to discovery of the underlying diagnosis of osteogenesis imperfecta (OI).

OI is an inherited disorder of connective tissue that affects bones, ligaments, dentin, and skin and is characterized by multiple fractures. An initial attempt to classify OI distinguished individuals who have fractures or a deformity at birth (OI congenita) from those who do not develop fractures or a deformity until later (OI tarda). At present, OI can be divided into four major groups, which differ in clinical presentation, inheritance, radiographic appearance, and biochemical abnormality.

Individuals who have types I and IV OI have a normal lifespan and are the ones likely to be misdiagnosed as abused children. During adolescence these patients experience a marked decrease in the number of fractures. Children who have types II and III OI have severe bone fragility and have findings that lead to diagnosis early in life. Half of all infants who have type II OI are stillborn; the others are babies of low birthweight who have deformed limbs and radiographic findings of multiple long bone fractures in various stages of healing, a situation pathognomonic of OI.

The child who has OI often will lack a history of injury severe enough to cause this kind of fracture normally. There may be a family history of "brittle bones" or of deafness (hearing loss secondary to otosclerosis is associated with OI), although usually it does not develop until the third decade of life.

Presentation

Blue sclerae, although pathognomonic of OI, are not always present. Distinctly blue in type I, the sclerae become less blue with age in patients who have types III and IV disease. The sclerae are thin and contain abnormal collagen. Other physical findings include hyperlaxity of ligaments, mild shortness of stature, opalescent dentin (yellow or gray-blue transparent teeth in type I), and kyphosis (types I and III). The thin dermis can lead to excessive sweating and abnormal temperature regulation. When trying to determine any abuse, look also for bruises, retinal hemorrhages, or evidence of intracranial hematoma.

Radiographic findings of fractures in various stages of healing, multiple posterior rib fractures, metaphyseal chip fractures, or spiral fractures of the humerus or femur often are associated with child abuse, but they all have been described in cases of OI. The osteopenia in this child commonly is found in OI, as are thinned cortices and a tendency for the healed fracture area to bow, causing deformities of the extremities.

Differential Diagnosis

Other conditions of bone can suggest child abuse, but radiologic findings can help in the diagnostic process. Hypophosphatasia involves a generalized decrease in bone density and bowing deformities of the extremities, but can be distinguished from OI by metaphyseal changes such as cupping and decreased mineralization at the growth plate. Osteoid osteoma has the distinctive radiographic finding of sclerotic bone around a radiolucent nidus of osteoid tissue. In infantile cortical hyperostosis (Caffey disease), radiographs reveal progressive cortical thickening.

Evaluation

The combination of frequent fractures, blue sclerae, and a family history with a dominant pattern leads to the diagnosis of OI type I. Laboratory confirmation of the diagnosis is provided by analysis of procollagen production in dermal fibroblastin culture.

Lesson for the Clinician

Remember that the presence of OI does not rule out the possibility of child abuse. The two are not mutually exclusive, and the child who has OI will be even more susceptible to injuries that result from inadequate supervision or deliberate trauma. At the same time, the clinician must be cautious about conclusions of abuse, if OI is suspected, until the results of specialist consultation and biochemical analysis are obtained.

Neeru Sehgal, MD, University of Rochester School of Medicine and Dentistry,
Rochester, NY

Bruises on the Lower Back and Buttocks

PRESENTATION

You are called to the telephone to speak with a social worker from a hospital near a seashore resort. A 19-month-old patient of yours has been brought to the emergency room with a fever. In the course of examining him, the physician noticed several bruises over the lower back and buttocks and suspects child abuse. Despite your inability to examine the child, you are able to supply information that explains the findings and makes further investigation unnecessary.

What is your differential diagnosis at this point?
Are there any elements of history or physical examination that would help you?
What additional diagnostic studies would you like performed?

DISCUSSION

Diagnosis

Babies of dark-skinned races and Asian heritage often are born having pigmented patches on their skin that can be confused with bruises, especially if one is not familiar with this phenomenon known as Mongolian spots. These gray or grayish-blue areas are found most commonly in the lumbosacral and buttock areas but can be widely disseminated; they can be solitary or multiple. Mongolian spots usually are large and homogeneous in color and never are tender. The melanin responsible for the spots is contained in melanocytes in the mid-dermis. These are benign patches that do not progress to melanoma; many disappear by age 5 years, and most are gone by age 10 years.

Heightened awareness of child abuse has made the recognition and documentation of Mongolian spots important. The child presented here had a Caucasian father and a Chinese mother and did indeed have Mongolian spots. Reassurance was given to the social worker that the hospital personnel were describing a benign skin finding. An African-American child seen in our emergency department had numerous pigmented areas over his back that raised the suspicion of abuse. Fortunately, his newborn hospital record documented the extensive Mongolian spots and clarified the situation.

Differential Diagnosis

Remember that bruises, although they can be large, usually are much smaller than Mongolian spots and express many more shades than the monotonous blue-gray of the spots. The color spectrum of bruises ranges from the blue-black or purple hue of the fresh injury through the stages of hemosiderin breakdown, leading to a yellow-green color.

Other conditions can mimic bruises and falsely suggest abuse. Urticaria pigmentosa is a form of mastocytosis that appears as multiple hyperpigmented areas, most commonly (but not exclusively) on the trunk. Sometimes the surface blisters and an actual hive forms, especially when the spot is rubbed (Darier sign). These lesions appear early in life, and many have disappeared by adolescence.

There is a Vietnamese and Chinese folk treatment known as coining, in which coins are coated with ointment and rolled or rubbed on the skin, causing linear, traumatic skin lesions, usually on the neck or chest. The intent is to treat illness, not to injure the child. A similar folk practice, known as cupping, will produce perfectly round areas of purpura—analogous to the human "passion mark"—by means of a heated cup that is placed on the skin and allowed to cool, thus exerting a negative pressure. This practice is a common ritual in southern and eastern Europe and Asia. Variations on this type of folk treatment include chope (candle suction), Chinese moxabustion, and the Latin American treatment for "fallen fontanelle" known as "ventosas."

Lesson for the Clinician

Documentation of lesions that can be confused with bruises is essential, as is knowledge of the cultural practices within one's patient population that might create the appearance of abusive behavior. Continued scrutiny of obvious bruises, as seen in patients who come in for unequivocal injuries, will provide an ongoing refresher course to help the physician sort out true bruises from imposters.

Certain disorders can create the appearance of child abuse where there may have been none, leading to accusations and complications that are not easily reversed. At the same time, the presence of one of these conditions does not rule out abuse; in some cases, the underlying disorder may increase the child's risk of abuse. There are also cases of abuse that masquerade as diseases. For example, an adult might be giving a sedating drug to a child, who appears to have a disorder of the central nervous system. The truth will be discovered by meticulous attention to the details of history and physical examination and by the physician's reluctance to accept what at first appears to be an obvious diagnosis.

Lawrence F. Nazarian, MD, Penfield, NY

Two Days of Vomiting and Diarrhea

PRESENTATION

A 28-month-old boy is sent to the pediatric emergency department, having had vomiting and severe diarrhea for 2 days. His stools were noted to be loose 48 hours previously, at which time he had a low-grade fever. His private pediatrician saw him and diagnosed an early viral gastroenteritis. The child's stools became watery and foul-smelling, and he began to vomit a clear, nonbilious fluid. The vomiting and diarrhea have persisted, and his temperature has increased as his activity level has diminished.

On physical examination, the boy lies quietly, although he does not appear to be in substantial distress. His temperature is 39.4 °C (103 °F), pulse is 140 beats/min, and weight is 6% lower than a recent weight at his pediatrician's office. He has slight tenderness on deep abdominal palpation. Findings on rectal examination are normal, as is the remainder of the physical evaluation. Abnormal laboratory findings include a serum carbon dioxide content of 13 mmol/L (13 mEq/L) (normal, 18 to 27 mmol/L [18 to 27 mEq/L]) and a white blood cell count of 23 x 10^9/L (23 x 10^3/mcL), with 72% neutrophils and 11% band forms.

Despite intravenous rehydration, his fever remains high and his activity level does not improve. His abdominal discomfort continues and the leukocytosis persists. A surgical consultant does not feel that the boy has a condition requiring surgery. An additional diagnostic test reveals the cause of his illness.

What is your differential diagnosis at this point?
Are there any elements of history or physical examination that would help you?
What additional diagnostic studies would you like performed?

DISCUSSION

Diagnosis

Pneumonia is a common disorder in children and can cause myriad unusual clinical presentations, such as acute abdominal pain or shoulder pain with a pleural effusion. This patient's clinical picture was that of vomiting and diarrhea, suggesting gastroenteritis and other intra-abdominal disorders. The only specific clues that suggested a bacterial process were the high spiking fever and the leukocytosis, both of which could have been caused by a bacterial enteritis. Urinalysis revealed no microscopic abnormalities.

The persistent spiking fever called for repeated physical examinations. By 12 hours of hospitalization, the child clearly had abdominal discomfort and was noted to have "splinted" respirations that were interpreted as being consistent with an intra-abdominal process. No other pulmonary symptoms or signs were present early in his hospitalization.

Re-examination later revealed a slight tachypnea and decreased breath sounds at the base of his right lung. A radiograph of the chest revealed a consolidation of the middle lobe of his right lung and a pneumonic process in his right lower lobe.

Antimicrobial therapy was initiated promptly; his fever resolved and his appearance improved markedly within 48 hours. A blood culture drawn on admission grew *Streptococcus pneumoniae* on the second day of hospitalization. His recovery continued, and the rest of his hospital course was uneventful.

Presentation

A child who has pneumonia may have few signs or symptoms that point specifically to a process in the chest; indeed, results of the chest examination may be normal. Experienced pediatricians know that when pulmonary signs do appear, they may be discerned better by observation than by auscultation. The child who is breathing abnormally may be appreciated best from across the room. Even a chest radiograph early in the course may show little in the way of abnormality, especially when the child is dehydrated. Rehydration can cause a dramatic change in radiographic findings.

Bacteremia is a relatively common accompaniment of pneumococcal pneumonia (23% to 30% of cases). A febrile young child who appears ill, especially if he has a leukocytosis, should be suspected of having bacteremia. Antigen detection and lung aspiration are other diagnostic techniques that can be used to diagnose pneumococcal pneumonia.

A right lower lobe pneumonia can cause diaphragmatic and abdominal irritation as well as ileus and can create a picture consistent with an acute abdominal process requiring surgery. The pediatrician who makes the correct diagnosis and spares the child an unnecessary operation does his patient (and the surgeon) a great service.

Treatment

Treatment of the child who has pneumococcal pneumonia traditionally has consisted of parenteral penicillin along with supportive therapies such as intravenous fluids and oxygen. In cases caused by susceptible strains of *S pneumoniae*, dramatic improvement in the patient's condition is the rule. Clinicians, however, must be aware of penicillin-resistant pneumococci, which are becoming more frequent. Because this resistance pattern varies with the geographic area, consultation with an infectious disease specialist who knows the local microbiologic climate makes sense when one is treating a serious pneumococcal infection. Similarly, sensitivity testing on the isolated strain of *S pneumoniae* has become important.

Oral second-generation cephalosporins have been recommended as a replacement for penicillin. However, differences in the antibiotic sensitivity of penicillin-resistant strains of pneumococci exist among cephalosporins. Vancomycin is the drug of choice for serious pneumococcal infections. Pneumococcal pneumonia can be life-threatening in children who have sickle cell disease.

Lesson for the Clinician

As this patient demonstrates, pneumococcal pneumonia can present a diagnostic challenge. The value of constantly re-examining a patient who is difficult to diagnose cannot be overemphasized.

Laurette Ho, MD, Bradley J. Bradford, MD, Mercy Children's Medical Center, Pittsburgh, PA

Sudden Onset of Headache Following a Cold

PRESENTATION

A 10-year-old boy is seen because of headache for 1 day. He was well until 10 days ago, when nasal congestion began. His cold symptoms seemed to worsen for several days but have subsided. The headache began suddenly yesterday afternoon when he returned home from school; his pain was in the frontal area and steady. He vomited once but did not experience dizziness. Still complaining of headache, he went to sleep early.

This morning, when awakened for school, his headache was worse, causing his mother to bring him to the office. He has never experienced a headache like this one. The boy has had no fever, and until this morning there has been no change in his appetite or activity. There have been no changes in his school performance recently, and no toxic or infectious exposures are known, except for his 12-year-old brother having had a mild upper respiratory tract infection last week. Both parents work full-time and were not home when the headache began.

On physical examination, he is cooperative but sleepy, answering appropriately but keeping his eyes closed throughout the examination. His temperature is 98.4 °F (36.9 °C), pulse is 72 beats/min, and blood pressure is 120/70 mm Hg. His pupils are equal and reactive, and the optic discs are sharp, although venous pulsations are not noted. He says that his entire head hurts, but denies tenderness when percussed over the frontal and maxillary areas. There is mild nuchal rigidity, but results of the neurologic examination otherwise are normal. His Glasgow coma score is 14.

What is your differential diagnosis at this point?
Are there any elements of history or physical examination that would help you?
What additional diagnostic studies would you like performed?

DISCUSSION

Diagnosis

On further questioning, the patient and his brother admitted to "roughhousing" after school; the patient had fallen from his upper bunk bed headfirst onto a wooden floor. Computed tomography revealed an epidural hematoma, and neurosurgical assistance was sought immediately.

Headaches are extremely common in childhood; as many as 75% of children experience headache in the first 15 years of life. The pattern of onset and duration as well as history and family history provide important clues to the etiology of the headache. The onset of intracranial hemorrhage generally is abrupt; often there is vomiting, and mental status changes frequently are seen. In most cases of intracranial bleeding in children, a precipitating traumatic event is followed by a variable combination of signs such as headache, depressed consciousness, seizures (focal or generalized), vomiting, and focal neurologic changes. In young children and infants, irritability or lethargy may be the only clues to the occurrence of bleeding.

Differential Diagnosis

Ruptured aneurysms and bleeding from arteriovenous malformations present with rapid onset of severe headache and rapid progression to coma and death if not surgically drained and, possibly, repaired. Blood in the subarachnoid space may lead to meningismus and fever, mimicking meningitis. Meningitis should be considered in any child who has an acute onset of headache, fever, and nuchal rigidity. Encephalitis may present with headache and fever with or without nuchal rigidity, and herpes simplex encephalitis in particular may mimic an intracranial hemorrhage by causing lethargy, focal neurologic findings, headache, a depressed level of consciousness, or irritability. In this patient, who had a history of recent upper respiratory tract infections, sinusitis should have been considered, but his cold had resolved, he did not have a persistent cough or congestion, and he was afebrile.

Headaches that are worse in the supine position or upon awakening and those that awaken the child at night are seen more commonly with intracranial tumors. The onset of symptoms usually is insidious, with progression in severity, but 0.5% to 3.5% of brain tumors present acutely because of bleeding into the tumor, and this abrupt presentation also can include headache and clouding of consciousness. Headache that comes on several hours to days after relatively minor blunt trauma to the back of the head, especially when there is associated vomiting and ataxia, is the typical presenting pattern of hematoma of the posterior fossa. Intracranial hemorrhage from head trauma in children is much more likely to be supratentorial, however.

Presentation
Subdural hematomas are more common in infants and epidural hematomas more common in older children. The typical clinical course in epidural hematoma of acute loss of consciousness followed by a lucent phase with subsequent lapse into coma is uncommon in children. Among children who present with intracranial bleeding after what appears to be relatively minor head trauma, structural abnormalities of the blood vessels (arteriovenous malformations and aneurysms) and defects in clotting (such as platelet abnormalities from leukemia or lupus erythematosus or coagulopathies as seen in von Willebrand disease) should be considered.

Evaluation and Treatment
If intracranial bleeding is suspected as the cause of headache in any child, a computed tomographic scan of the head is the diagnostic choice, and neurosurgical consultation is critical. In head injuries and vascular lesions that involve acute hemorrhage, rapid diagnosis is crucial, and early surgical intervention can be lifesaving.

Lesson for the Clinician
This case illustrates the importance of persistence in obtaining a complete history. Other children may have knowledge about antecedent events that are crucial in the management of the patient but may be reluctant to speak up for fear of getting themselves or the patient into trouble.

Lynn C. Garfunkel, MD, University of Rochester School of Medicine and Dentistry, Rochester, NY

Update: When the clinician suspects an acute intracranial hemorrhage, computed tomography remains the imaging procedure of first choice. When investigating the cause of subacute or chronic headaches and when looking for vascular lesions or tumors, more useful information may be obtained from magnetic resonance imaging.

Constant Nasal Congestion

PRESENTATION

You are seeing a 16-year-old boy who has had nasal congestion that began a few months ago. The congestion was intermittent at first but has become constant. He denies sneezing, itchy eyes, or other respiratory difficulty.

His mother is concerned because he often is awakened by his congestion. He frequently is irritable in the mornings, and she believes the sleep disturbance is responsible for the decline in his grades, which had been very good. Except for one uncle, no family members have complained of allergies.

He is a slim boy whose pulse is 90 beats/min, blood pressure is 136/80 mm Hg, and temperature is 37.1°C (98.8°F). Physical examination otherwise is normal except for mildly reddened, edematous nasal mucous membranes that have a small amount of thin, white mucoid discharge. His sinuses are not tender, and findings on sinus transillumination are normal.

What is your differential diagnosis at this point?
Are there any elements of history or physical examination that would help you?
What additional diagnostic studies would you like performed?

DISCUSSION

Differential Diagnosis

Nasal congestion is a commonly expressed complaint in a pediatrician's office. Clinicians usually think initially of an upper respiratory tract infection or allergic rhinitis. Congestion lasting months, however, cannot be attributed to a common upper respiratory tract infection, and allergic symptoms are unlikely to last for months without some period of remission. In addition, both of these diagnoses often are associated with nighttime cough. Sinusitis in childhood and adolescence has received much recent attention and should be considered. Sinusitis, however, is unlikely without daytime cough and usually causes some physical findings.

The prudent clinician will question the patient about the use of drugs, both illicit and legal, including over-the-counter medications. Rhinitis medicamentosa associated with the use of nasal sprays should be kept in mind. The sympathomimetic amines contained in the sprays initially constrict the vessels of the nasal mucosa, but a rebound congestion follows as the vasoconstrictive effect diminishes.

Similar effects can occur with nasal inhalation (insufflation) of cocaine, which has a vasoconstrictive effect. Discontinuation of the use of cocaine is followed by a rebound hyperemia with associated edema and rhinorrhea. Patients often compound this phenomenon by using over-the-counter nasal decongestants that temporarily relieve the symptoms but contribute to a vicious cycle of congestion, constriction, hyperemia, and congestion.

Presentation

Cocaine use can cause throat and mouth dryness and diminished senses of taste and smell. The ongoing congestion also interferes with sound sleep. The patient often

wakes throughout the night because of the stuffy nose. This sleep disturbance contributes to morning irritability, which also can result from the direct insomnia-induc-
ing effects of cocaine. The nasal septum can be damaged and ultimately perforated
by the chronic ischemia.

In addition to the clinical pattern of chronic cocaine use, the clinician must be
aware of the symptoms and signs of cocaine overdose: dry mouth, nausea, vomiting, dilated pupils, excessive sweating, increased talking, paresthesias, flushing, elevated temperature, and respiratory failure.Neurologic signs of overdose include
seizures, hyperactive reflexes, and tremor. Psychiatric manifestations can occur in
the form of toxic psychosis, paranoid behavior, anxiety, delusions, hallucinations,
irritability, and picking at the skin. Cardiac effects include tachycardia, angina,
arrhythmia, hypertension, and cardiovascular collapse. This patient had a borderline high systolic blood pressure and mildly elevated pulse rate. Unless he had used
cocaine recently, these findings are more likely due to anxiety, perhaps related to
fear of having his habit discovered.

Treatment
Treatment of cocaine toxicity is supportive, with specific treatment only for arrhythmias, seizures, and psychosis.

Lesson for the Clinician
Lest you think there is no cocaine use in your area, be aware that a 1991 tally of
national surveys of high school students showed that 1% to 4% of the students
reported using cocaine in some form during the 60 days prior to the survey.

Elizabeth R. Marino, MD, New Jersey Medical School, Newark, NJ

Fever and Lethargy Progressing to Unresponsiveness

PRESENTATION

An 8-month-old African-American boy has experienced fever and poor feeding for 3 days. He has been lethargic today. When he develops jerking of his left arm and becomes unresponsive, his parents rush him to the emergency department.

History reveals that the child was born at term and has developed normally. He has received no vaccinations because of multiple family moves. At 6 months of age, he developed fever and poor feeding, was found to have pneumococcal meningitis, and was treated with penicillin G. Results of a computed tomographic (CT) scan of his head were within normal limits, and he was discharged home with no apparent sequelae. His parents did not bring the infant back for a follow-up visit, but they report that he has been healthy until 3 days ago.

On physical examination, the child is unresponsive to painful stimuli and has a temperature of 41.1°C (102.4°F). During the examination he develops focal seizures and becomes apneic for 30 seconds, requiring intubation. A lumbar puncture reveals 12 erythrocytes and 56 white blood cells per cubic millimeter of cerebrospinal fluid (CSF), a glucose level of 0.111 mmol/L (2 mg/dL), and a protein level of 2.95 g/L (295 mg/dL). Stain of the CSF shows sheets of Gram-positive cocci in pairs. Both blood and CSF cultures later grow pneumococci sensitive to penicillin.

The child is treated with penicillin G, but he responds poorly, requiring assisted ventilation and suffering progressive loss of neurologic function. CT scan and magnetic resonance imaging (MRI) show ventriculomegaly with extreme loss of brain tissue due to a diffusely infarcted brain. A shunt is placed to treat obstructive hydrocephalus. On discharge from the hospital, the baby is in a vegetative state and dies 1 month later following an apneic episode. Tests performed during this admission reveal the cause of his recurrent meningitis.

What is your differential diagnosis at this point?
Are there any elements of history or physical examination that would help you?
What additional diagnostic studies would you like performed?

DISCUSSION

Differential Diagnosis

This infant had recurrent bacterial meningitis with fatal results. The differential diagnosis of recurrent meningitis includes human immunodeficiency virus (HIV) infection, congenital asplenia, congenital CSF fistula due to an anatomic defect, and primary immunodeficiency.

This patient had no risk factors for HIV infection or other signs of that condition, such as failure to thrive, lymphadenopathy, or hepatosplenomegaly. HIV testing by enzyme-linked immunosorbent assay and by polymerase chain reaction was performed, and results of both tests were negative.

Congenital asplenia is associated with Ivemark syndrome, which includes bilateral trilobed lungs; a symmetric, centrally located liver; and complex congenital heart disease. This boy did not have any of these features. Peripheral blood smear did not show any Howell-Jolly or Heinz bodies, which are found in asplenia, and a liver-spleen scan was within normal limits, ruling out that condition.

Congenital CSF fistula causes recurrent bacterial meningitis by allowing direct entry of bacteria into the CSF from a defective cribiform plate. High-resolution CT scan and MRI performed to rule out congenital CSF fistula did not show any anatomic defect in this boy. A careful search of his spine with a magnifying glass failed to reveal any portals of entry into the spinal canal.

Complement deficiency should be considered in anyone experiencing recurrent bacterial infections because the complement system plays an important role in the inflammatory response and host defenses. C2 and C3 deficiencies are both autosomal recessive in inheritance and associated with serious bacterial infections. C2 deficiency has been associated with repeated pneumococcal infections. Deficiencies of terminal components C5 to C9 are associated with repeated meningococcal or disseminated gonococcal infections. This child's total hemolytic complement activity was normal. Results of C2, C3, and C4 assays were within the normal range for his age, ruling out a complement deficiency.

Primary congenital immunodeficiency states such as X-linked (Bruton) agammaglobulinemia and severe combined immunodeficiency present with recurrent meningitis due to the absence of humoral or combined humoral and cellular immunity, respectively. This patient did not have any viral or fungal infections and was well up to 6 months of age, a course inconsistent with severe combined immunodeficiency. T-cell studies showed CD3, CD4, and CD8 values that were normal for the child's age. The CD4/CD8 ratio also was in the normal range. Mitogen stimulation studies for lymphocyte proliferation using phytohemagglutinin and concanaualin A showed good response. Thus, the determination of intact T-cell function ruled out severe combined immunodeficiency.

Diagnosis

Immunoglobulin (Ig) levels were as follows: IgG, 0.8 g/L (80 mg/dL) (normal range, 1.72 to 10.69 g/L [172 to 1,069 mg/dL]); IgA, 0.08 g/L (8 mg/dL) (normal range, 0.11 to 1.06 g/L [11 to 106 mg/dL]); IgE, not detected (normal range, 0 to 0.23 g/L [0 to 23 mg/dL]); IgD, not detected (normal range, 0 to 0.8 g/L [0 to 80 mg/dL]); and IgM, 0.05 g/L (5 mg/dL) (normal range, 0.3 to 1.26 g/L [30 to 126 mg/dL]). CD 19 and CD 20 (both markers of B cells) were absent, and isohemagglutinin titers were undetectable. Gene mapping showed an abnormal gene mapped to q22 on the X chromosome.

The combination of low immunoglobulin levels and the chromosomal abnormality established the diagnosis of X-linked agammaglobulinemia, an X-linked recessive disorder. The abnormal gene is located at the q22 locus on the long arm of X chromosome. The defective gene has been identified as a member of the Src family of proto-oncogenes, which encode protein tyrosine kinases. This abnormal gene results in the inability of a specific tyrosine kinase known as BTK to perform normal intracellular signaling in the production of immunoglobulin by B cells.

Most boys who have X-linked agammaglobulinemia remain asymptomatic until 6 months of age because of the protection afforded by maternally transmitted IgG antibodies. Thereafter, they repeatedly acquire infections caused by extracellular organisms such as pneumococci, streptococci, and *Haemophilus* sp. Chronic fungal infections are not usual, and viral infections are handled normally, except for those caused by hepatitis viruses and enterovirus.

Presentation
In 60% of patients, the presenting manifestations are pulmonary infections and infections of the ears, nose, and throat. Meningitis has been reported as an initial problem in 10% of patients. The remaining patients present with pyoderma or arthritis. One can speculate as to whether it might be worth measuring immunoglobulin levels on all infants who have bacterial meningitis to detect the rare child who has a deficiency.

X-linked agammaglobulinemia should be suspected if serum concentrations of immunoglobulins are far below the 95% confidence limits for the patient's age compared with appropriate controls (usually 2 g/L [200 mg/dL] of total immunoglobulin). Hypoplasia of adenoids, tonsils, and peripheral lymph nodes can occur. Lymph node biopsy reveals absent germinal centers, and plasma cells are rarely present.

Treatment
Treatment includes aggressive management of infections by using broad-spectrum antibiotics and administering intravenous immune globulin monthly. These patients should not receive live viral vaccines because they cannot respond with appropriate antibody production and instead are likely to develop clinical disease. They also are at risk of contracting clinical disease from live vaccines excreted by close contacts, such as polio from the live vaccine virus excreted in the stool of siblings. The mortality rate in patients who have this condition is approximately 10% by the age of 30 years. Causes of death include infections and chronic pulmonary disease. Lymphoproliferative malignancy develops in 6% of patients who have X-linked agammaglobulinemia.

An additional X-linked primary immunodeficiency is Wiskott-Aldrich syndrome, which is characterized by eczema, thrombocytopenia, and recurrent infection. Although immunoglobulin levels (particularly IgM) are low, they are not as low as the levels found in patients who have X-linked agammaglobulinemia.

Lesson for the Clinician
Disorders of the immune system are not common but must be considered in children who have severe or recurrent infections.

Smita Kumar, MD, Bindu Bennuri, MD, The Brooklyn Hospital Center, Brooklyn, NY

Right Leg and Left Shoulder Pain Following a Car Accident

PRESENTATION

A 10-year-old boy is brought to the emergency department by ambulance from an automobile accident. He was seated in the back seat with a seatbelt fastened appropriately when the automobile was struck while stopped at an intersection. Witnesses state that he did not lose consciousness, but he has no recollection of the accident. He is strapped to a backboard and has a hard cervical collar in place. An intravenous line has been placed in his right arm.

On physical examination, the boy appears cooperative and complains of pain in his right leg and left shoulder. His blood pressure is 100/60 mm Hg, pulse is 150 beats/min, and temperature is 37.2°C (98.96°F) orally. After his airway, breathing, and circulation are judged to be satisfactory, radiographs of his cervical spine are obtained and are normal. Further examination reveals a normal sensorium, clear and unlabored breath sounds, and normal heart sounds. There is mild diffuse tenderness of the chest. The abdomen is mildly tender but not distended, and normal bowel sounds are present. Slight bruising is noted on the abdomen in a distribution that reflects the position of the seatbelt. The right thigh is tender, but a radiograph reveals no evidence of fracture. The left leg and both arms have normal range of motion.

What is your differential diagnosis at this point?
Are there any elements of history or physical examination that would help you?
What additional diagnostic studies would you like performed?

DISCUSSION

Diagnosis

The spleen is the most commonly injured abdominal organ. Most injuries to the spleen occur as a result of motor vehicle accidents, although other forms of blunt abdominal trauma, such as falls, bicycle accidents, and sports injuries, may lead to splenic laceration or rupture. Because of the highly vascular nature of the spleen, injury often leads to blood loss into the peritoneal cavity. In cases of severe splenic injury, this blood loss may cause hemodynamic instability.

Presentation

Either diffuse or focal (usually left upper quadrant) abdominal tenderness may accompany injury to the spleen. Although abdominal tenderness after trauma is the hallmark of splenic injury, such tenderness is not always present. The abdomen may be firm to palpation due to peritoneal irritation from intraperitoneal hemorrhage, but it often is soft when bleeding is mild to moderate. Blood collecting in the left upper quadrant of the peritoneal cavity may cause diaphragmatic irritation and referred left shoulder pain.

Keys to recognizing splenic injury include external signs of trauma to the abdomen (such as seatbelt marks or bruises from a direct blow) and signs of early hemodynamic instability (in this case, tachycardia); one also should suspect splenic injury when there has been trauma of significant force, as in a motor vehicle accident. Diagnostic evaluation for injury to the spleen should be carried out in any traumatized patient who has a declining hematocrit, inexplicable requirements for intravenous fluids or blood, or multiple injuries that interfere with reliable examination of the abdomen.

Diagnosis and Treatment

Management of suspected injury to the spleen depends on the extent of associated injuries and the degree of hemodynamic instability. In cases of multiple trauma, where acute surgical management of other injuries is indicated, rapid diagnosis of intra-abdominal trauma is desirable prior to administration of anesthesia. Nasogastric intubation is recommended to remove gastric contents and decompress the stomach, facilitating examination and reducing the risk of aspiration. The presence of blood in the gastric secretions suggests upper gastrointestinal injury. In most cases of suspected splenic injury, stabilization of the patient, including volume support, followed by double contrast (intravenous plus oral) abdominal computed tomographic (CT) scan is the appropriate course. In the unstable patient, prompt surgical consultation and diagnostic peritoneal lavage (DPL) may elucidate the presence of significant intraperitoneal hemorrhage more quickly. In the hemodynamically stable patient, DPL is too sensitive a test and often is positive in cases of mild-to-moderate splenic injury. CT scan offers more detailed information for planning the management of the injury and may obviate the need for laparotomy that might follow a positive DPL.

Management of splenic injury has evolved toward more conservative therapy, especially in children, as recognition of postsplenectomy sepsis has focused attention on the risks of splenectomy. Presently, up to 80% of splenic injuries in children are managed nonoperatively with bedrest, fluid support, and careful observation in the hospital. Monitoring in an intensive care unit is recommended for the first 24 to 48 hours. Occasionally, blood transfusion is necessary. In the hemodynamically unstable child, surgery is indicated. In those cases, splenorrhaphy, partial splenectomy, and splenectomy with autotransplantation of splenic tissue are the preferred surgical approaches when possible.

John S. Andrews, MD, Catherine DeAngelis, MD, Johns Hopkins University School of Mediine, Baltimore, MD

Lethargy and Vomiting

PRESENTATION

A 13-month-old girl is brought to the emergency department because of lethargy and vomiting. The child was well and playful until 2 days ago, when she was noted to have become listless. Three hours later she began to vomit. After eight episodes of nonbilious, nonbloody vomiting, she was even more lethargic.

Her mother denies noting any upper respiratory tract infection, fever, abdominal pain, seizure, loss of consciousness, accidental ingestions, or trauma. The child's last stool was yesterday and was normal. Although born at 32 weeks' gestation, she experienced no complications and has been well. She is receiving no medications, has no allergies, and is fully immunized.

The physical examination reveals a weak, listless girl who has decreased muscle tone. Her temperature is 37.8°C (100.1°F), pulse is 96 beats/min, and respirations are 20 breaths/min. She has no focal neurologic findings. Findings on the remainder of the examination, including evaluation of the abdomen, are normal.

Results of a complete blood count and differential, blood urea nitrogen, and serum levels of electrolytes, creatinine, and glucose are normal. Urinalysis after intravenous fluid administration reveals a specific gravity of 1.010; ketone level of 150 mg/dL; and no glucose, protein, or blood.

The patient is admitted for fluid therapy with an initial diagnosis of acute gastroenteritis and dehydration. Two hours after admission, she has an episode of bilious vomiting. Results of the physical examination remain unchanged. Her abdomen is soft and not distended, with normoactive bowel sounds. No masses or organomegaly are noted.

The combination of lethargy and vomiting prompts her physicians to obtain an abdominal radiograph, the results of which provide clues to the diagnosis.

What is your differential diagnosis at this point?
Are there any elements of history or physical examination that would help you?
What additional diagnostic studies would you like performed?

DISCUSSION

Diagnosis

A plain radiograph of the abdomen that was obtained on admission revealed marked gaseous distension of a few loops of proximal jejunum. The colon showed small amounts of bowel gas. Sixteen hours after admission, the child developed loose, bloody stools and mild abdominal distention. A repeat radiograph revealed increased distension of bowel loops, with multiple air-fluid levels, a picture consistent with intestinal obstruction primarily involving the small bowel.

Barium enema documented an intussusception. After an unsuccessful attempt at reduction by enema, laparotomy revealed an ileocecal intussusception with erythema and viable bowel. Emergency reduction and appendectomy were performed.

Intussusception is the result of invagination or telescoping of a portion of proximal intestine into the adjacent distal bowel. Most commonly it involves the ileocecal valve (95% of cases) and is a frequent cause of intestinal obstruction. The intus-suscepted mass can obstruct the intestinal lumen quickly, causing distension and rushes of peristalsis more proximal to the mass.

Etiology

Although there is no identifiable etiology in more than 90% of cases, a number of conditions are associated with intussusception. Viral illnesses or other infections such as measles or gastroenteritis may cause swelling of the lymphoid tissue (Peyer patches) of the bowel. In approximately 2% to 8% of cases, there is a definite lead point, such as a Meckel diverticulum, intestinal polyps, enteric duplications, ectopic or nodular pancreas, or lymphoma. Patients who have Henoch-Schönlein purpura, cystic fibrosis (CF), leukemia, abdominal trauma, or hemophilia may have lead points due to hemorrhage, localized swelling, or hypertrophied mucosal glands, which are seen in CF.

Presentation

The classic picture involves a previously healthy infant between the ages of 6 and 24 months who presents with a triad of brief, colicky, intermittent abdominal pain that causes flexion of the hips and knees; vomiting; and bloody stools or rectal bleed-ing. The abdominal pain is due to the peristaltic rushes against the mass. The pain resolves, and the child may appear completely normal. The abdominal examination likewise may reveal no abnormalities. After multiple episodes of pain, vomiting develops in 80% of cases. Initially, the vomitus may be clear, but it then becomes bilious and even may be feces-stained, as the obstruction ensues.

The initial bowel movement may be normal (usually formed by stool present in the rectum prior to the intussusception). As the mesentery of the invaginating bowel becomes compressed, it causes venous obstruction and intestinal mucosal ischemia, which lead to leakage of blood and mucus into the intestinal lumen. This material causes the bright or dark red, bloody, "currant jelly" stools. It takes several hours for these stools to develop, making them a relatively late sign of intussus-ception. Clinicians should realize that some children who experience intussusception may pass no stool at all in the initial stages of their illness.

The physical examination initially may reveal a benign abdomen, with abdomi-nal tenderness developing later over the site of intussusception. A sausage-shaped mass in the area of the right upper or middle abdomen may be palpated in as many as 95% of patients, but the absence of a mass does not mean intussusception is not present. Abdominal distension is a later sign that develops as obstruction occurs. The rectal examination may reveal blood, a mass, or an empty rectal ampulla.

The presentation may not always be typical. Altered states of consciousness, apa-thy, and lethargy (which were prominent in this child) may be the only initial signs. The lethargy is thought to be due to endogenous opioids that are released follow-ing bowel ischemia. The mental status changes can be so pronounced that they sug-gest meningitis. It is not unusual for a patient who ultimately is diagnosed as hav-ing intussusception already to have undergone lumbar puncture. Patients also may develop high fever. The diagnosis is difficult to make unless the physician keeps intus-susception in mind.

Evaluation and Treatment

A plain radiograph of the abdomen may reveal signs of obstruction, such as distended loops of bowel and air-fluid levels. A "mass effect" or nonspecific intestinal gas pattern also may be seen. Radiologic signs of obstruction, however, are more likely to occur later in the course of the illness. Intussusception should not be ruled out if the initial radiograph is normal.

The key to diagnosis and a primary step in managing the patient who has intussusception is contrast enema. Contrast materials include barium, water-soluble contrast such as Gastrografin®, and air. On barium enema, the intussusception typically will have a "coiled spring" appearance. An intravenous line and nasogastric tube should be inserted for decompression before obtaining the contrast enema, and the operating room should be prepared for emergency surgery. Whenever the patient's condition suggests the possibility of an operation, consultation with a surgical colleague early in the course will provide diagnostic help and facilitate preparation for surgery.

Because of its better safety record and efficacy, air is the currently preferred contrast medium for reduction of intussusception, although barium and water-soluble contrast have been used. The only absolute contraindications to pressure reduction are peritoneal signs of inflammation, free air in the abdomen, and a clinical picture of toxicity. Intestinal obstruction is a relative contraindication.

Reduction by radiographic contrast is achieved in 85% of the cases. If reduction is unsuccessful, surgical correction is performed. Recurrence rates are similar with hydrostatic reduction and surgical reduction (5% and 3%, respectively).

This patient had the unusual complication of hypertension, having preoperative blood pressures in the range of 130 to 150 mm Hg systolic and 80 to 110 mm Hg diastolic and no difference between upper and lower extremities. There have been fewer than five reported cases of intussusception associated with transient hypertension. In all cases, the hypertension resolved within a few days postoperatively, as it did in this child. She was discharged from the hospital on the seventh postoperative day.

Differential Diagnosis

The differential diagnosis of intussusception includes gastroenteritis because the child usually presents with vomiting and colicky pain. A major difference between the two conditions is that the abdominal pain of intussusception is more likely to be intermittent. Any patient who has signs and symptoms of intestinal obstruction, intermittent colicky pain, currant jelly or guaiac-positive stools, or a sausage-shaped abdominal mass should undergo a radiographic contrast enema.

Also included in the differential diagnosis of abdominal distress and hypertension are pheochromocytoma, neuroblastoma, and Henoch-Schönlein purpura.

The possibility of ingestion of a toxic substance should be considered in any child who exhibits lethargy and vomiting. Alcohol, barbiturates, benzodiazepines, and opiates must be considered. If hypertension also is present, potential causative substances are cocaine, amphetamines, ephedrine and pseudoephedrine, phencyclidine, and antihistamines. Findings on physical examination and laboratory tests will allow the clinician to identify or rule out specific substances.

One case of cocaine-induced intussusception has been reported. Cocaine colitis results in hemorrhagic diarrhea, abdominal distension, and vomiting. Cocaine-induced vascular injury causes mucosal inflammation, ischemia, and bleeding, which could create a lead point for intussusception.

Central nervous system disorders also must be considered. Increased intracranial pressure usually presents with headache, vomiting, and papilledema, with lethargy occurring later.

Prior to the change in this patient's clinical picture, these additional conditions were considered. Urine toxicology, abdominal ultrasonography, lumbar puncture, and computed tomography of the head were performed, and all results were normal.

Lesson for the Clinician
This case is of special interest because abdominal pain was not a prominent feature of the clinical course, as it usually is in intussusception. It reminds us that the combination of intestinal signs and lethargy may be caused by intussusception.

Patricia D. Morgan-Glenn, MD, New Jersey Medical School/
St. Michael's Medical Center, Newark, NJ

Jaundice and Tea-colored Urine

PRESENTATION

A 14-year-old girl comes to the emergency department because of a 2-day history of jaundice and tea-colored urine. Two weeks earlier, she had experienced fatigue and malaise. Subsequently, she developed fever, sore throat, neck stiffness, and headache. There is no history of recent travel or contact with ill people. She has been taking amoxicillin for the past 2 days.

Physical examination reveals a temperature of 38.9°C (102°F) and a heart rate of 110 beats/min. The girl is pale and jaundiced, has obvious scleral icterus, but does not appear to be toxic. Her oropharynx appears normal, but several cervical lymph nodes are palpable. Abdominal examination reveals a tender spleen palpable 3 cm below the left costal margin; the liver is not palpable.

Results of laboratory investigation include a white blood cell count of 10.8 x 10⁹/L (10.8 x 10³/mcL) with 25% atypical lymphocytes. Hemoglobin is 1.04 mmol/L (6.7 g/dL), with a mean corpuscular volume of 91 fL, and the smear shows normochromic, normocytic red blood cells that demonstrate polychromasia. The unconjugated bilirubin level is 59 mcmol/L (3.5 mg/dL); results of other liver function tests are within normal limits. Urinalysis reveals the presence of hemoglobin and urobilinogen. The result of a direct antiglobulin (Coombs) test is positive, and cold agglutinins are present. A further test confirms the underlying diagnosis.

What is your differential diagnosis at this point?
Are there any elements of history or physical examination that would help you?
What additional diagnostic studies would you like performed?

DISCUSSION

Diagnosis

Studies of the heterophile antibody and Epstein-Barr virus (EBV) - specific antibodies were positive, confirming the diagnosis of infectious mononucleosis (IM). Clinical IM is caused by EBV in 90% of cases. Although malaise, fever, lymphadenopathy, splenomegaly, and exudative pharyngitis are the classic findings in an adolescent who has IM, jaundice occurs in 5% to 10% of patients. The jaundice usually is caused by a mild hepatitis that resolves without treatment and is associated with elevation of serum transaminase levels. In this case, the jaundice was not associated with hepatomegaly or laboratory evidence of hepatitis. These findings, combined with pallor, splenomegaly, and dark urine, suggested a hemolytic process.

Autoimmune hemolytic anemia is a rare but important complication of IM. The estimated prevalence is 3% to 5%. The hemolysis results from production of anti-red cell antibodies, usually of the anti-i system, but not exclusively. Also, up to 50% of patients who have IM develop cold agglutinins of anti-i specificity, but not all patients who have this finding develop hemolysis. It is not known why only some patients are afflicted. The phenomenon of hemolysis occurs 1 to 2 weeks into the illness and resolves spontaneously approximately 1 month later. The anemia is usually mild, but some patients experience a life-threatening reduction in hemoglobin levels that requires treatment.

Evaluation

When investigating anemia of acute onset, it is essential to proceed in an organized manner and to order the appropriate investigations, especially if transfusion is being considered. Examination of the blood smear and urinalysis is useful in focusing the differential diagnosis. In this case, the normocytic, normochromic nature of the red blood cells, the presence of polychromasia, and the presence of hemoglobin and urobilinogen in the urine strengthened the case for a hemolytic process.

Reticulocyte count and haptoglobin level should be measured as indicators of hemolysis. Unconjugated bilirubin level and direct Coombs test should be included in the evaluation.

A positive direct antiglobulin test indicates that the hemolytic process is immune-mediated. The immune hemolytic anemias are either alloimmune (such as hemolytic disease of the newborn) or autoimmune, often associated with infections (as in this case), drugs, connective tissue disorders, or oncologic conditions.

Treatment

Most cases of acute hemolytic anemia in IM are self-resolving and require no treatment. Occasionally, patients who are hemodynamically unstable require intervention. There are anecdotal reports that therapy with steroids (prednisone 1 to 2 mg/kg for 1 week) has improved symptoms significantly, but no controlled trials have confirmed this finding. It should be mentioned that transfused red blood cells are destroyed rapidly in autoimmune hemolytic anemia, so transfusion is not recommended.

Sharon Bates, MD, Jeremy Friedman, MB, The Hospital for Sick Children, Toronto, Ontario, Canada

Jaundice and Tea-colored Urine

PRESENTATION

A 6-year-old Chinese boy is brought to the emergency department with a 2-day history of jaundice and tea-colored urine. He has experienced lethargy and anorexia for several days preceding this visit. There is no history of recent travel, fever, or infections. He is not taking any medications and is otherwise well. There is no family history of jaundice or anemia. He had been born at 35 weeks' gestation and received treatment for neonatal jaundice.

On physical examination, the boy appears pale but not distressed or toxic. He has mild scleral icterus. No lymphadenopathy or hepatosplenomegaly is noted, and no rashes are present. He has a tachycardia with a soft ejection systolic flow murmur. Laboratory evaluation reveals a hemoglobin of 0.85 mmol/L (5.5 g/dL) with normal white blood cells and platelets. The reticulocyte count is 20%, and a blood smear shows normochromic, normocytic red cells, with anisocytosis, poikilocytosis, and occasional bite cells. His unconjugated bilirubin is 30 mcmol/L (1.8 mg/dL), and results of liver function tests are normal. The plasma haptoglobin is significantly decreased, and the direct antiglobulin (Coombs) test is negative. His urine is positive for both hemoglobin and urobilinogen. One additional test confirms the diagnosis.

What is your differential diagnosis at this point?
Are there any elements of history or physical examination that would help you?
What additional diagnostic studies would you like performed?

DISCUSSION

Diagnosis

The hemolysis experienced by this child was caused by an intrinsic erythrocyte defect, which was proven when the glucose-6-phosphate dehydrogenase (G6PD) quantitative assay was found to be 1.6% of normal.

G6PD is the most common metabolic disease of red blood cells and is estimated to affect 130 million people worldwide. Because synthesis of red blood cell G6PD is determined by genes borne on the X chromosome, diseases involving this enzyme occur more frequently in males. It is most common in Mediterranean, African, and Asian ethnic groups. G6PD is estimated to affect 10% to 15% of African-Americans. The majority of patients are asymptomatic until presented with an oxidative stress that precipitates a crisis. However, patients experiencing a continuous, low-grade hemolysis have been described.

G6PD is an enzyme in the pentose phosphate pathway required to reduce nicotinamide adenine dinucleotide phosphate (NADPH). This compound is essential for the production for glutathione, the most important cellular agent protecting against oxidative damage.

Presentation

The classic manifestation of G6PD deficiency is an acute hemolytic crisis. These crises are triggered by exposure to a substance that has oxidant properties. Such triggers include mothballs (naphthalene), fava beans, infections, and drugs (eg, antimalarials, sulfonamides, nitrofurans, vitamin K, aspirin). After 1 or 2 days, the patient experiences the acute onset of intravascular hemolysis, manifested first by lethargy or irritability, and followed by the subsequent development of jaundice, pallor, and tea-colored urine. Common symptoms and signs include fever, nausea, and abdominal or back pain; hepatosplenomegaly frequently occurs. The hemoglobin level is low, with bite cells and Heinz bodies (denatured hemoglobin as a result of the oxidative damage) sometimes present on the peripheral blood film. The haptoglobin level also is low, and both hemoglobinemia and hemoglobinuria occur, which demonstrates the intravascular nature of the hemolysis. The crisis usually is self-limiting and requires no treatment. The hemolysis preferentially affects the oldest red blood cells that have the least G6PD activity; once the bone marrow releases younger cells with relatively more G6PD, the crisis aborts.

An interesting finding is that only 25% of patients who have G6PD experience a hemolytic crisis after ingesting fava beans. Those affected generally have the G6PD Mediterranean variant (G6PD B-) and are usually Italian, French, or Chinese. African-American patients, who have a different genotype (G6PD A-), rarely are affected by favism.

Neonatal jaundice and chronic nonspherocytic hemolytic anemia are other less common presentations of this deficiency. Neonatal jaundice is more common in the G6PD B- (Mediterranean) variant and usually develops on the second day of life. Often there is no exposure to an offending agent. Chronic nonspherocytic hemolytic anemia occurs chiefly in northern European males.

Evaluation

The diagnosis of G6PD deficiency usually is obvious if there is an appropriate history. A negative direct Coombs test will rule out an immune cause for the hemolysis. The diagnosis is confirmed by a quantitative assay for G6PD activity. This determination often must be repeated several months after the acute episode because the increased number of immature red blood cells during the crisis may elevate the G6PD activity falsely. By direct measurement, enzyme activity in affected persons is 10% of normal or less.

Lesson for the Clinician

In this case, the diagnosis was not immediately obvious because the family denied any exposure to inciting agents. The ingestion of fava beans 2 days before the symptoms occurred became evident only when a sample of the beans was shown to the family, who knew the bean only by its Chinese name. Acute hemolytic crises can be prevented with appropriate education. The importance of visually demonstrating those items to avoid cannot be underestimated.

Sharon Bates, MD, Jeremy Friedman, MB, The Hospital for Sick Children, Toronto, Ontario, Canada

Scrotal Pain Following Trauma

PRESENTATION

A 12-year-old boy is seen several hours after the onset of rather severe scrotal discomfort. The pain began shortly after the gym class in which an errant basketball pass struck him squarely in the scrotal area. He is in obvious pain, complains of nausea, and vomited on the car ride to your office.

On physical examination, there is swelling and erythema of the left hemiscrotum, and any movement or palpation of the left testis causes great pain; gentle elevation of the testis brings no pain relief. The testis is of firm consistency and quite tense. A cremasteric reflex cannot be elicited on the left side.

What is your differential diagnosis at this point?
Are there any elements of history or physical examination that would help you?
What additional diagnostic studies would you like performed?

DISCUSSION

Diagnosis

Acute scrotal pain is the cardinal symptom of torsion of the testicle, and prompt diagnosis and appropriate surgical intervention is essential to prevent loss of the testis. Do not be misled by preceding trauma in considering this diagnosis. Scrotal trauma in some instances may play a role in the etiology of the torsion. A history of direct scrotal trauma certainly should not rule out this entity; rather, it should increase suspicion for torsion if scrotal pain persists after the trauma.

Differential Diagnosis

The differential diagnosis of the acute scrotum includes not only torsion of the testis and traumatic injuries, but also torsion of the appendix testis, incarcerated hernia, acute hydrocele, inguinal lymphadenitis, acute epididymitis, scrotal abscess, Henoch-Schönlein purpura, and leukemic infiltrate of the testis.

If the boy is sweaty and in acute pain, with nausea, vomiting, testicular retraction, and absent ipsilateral cremasteric reflex, acute testicular torsion must be the primary diagnostic consideration, and urgent surgical consultation is mandatory. However, if the acute tenderness can be localized to an exquisitely tender nodule near the upper pole of the testis, the remainder of the testis is relatively less tender, and the cremasteric reflex is present on that side, then testicular torsion is much less likely, and suspicion is high for a torsion of the appendix testis, a diagnosis that is usually manageable with analgesics. Diffuse scrotal pain radiating along the spermatic cord into the flank, with temperature elevation and often with associated symptoms of urgency, frequency of urination, and dysuria, strongly suggests the diagnosis of epididymitis, especially when the cremasteric reflex is present and the pain is relieved by lifting the scrotum.

Evaluation

When a definitive diagnosis cannot be discerned from the history and physical examination, as is the case in approximately one third of boys who have acute scrotal swelling and pain, the patient should be referred immediately to the urologist for diagnostic studies. Although the Doppler stethoscope is rapid, noninvasive, and usually readily available, the rate of error is significantly high. High-resolution ultrasonography accurately depicts the anatomy of the area but lacks the ability to detect blood flow, making it not particularly helpful in evaluating the acute scrotum. Nuclear imaging using technetium 99m pertechnetate is highly reliable in determining the presence or absence of blood flow and has been proven to be successful in the differential diagnosis of torsion versus nontorsion. This technique frequently has avoided unnecessary surgery, but it involves ionizing radiation and often is not available on a 24-hour basis.

The development of high-resolution color Doppler ultrasonography has afforded diagnostic information that previously was available only through surgical exploration. This technique combines the anatomic imaging of high-resolution ultrasonography with accurate imaging of intratesticular blood flow. It is noninvasive, does not involve ionizing radiation, and can be performed in far less time than a radionuclide scan. When available and when performed by an experienced examiner, this imaging method is the procedure of choice in evaluating the acutely painful scrotum of uncertain etiology.

Lesson for the Clinician

Early recognition of the signs and symptoms of testicular torsion, with appropriate prompt referral to the pediatric urologist for management, is mandatory and will help salvage a viable testis when at all possible.

John L. Green, MD, Rochester, NY

"My Throat is Closing Up"

PRESENTATION

A 17-year-old girl is seen in the emergency department because of dyspnea and the feeling that "my throat is closing up." She says that she is allergic to food coloring and that she ate flavored potato chips a few hours earlier. She self-diagnosed her food coloring allergy based on five episodes of similar symptoms over the past 2 months. She had been seen in different emergency departments, treated for anaphylaxis, and released. Before these episodes she had no known allergies. At her last visit, cetirizine and diphenhydramine had been prescribed as well as an epinephrine autoinjector. Skin testing is scheduled for the coming month.

Her respiratory rate is 28 breaths/min, pulse is 120 beats/min, and blood pressure is 108/60 mm Hg. Air entry is decreased, and wheezes are heard in all lung fields. Her face is red, but there is no urticaria. Oxygen saturation is 0.85 (85%). Because she improves only slightly with subcutaneous epinephrine, intravenous diphenhydramine and hydrocortisone, and aerosolized salbutamol, she is admitted to the hospital.

Additional history reveals a 2-month course of variable intermittent symptoms consisting of a "mushy" voice, a drooping left eye lid, generalized weakness, and one episode of diplopia. On re-examination she is noted to have facial weakness, left ptosis, and generalized muscle weakness that worsens with repetitive movements. A pharmacologic test confirms the diagnosis.

What is your differential diagnosis at this point?
Are there any elements of history or physical examination that would help you?
What additional diagnostic studies would you like performed?

DISCUSSION

Diagnosis

An edrophonium (Tensilon) test was positive and confirmed the diagnosis of myasthenia gravis. The acute respiratory symptoms that prompted this patient to seek care were due to aspiration episodes caused by weakness of her pharyngeal muscles. Allergy skin testing was negative.

In the pediatric population, myasthenia gravis is a condition that presents most commonly in late adolescence. Neonates born to mothers who have myasthenia gravis also may manifest the disorder.

Presentation

The characteristic features of myasthenia gravis beyond the newborn period are weakness, diplopia, and ptosis. The weakness characteristically worsens with repetitive activity. Fifteen percent of patients will have only ocular manifestations without other muscle weakness. Because symptoms develop insidiously, patients often will attribute their complaints erroneously to other causes, as with this patient, who blamed her respiratory symptoms on food allergy. Clinical effects result from an autoimmune depletion of nicotinic acetylcholine receptors at the muscle motor endplate. The trigger for the autoimmune event is unknown and remains the subject of intense investigation.

Evaluation

Diagnosis is made by a positive edrophonium test. The physician has the patient perform a repetitive activity until fatigued and then injects first a test dose and finally a full dose of edrophonium while observing for a return of muscle strength. Ideally, the test should be performed in double-blind fashion and videotaped to avoid a placebo effect and to provide an objective record of the results. Edrophonium, an anticholinesterase that has an onset of action of 30 seconds and a duration of action of about 5 minutes, inhibits the normal destruction of acetylcholine at the motor endplate, making more acetylcholine available to stimulate the reduced number of receptors and improve motor strength. Electromyographic studies often help in confirming the diagnosis, especially if results of edrophonium testing are equivocal.

Approximately 12% of patients who have myasthenia gravis have an associated thymoma, which is a locally invasive tumor that requires complete excision. Computed tomography or magnetic resonance imaging of the anterior mediastinum is imperative when evaluating a patient for myasthenia gravis to identify a thymoma.

Treatment

Several strategies are used to treat myasthenia gravis. The first approach is to improve muscle strength directly, which may be accomplished with a long-acting anticholinesterase, pyridostigmine. Pyridostigmine is administered orally and results in fair improvement in muscle strength, but effectiveness declines over months.

The second strategy involves reducing the antibody load, which allows for nicotinic receptor repopulation and return of muscle strength. Antibodies may be reduced by plasma exchange transfusion (plasmapheresis) or administration of intravenous immune globulin. Both methods improve symptoms rapidly, but improvement is short-lived, lasting a few months at best. Long-term remission usually is achieved by thymectomy followed by immunosuppressive therapy that results in a sustained reduction of antibody.

Immunosuppressants employed to treat myasthenia gravis include corticosteroids, azathioprine, and cyclosporine. Steroids are the most effective, but they are associated with the most adverse effects and may cause a transient worsening of symptoms in almost 50% of treated patients.

Any respiratory infection in a patient who has myasthenia gravis and is not in remission should be managed as a life-threatening emergency. Increased use of respiratory muscles because of tachypnea and coughing may lead to respiratory muscle fatigue and respiratory failure in hours. For these patients, admission to an intensive care unit should be considered and prompt consultation with a neurologist obtained.

Prognosis

The current prognosis for patients who have myasthenia gravis is encouraging. Following thymectomy, most patients are maintained free of symptoms on single-agent immunosuppressive therapy. Once the patient is in remission, pyridostigmine may be tapered and, in most cases, discontinued.

Barry A. Love, MD, Montreal Children's Hospital, Montreal, Quebec, Canada

Bilious Vomiting and Distended Abdomen in a Neonate

PRESENTATION

A 3,884 g boy is born to a healthy 30-year-old woman. The mother has negative serology for syphilis and is hepatitis B antigen-negative. She has blood type O+; the baby's type is A+, and he has a positive direct Coombs test.

Initial physical examination reveals a vigorous baby who has a grade I/VI systolic murmur along the left sternal border; his blood pressure is 64/39 mm Hg. The remainder of the examination is normal. At 1 day of age, the murmur is no longer audible and the baby is doing well.

On the second day of life, the baby, who has been drinking a cow milk formula well, vomits several times, bringing up a bilious fluid. His abdomen becomes distended, and his bowel sounds are hypoactive. Nursing notes reveal only a "smear of meconium" since birth.

Intravenous fluids are started, a nasogastric tube is passed, and 6 mL of green fluid are aspirated from the baby's stomach. Complete blood count, serum electrolyte levels, blood urea nitrogen, serum creatinine, and blood glucose level are normal. The total bilirubin is 81.6 mcmol/L (4.8 mg/dL). A plain abdominal radiograph reveals a large amount of gas in dilated loops of bowel and the stomach; no gas is in the rectum. An additional study reveals the cause of the baby's distress.

What is your differential diagnosis at this point?
Are there any elements of history or physical examination that would help you?
What additional diagnostic studies would you like performed?

DISCUSSION

Diagnosis

The baby had an "unprepped" barium enema that showed a narrow rectal segment with dilatation of the segment proximal to the narrow area, characteristic of Hirschsprung disease. A loop sigmoid colostomy relieved this obstruction.

Hirschsprung disease (congenital aganglionic megacolon) is a motility disorder of the bowel that results from an absence of parasympathetic ganglion cells in part of the colon. Aganglionosis is thought to be due to the arrest of the caudal migration of cells from the neural crest that are destined to develop into the gut's intramural plexuses. The narrowed aganglionic segment extends from the internal anal sphincter proximally for a variable distance, with the defect being in the sigmoid colon 85% of the time. On rare occasions, the entire colon or even the entire intestine may be involved.

Hirschsprung disease occurs in 1 in 5,000 births, is multifactorial in origin, and has a 4:1 male predominance, except in long-segment aganglionosis, which is twice as common in females. It has been associated with other congenital conditions and various syndromes, including Down syndrome, Waardenburg syndrome, and myelomeningocele. It rarely is seen in preterm infants. Although the majority of patients are diagnosed in the first month of life, Hirschsprung disease is detected later in life in some children, who will have a long-standing history of incompletely passing stool. In contrast to the pattern seen in the more common functional constipation, patients who have Hirschsprung disease almost never demonstrate encopresis or pass huge bowel movements.

Presentation

The most common sign of Hirschsprung disease is constipation. Any infant who fails to pass meconium in the first 48 hours of life should be suspected of having this condition. Other signs include abdominal distention and pain, the vomiting of bile, refusal to eat, and growth failure. When dealing with an infant who has such a clinical picture, the clinician also must consider cystic fibrosis with meconium ileus, infection, hypothyroidism, volvulus, imperforate anus, intestinal atresia, malrotation, and other malformations of the gut.

On rectal examination, no stool is found in the rectal ampulla, which is a characteristic of Hirschsprung disease. Digital examination, rectal tube insertion, or enema administration may result in the passage of retained fecal material with apparent relief of symptoms.

Evaluation

A plain abdominal radiograph often demonstrates dilatation of the colon proximal to the aganglionic segment, with no gas or stool evident in the rectum. Anorectal manometry may help in the diagnosis. Failure of reflex relaxation of the internal sphincter in response to rectal distension distinguishes Hirschsprung disease from chronic constipation in early infancy.

An unprepped barium enema reveals the characteristic narrowing of the distal rectal or rectosigmoid segment below a dilated proximal segment of bowel. In doubtful cases, mucosal suction biopsy is the appropriate initial procedure, but absence of ganglion cells does not establish the diagnosis, and a full-thickness biopsy of the rectum then is required.

Treatment

Treatment of Hirschsprung disease involves resection of the aganglionic bowel and reanastomosis of the proximal normal bowel to the normal anal canal. Colostomy usually is performed first, followed by a pull-through procedure when the infant reaches 6 months of age or 8.1 kg; this varies with surgical judgment. Some physicians believe that patients diagnosed at 10 months of age or older who have not had complications are candidates for the pull-through procedure without requiring a prior fecal diversion procedure.

The most feared complication of both delayed diagnosis and surgery is enterocolitis, which is the most frequent cause of death in Hirschsprung disease.

Vincent J. Menna, MD, University of Pennsylvania Health System,
Doylestown, PA

Decreased Growth Rate and Slightly Thickened Wrists in an Infant

PRESENTATION

A 9-month-old African-American boy is brought to you in early April for a health supervision visit. Born after an uncomplicated pregnancy and delivery, he has been healthy at all previous visits and was noted to have normal growth and development when last seen at 6 months of age.

At this visit, the baby's length has dropped from the 50th to the 5th percentile, while his weight and head circumference remain at the 50th. He is breastfed and eats small amounts of chopped fruits and vegetables. His parents give him no foods that contain artificial ingredients, and he receives no supplemental vitamins. The baby's stools are normal in pattern and consistency, and he has had no recent illnesses. His mother eats a well-balanced diet but does not like milk.

On physical examination, the infant is noted to have slightly thickened wrists. Otherwise, results of his examination are unremarkable, including normal developmental and neurologic evaluations. Further testing with simple methods establishes the cause of his striking reduction in growth rate.

What is your differential diagnosis at this point?
Are there any elements of history or physical examination that would help you?
What additional diagnostic studies would you like performed?

DISCUSSION

Diagnosis

Because the history and physical findings in this child suggested rickets, radiographs of his wrists were taken and showed cupping and fraying of the distal radius and ulna bilaterally. His serum calcium level was 1.75 mmol/L (7.0 mg/dL) (normal, 2 to 2.6 mmol/L [8.0 to 10.5 mg/dL]), phosphorus level was 1.16 mmol/L (3.5 mg/dL) (normal, 1.25 to 2.05 mmol/L [3.8 to 6.2 mg/dL]), and alkaline phosphatase level was 930 U/L (normal, 150 to 400 U/L). The serum 25-hydroxyvitamin D level was 5 ng/mL (normal, 9 to 52 ng/mL). Results of renal function tests were normal. The diagnosis of rickets was confirmed by characteristic changes on radiographs of the wrists, low serum calcium and phosphorus levels, a markedly elevated serum alkaline phosphatase level, and a low serum level of 25-hydroxyvitamin D. This child's condition was caused by insufficient vitamin D, which, in turn, was due to a combination of seemingly innocent factors: exclusive breastfeeding, dark skin, little exposure to sun, and no vitamin supplementation.

Vitamin D plays a key role in the homeostasis of serum calcium and phosphorus and in bone mineralization. Its bioavailability depends on absorption from the intestine as well as conversion of a provitamin in the skin by ultraviolet light. It then is changed into its active form in the liver and kidney.

Active vitamin D has three primary sites of action: intestine, kidney, and bone. It increases absorption of calcium and phosphate from the intestine and enhances reabsorption of phosphate in the renal tubules. In addition, vitamin D acts directly on bone, promoting breakdown of older bone and mineralization of new bone. Vitamin D, parathyroid hormone, and calcitonin act together to regulate body fluid levels of calcium and phosphate and to control bone formation.

Inadequate vitamin D in children can lead to a number of problems, including rickets, poor growth, and even hypocalcemic tetany. The term rickets refers to the clinical manifestations of abnormal mineralization of bone. In children, the sequelae are most notable in growing bone, particularly in the growth plates, where disorganized, nonmineralized cartilage appears. Rickets occurs when, in the face of low serum vitamin D, the body attempts to maintain a normal serum calcium level to maintain vital cell function.

When vitamin D levels drop, calcium absorption from the intestine is reduced. A slightly lowered serum calcium level stimulates increased parathyroid hormone secretion, which leads to mobilization of calcium and phosphorus from the bone. The serum calcium level is maintained relatively well, but the serum phosphorus level drops because of reduced reabsorption within the kidney, and serum alkaline phosphatase levels increase due to vigorous osteoblastic activity. Changes in the bones occur, particularly in fast-growing bones such as the skull, extremities, and rib cage.

Presentation

Patients who have rickets present in a number of ways, depending on the severity and duration of illness as well as the age of the child. They may have growth failure, weakness, lethargy, tetany, and seizures due to hypocalcemia as well as the characteristic bony deformities. Physical examination of the head (particularly in infants) may reveal a "bossing" deformity and a "ping-pong ball" tactile sensation when the examiner presses on the occiput or posterior parietal bones (craniotabes). Examination of the chest may reveal palpably enlarged costochondral junctions called the rachitic rosary. An indentation sometimes is found at the insertion of the diaphragm and is caused by softened lower ribs; this finding is known as Harrison groove. The wrists and ankles may be thickened due to epiphyseal enlargement. In toddlers, pressure from ambulation can cause bowing of the legs and an accentuated lumbar lordosis.

Evaluation

Laboratory and radiographic findings are helpful in making the diagnosis. Serum levels of phosphorus and calcium can be normal, but commonly are deceased, depending on the parathyroid hormone response and mobilization from the bone. A marked elevation of alkaline phosphatase occurs in all patients by the time clinical signs are apparent. A low, sometimes undetectable level of serum 25-hydroxyvitamin D confirms the diagnosis. Radiographic changes can be seen most easily in areas of active growth, such as the costochondral junctions, distal femur, proximal and distal ends of the tibia, and wrist. Early in the course of the disease, axial widening and decreased mineralization appear at the growth plates. As the disorganized cartilage mass increases, widening, cupping (concave deformity), and fraying of the metaphysis may become evident. In severe disease, widespread demineralization of the bones (osteopenia) and fractures can occur.

Risk Factors

Infants at increased risk of developing vitamin D-deficient rickets include those experiencing limited sun exposure who have inadequate amounts of vitamin D in their diets. Generally, just a short exposure to the sun can raise vitamin D levels significantly. However, melanin in the skin, glass windows, clothing, and sunscreen all will decrease the amount of ultraviolet light that is absorbed, resulting in reduced production of the vitamin. Thus, rickets may occur in dark-skinned infants during winter months as well as in children who live in sunnier climates but are swaddled in clothing or kept indoors.

Only a limited number of foods contain vitamin D, including fatty fish and fish oils, eggs, and liver. Currently, fortified cow milk and infant formulas provide the primary sources of dietary vitamin D in the United States. In fact, vitamin D-deficient rickets has occurred much less commonly in this country since routine fortification of milk was instituted. Human milk, on the other hand, contains variable amounts of vitamin D, depending in part on maternal milk consumption and sun exposure. In some cases, human milk may not be an adequate source of vitamin D after the first few months.

Treatment

Treatment of rickets consists of oral vitamin D therapy. Initially, calcium also should be administered orally to avoid transient hypocalcemia, which sometimes can accompany abrupt initial bone remineralization ("hungry bone" syndrome). Both a single large dose of vitamin D and repeated smaller doses over several months have been used successfully to heal the rachitic process in 2 to 3 months. One standard regimen is the administration of 1,000 to 2,000 U of vitamin D each day for 6 weeks. Blood levels of calcium, phosphorus, and alkaline phosphatase should be monitored closely during the initial phases of treatment. In response to therapy, the alkaline phosphatase level should begin to normalize within 4 weeks, although it may take several months to return fully to normal. Serial wrist radiographs show progressive improvement of bone mineralization and organization over several months, but are not necessary to document the response to therapy. Lack of response to therapy raises issues of compliance as well as the possibility that the rickets may have an etiology other than vitamin D deficiency.

Lesson for the Clinician

Although healthy children may cross growth percentiles gradually during infancy, based on their genetically determined growth patterns, rickets should be suspected in those who have unusually poor growth and are at risk for vitamin D deficiency. To prevent rickets, pediatricians must explore each patient's risk factors by taking a history about sun exposure and dietary sources of vitamin D. These issues should be discussed with the family early in infancy because rickets often develops over many months during the first year of life. Pediatricians should consider early vitamin D supplementation for children identified to be at increased risk to avoid this preventable disease.

Eve R. Colson, MD, University of Connecticut School of Medicine,
Farmington, CT; Neil Herendeen, MD, Peter Szilagyi, MD,
University of Rochester School of Medicine and Dentistry, Rochester, NY

Hypoxia and Paroxysmal Cough

PRESENTATION

A 5-month-old girl is admitted to the pediatric intensive care unit in January because of profound hypoxia. She has had a paroxysmal cough for 2 months and has lost 0.45 kg in the past month. At 1 month of age she had been hospitalized because of bloody stools, which resolved on a lactose-free, casein hydrolysate formula. She has had diaper dermatitis several times. The infant is exposed to cigarette smoke at home.

Physical examination reveals a distressed, thin infant whose weight is in the 5th percentile and head circumference in the 50th; both were above the 50th percentile at birth. She is breathing at 70 to 80 breaths/min with subcostal and intercostal retractions; rales are heard. Her oxygen saturation by pulse oximetry is 0.40 (40%), and it improves with oxygen administration. The baby's spleen is palpable 1 cm below the left subcostal margin.

Chest radiography reveals hyperinflation, multifocal parenchymal densities consistent with atelectasis or pneumonia, and diffuse perihilar densities. Results of echocardiography are normal. Her white blood cell count is 15.7×10^9/L (15.7×10^3/mcL), with 75% segmented neutrophils and 11% lymphocytes. Immunofluorescence tests for pertussis, Chlamydia, and viruses (respiratory syncytial, parainfluenza, influenza, and adenovirus) are negative, as are cultures of blood and tracheal aspirate. Sweat chloride and alpha-1 antitrypsin levels are normal. A Mycoplasma immunoglobulin M (IgM) titer is positive.

The baby requires ongoing mechanical ventilation because of poor oxygenation and does not improve on antibiotic and bronchodilator therapy. Her temperature fluctuates between $37°C$ and $39°C$ ($98.6°F$ and $102.2°F$). She develops rotavirus gastroenteritis, oral thrush, and diaper dermatitis.

What is your differential diagnosis at this point?
Are there any elements of history or physical examination that would help you?
What additional diagnostic studies would you like performed?

DISCUSSION

Diagnosis

After several weeks of hospitalization, human immunodeficiency virus (HIV) antibody testing done by enzyme-linked immunosorbent assay (ELISA) was positive; the result was confirmed by the Western blot test.

These screening tests cannot establish the diagnosis of HIV infection in infants younger than 15 months because the presence of antibody simply may reflect passive transfer of maternal antibody. Therefore, definitive HIV polymerase chain reaction and p24 antigen (an HIV core antigen) testing were performed and also were positive. The infant's white blood cell count was 8.9×10^9/L (8.9×10^3/mcL) with 7% lymphocytes. The absolute number of CD4 lymphocytes was 45/mL (normal value for this age, 1,750 cells/mL).

Bronchoalveolar lavage culture was positive for *Mycoplasma hominis* and respiratory syncytial virus, but did not reveal *Pneumocystis carinii*, fungi, or acid-fast bacilli. Developmental assessment placed the child within the range of a 1- to 3-week-old infant. A computed tomographic scan of her brain showed bilateral cerebral hemispheric atrophy with ventriculomegaly. Prompt treatment with dual-drug antiretroviral therapy was instituted.

HIV infection has become the leading cause of death in men and the fourth leading cause of death in women in the 25- to 44-year-old age group. HIV infection in infants is acquired primarily by perinatal transmission from infected mothers. Diagnosis of HIV infection in the pregnant mother should lead to her treatment with zidovudine after the third trimester and delivery and treatment of the infant for the first 6 weeks of life. This intervention requires coordination between pediatrician and obstetrician, but it can reduce the risk of infection in the baby from approximately 26% to 8%. Detection before birth also allows prohibition of breastfeeding, which can lead to infection of the infant.

Presentation

The Centers for Disease Control and Prevention (CDC) published a new classification system for HIV infection in children in 1994. The average incubation period for perinatal acquired immunodeficiency syndrome (AIDS) is 12 months. There are two distinct patterns of disease. The first presents early, between 4 and 8 months of age, with a wasting syndrome, encephalopathy, and *Pneumocystis carinii* pneumonia (PCP). The other is a later illness, with lymphoid interstitial pneumonitis, hepatosplenomegaly, lymphadenopathy, and parotid gland enlargement. Recurrent bacterial infections are common in both disease patterns.

Problems with growth and development may be the initial signs of HIV infection in infants, and the general pediatrician may be the first to recognize them. Failure to thrive must be recognized early so that adequate nutritional support can be provided. HIV encephalopathy may manifest as motor, speech, and cognitive delays or as regression in already attained developmental milestones. A computed tomographic scan of the head may show cerebral atrophy and calcifications in the basal ganglia.

Pulmonary disease is an important aspect of HIV infection. PCP is a leading cause of mortality in children who have AIDS and is characterized by fever, cough, dyspnea, hypoxia, increased arterial-to-alveolar gradient, and radiographic findings of diffuse interstitial changes, air space filling, and air bronchograms. The diagnosis is established by detecting the organism in specimens obtained by bronchoalveolar lavage, open lung biopsy, or tracheal suction. The incidence of PCP among infants has not declined over the years, emphasizing the importance of diagnosing HIV infection early and providing early prophylaxis for this fatal but preventable disease.

Lymphoid interstitial pneumonitis is a slowly progressive pulmonary disease that causes cough, tachypnea, wheezing, hypoxemia, generalized lymphadenopathy, salivary gland enlargement, and digital clubbing (in advanced disease). Children infected with HIV also are prone to recurrent pneumonia.

Differential Diagnosis

Persistent or recurrent cough of more than 3 weeks' duration occurs commonly in children. The most likely causes are recurrent viral upper respiratory tract infections and reactive airway disease. Other etiologies include allergies, sinusitis, irritation (as from smoke), foreign body aspiration, chlamydial infections, pertussis, tuberculosis, cystic fibrosis, immotile cilia syndrome, congenital abnormalities, and immunodeficiency.

This case demonstrates many aspects of perinatal HIV infection, including failure to thrive, encephalopathy, pulmonary disease, and dermatitis. Children also can present with cardiac problems, hematologic abnormalities, tumors, chronic diarrhea, persistent fever, and recurrent infections caused by bacteria, viruses, or fungi.

Lesson for the Clinician

Early recognition of HIV infection in infants is important for several reasons. Detection will allow the institution of antiretroviral drug therapy that may delay disease progression as well as timely prophylaxis for PCP, which is recommended for babies 1 to 4 months old whose mothers are HIV-positive and babies 1 to 12 months old who are proven or suspected to be HIV-positive. (In older children, prophylaxis is started when the CD4 lymphocyte count drops below certain levels.) Also, a multidisciplinary team approach for management of the child and support of the family is important and is best established as soon as possible. Detection of HIV in pregnant women is crucial so that prophylactic treatment can be used to provide infants a dramatically increased chance of escaping infection.

Meena Kalyanaraman, MD, Maria Patterson, MD, PhD, Michigan State University, East Lansing, MI

Poor Growth in an Adopted Child

PRESENTATION

A 6½-year-old Haitian-American girl is brought to the emergency department because of poor growth. She was born in Haiti and abandoned at a hospital, having severe diarrhea and dehydration when 6 months old. She was brought to the United States and adopted by her current parents at 11 months of age. At 21 months, she was growing poorly but was lost to follow-up for 2 years. When seen at 4 years, she was below the 5th percentile for height and weight, had a bone age of 2 years, and had normal thyroxine and thyroid-stimulating hormone levels. Again she was lost to follow-up. Apparently she has been otherwise healthy except for a mild learning disability and occasional diarrhea.

On physical examination, she is active, alert, and playful, but appears cachectic, having severe muscle wasting and a protuberant abdomen. Her height is 77 cm, weight is 7.9 kg, and head circumference is 44.5 cm; all measurements are well below the 5th percentile. Her skin is dry, and her liver edge is palpable 8 cm below the right costal margin.

Further history reveals that her current adoptive parents want to put her back up for adoption because she "eats like an animal" and exhibits bizarre behavior, such as going through trash for food, smearing feces, and drinking bubble bath. She is such a "disgrace" to the family that they make her eat in her room. The parents have two other biologic children who are well behaved and "normal."

An extensive evaluation reveals the following abnormal results: bone age of 2 years (more than 2 standard deviations below the mean), white blood cell count of 2.6×10^9/L (2.6×10^3/mcL), hematocrit of 0.31 (31%), elevated liver enzyme levels, and positive Mantoux test.

What is your differential diagnosis at this point?
Are there any elements of history or physical examination that would help you?
What additional diagnostic studies would you like performed?

DISCUSSION

Diagnosis

Failure to thrive (FTT) is defined as inadequate weight gain, as judged by standardized growth charts. Often, linear growth is poor and other signs of undernutrition are present. Some authors have suggested that the term "growth deficiency" is more appropriate because it is more general and does not imply any specific diagnosis. Whichever term is used, one useful definition of this condition states that the weight must be below the 5th percentile or the patient's growth line must decline across two or more major percentile lines. As always, a good history is essential for proper diagnosis and should cover perinatal events, illnesses, development, nutrition, behavior, and psychosocial factors. Having data on the growth patterns of the parents also is important.

Disease Classification

Traditionally, FTT is divided into organic and nonorganic types, although children who have this problem often suffer from multiple problems, some organic and some nonorganic, that work together to the child's detriment. For example, a chronic illness may make a child irritable and hard to deal with, adversely influencing the way the rest of the family relates to him or her. In this patient, as should be done for all children who are growing poorly, both types of etiologic factors were considered.

Nonorganic causes in which inadequate nutrition is the central feature constitute the vast majority of FTT cases. Therefore, a detailed history of eating habits, content of the diet, home situation, and child-parent interaction is essential. If specific problems cannot be identified, hospitalization may be necessary. While the child is in the hospital, the number of calories he or she consumes can be counted, and the child's eating habits as well as the interactions between child and parents can be observed by the doctors and nurses. Weights are obtained daily. If the patient gains weight in the hospital without difficulty, a social cause of the FTT is most likely. Clinicians must remember that children younger than 6 months of age will gain weight more quickly than older children; thus, an older child may need a longer period of observation.

Organic causes cover a wide spectrum of etiologies. Sometimes the causative mechanism is failure to ingest and retain enough calories, as in gastroesophageal reflux or cerebral palsy. In other patients there is a greatly increased caloric need, as in congenital heart disease, bronchopulmonary dysplasia, malignancy, hyperthyroidism, or infection. Still other causes of FTT result from the inability to use calories, as in gastrointestinal disorders (celiac disease, inflammatory bowel disease, parasitic infections, cystic fibrosis), endocrine disorders (diabetes mellitus, growth hormone deficiency), renal disorders (renal tubular acidosis), and metabolic disorders involving the absorption and breakdown of fats, proteins, and carbohydrates.

Evaluation
The variety of etiologies for FTT suggests why a "shotgun" evaluation is both futile and costly. A helpful general screening includes obtaining a complete blood count, urinalysis, blood urea nitrogen, and stool analysis for ova and parasites as well as reducing substances. A radiograph of the chest and sweat test also should be considered, but the decision to obtain any laboratory studies should be influenced by the specific features of the patient's situation. In this child, the evaluation focused on the gastrointestinal system because of the history of diarrhea and the findings of an enlarged liver.

Treatment
This patient eventually was diagnosed as having psychosocial dwarfism, a condition in which growth hormone production is impaired in response to stress. Her adoptive parents were shown to have neglected her. Her abnormal laboratory values were explained by caloric deprivation, which had caused the suppression of blood counts and fatty infiltration of the liver. After her hospitalization, the child was placed with a foster family, where she soon gained weight and grew nicely.

Lesson for the Clinician
This case reinforces the value of careful observation—often in the hospital—before launching an extensive laboratory investigation.

Holly Swanson, MD, Maine Medical Center, Portland, ME

Seizure in an Infant Who Has Gastroesophageal Reflux

PRESENTATION

The mother of a 2-month-old infant calls you after hours, concerned that her son might be having a seizure. You know her well because you have seen the child several times recently for feeding difficulties. Last week he was diagnosed at a tertiary care center as having gastroesophageal reflux and was placed on ranitidine and metoclopramide. The mother reports that he has been acting strangely for the past 30 minutes, with stiffening of all extremities, an unusual cry, and a lack of normal responsiveness. A nurse who is a neighbor corroborates the mother's story and believes that the child is having a seizure. She adds that the child's breathing is somewhat irregular and that he is pale, although he is not cyanotic. You advise the mother to call an ambulance to take him to the hospital.

On arrival at the emergency department, the infant is unresponsive, stiff, and pale. His heart rate is 210 beats/min, respirations are 32 breaths/min with grunting, and pulse oximetry is 0.88 (88%) in room air. His temperature and blood pressure are normal. He is given oxygen and intravenous diazepam, which causes a slight improvement in the tachycardia and rigidity. After another dose of diazepam, he is more relaxed and more responsive, and his cry sounds normal. A full evaluation for seizures is initiated.

What is your differential diagnosis at this point?
Are there any elements of history or physical examination that would help you?
What additional diagnostic studies would you like performed?

DISCUSSION

Diagnosis

Seizures in infants can present in unusual ways as neural pathways that are not complete at birth begin to mature. The consensus of the parents, nurses, and physicians who evaluated this child initially was that he was in the throes of status epilepticus. When the acute event was over, however, and a more complete history was obtained, it was revealed that the infant had demonstrated eye-crossing and tongue protrusion (initially thought to be tongue thrusting) during the episode as well as an agitated cry not usually noted during seizures. It was unclear whether he had been unresponsive, as would be expected during a seizure, or whether his rigidity had prevented him from responding to stimuli.

Results of subsequent electroencephalography (EEG) and computed tomographic (CT) scan of his head were normal, as was a full sepsis evaluation, including lumbar puncture, drug screen, and measurements of electrolytes, glucose, and ammonia. It was the consulting neurologist's opinion that the baby had not had a seizure because the EEG was completely normal less than 24 hours after the episode and because there were too many features of the episode not typical of a seizure.

The diagnosis of dystonic reaction to metoclopramide was made. The child's apparent clinical response to anticonvulsants was believed to be a coincidence, although it has been shown that diazepam—given in this case for seizure control—also can have a beneficial effect in treating dystonic reactions to drugs. (Current clinical practice favors lorazepam as the preferred benzodiazepine for seizure control.)

The antireflux medications were discontinued, and the infant recovered uneventfully without further episodes. Mechanical antireflux measures had been mentioned during the baby's initial evaluation but had not been stressed; the focus had been on drug therapy. When the mechanical measures were applied consistently, the child's spitting-up subsided considerably.

Although extrapyramidal reactions to drugs usually are associated with overdosage, several agents can cause adverse effects at therapeutic doses in children. These drugs include metoclopramide, phenothiazines, and other medications that have anticholinergic effects. Metoclopramide is one of the most common offenders. The overall incidence of extrapyramidal effects associated with this drug is 0.2%, but very old and very young patients are affected more commonly, with an incidence as high as 10%. These side effects usually occur within a few days after initiation of the medication, as in this case, and are more common at higher doses. The reactions usually are short-lived if the drug is discontinued promptly. Occasionally, delayed extrapyramidal effects may occur after a single overdose, and in some cases the cause may have been only a small dose, complicating the search for an etiology.

Treatment

Treatment of extrapyramidal side effects caused by metoclopramide is similar to that for phenothiazine-induced movement disorder and consists of intravenous or intramuscular administration of diphenhydramine or benztropine mesylate. In children, diphenhydramine usually is used. The dosage is 1 mg/kg initially, which may be repeated if there is no effect. Occasionally, doses up to 5 mg/kg are required. Although diphenhydramine is approved only for children weighing more than 10 kg, it probably is safe for smaller infants as well. However, supporting data are not available. Diphenhydramine is contraindicated in preterm infants and newborns because it may cause seizures. Benztropine is not approved for children younger than 3 years, and this agent has been noted to cause dystonic reactions. Close monitoring of these drug side effects is important during and for a few hours after treatment because dystonic reactions occasionally are accompanied by fluctuations in blood pressure and disturbances of cardiac rhythm.

Lesson for the Clinician

The dose of metoclopramide given to this infant for 5 days prior to the episode was at the high end of the normal range. The mother denied mismeasuring the medication or giving any extra doses. This response, therefore, fit the pattern of a typical adverse reaction to metoclopramide. The baby's symptoms did not recur after the initial event was completed, and he exhibited no arrhythmias or changes in blood pressure. In this case, the thinking of the physicians became less rigid around the same time that the patient did.

Christopher J. Stille, MD, Connecticut Children's Medical Center, Hartford, CT

Gradual Loss of Sight

PRESENTATION

An 11-year-old Asian girl comes to the emergency department because of visual loss. Two months ago she was seen at another hospital because of a painful stiff neck with worsening pain on rotation of her head to the left. Radiographs of her cervical spine were normal, and she was discharged with a diagnosis of muscle spasm, for which ibuprofen was recommended. Subsequently, she experienced gradual changes in her vision but did not mention the problem until several days ago, when she noticed that she no longer could read her homework because her vision was blurry.

Her history includes noncompliance in wearing glasses prescribed at age 5 years. The patient's mother feels that she has not gained weight properly, and friends have noticed that she seems apathetic.

This thin girl appears in no distress. Her temperature, pulse rate, blood pressure, and respiratory rate are normal. She is at Sexual Maturity Rating (Tanner) stage 1. Her pupils are equal, round, and reactive to light, and her extraocular movements are intact. She has incomplete convergence and a slight ptosis of her left eye. Her visual acuity is 20/80 in each eye, and there is a subtle visual field defect in the upper and nasal quadrants of both eyes. Her optic disc margins are indistinct. The remainder of her cranial nerve functions are normal. She has normal muscle tone and symmetric, 2+ deep tendon reflexes. Her neck is supple without pain on movement, deformity, or palpable thyroid. Results of the examination of her head, back, heart, lungs, and abdomen are normal.

A thorough skin examination and one radiologic study confirm the diagnosis.

What is your differential diagnosis at this point?
Are there any elements of history or physical examination that would help you?
What additional diagnostic studies would you like performed?

DISCUSSION

Diagnosis

A complete skin examination revealed inguinal freckling and numerous café-au-lait spots—some as large as 5 cm—on the backs of the girl's legs. A computed tomographic scan of her head revealed a large suprasellar mass at the area of the optic chiasm. These findings confirmed the diagnosis of neurofibromatosis type 1 (NF-1). The child was admitted for removal of the brain mass, which was found on pathologic examination to be a juvenile pilocytic astrocytoma. The cause of her initial neck complaints was not evident; they may have been related to unnatural positioning of her head in an attempt to compensate for the visual changes.

Evaluation

Neurofibromatosis is one of several disorders known as phakomatoses, which are characterized by their tendency to cause neurocutaneous lesions. There are at least eight forms of the disease. The most common is NF-1, which accounts for 80% of cases. The prevalence of NF-1 is about 1 in 3,000 in the general population. It is inherited in an autosomal dominant fashion, although as many as 50% of patients may have developed the disorder through a spontaneous mutation. Although its penetrance is virtually 100%, patients who have NF-1 can present with a broad spectrum of symptoms, from very mild disease that primarily involves skin lesions to severe disease that involves the development of both neurofibromas in vital organs and malignant tumors.

The gene for NF-1 has been localized on chromosome 17. It is believed that the gene normally encodes for a tumor suppressor; hence, mutations in its sequence are believed to lead to the increased incidence of malignant tumors associated with the disorder. Among the tumors that occur with increased frequency in patients who have NF-1 are optic gliomas, astrocytomas, malignant peripheral nerve sheath tumors, several forms of leukemia, and rhabdomyosarcoma.

The diagnostic features of NF-1 are as follows, with the presence of two or more necessary to make the diagnosis:

- Six or more café-au-lait macules whose greatest diameter is more than 5 mm in prepubertal patients and more than 15 mm in postpubertal patients.
- Two or more neurofibromas of any type or one plexiform neurofibroma.
- Freckling in the axillary or inguinal region.
- Optic glioma.
- Two or more Lisch nodules (hamartomas of the iris) detected by slitlamp examination.
- A distinctive osseous lesion, such as sphenoid dysplasia or thinning of long-bone cortex, with or without pseudoarthrosis.
- A first-degree relative who has NF-1 according to these criteria.

Many of these lesions develop subtly, with periods of rapid growth in adolescence and during pregnancy.

Differential Diagnosis

The complaint of visual loss in a child always should be taken seriously. The differential diagnosis includes diseases that involve the eye, such as iritis or retinal detachment, as well as conditions of the central nervous system, such as basilar migraine, disease of the occipital lobe, or tumor of the optic chiasm, as in this girl.

Presentation

The presentation of NF-1 is highly variable. The presence of café-au-lait spots is one of the most common signs. These well-circumscribed, light brown macules are found in 10% of all individuals and often are not a sign of any disorder. The presence of six or more of these lesions, however, should raise the suspicion of NF-1 and prompt further investigation. It must be noted that café-au-lait spots also are associated with other disorders, including ataxia telangiectasia, tuberous sclerosis, Albright syndrome, Bloom syndrome, Russell-Silver syndrome, multiple lentigines, Fanconi anemia, and Turner syndrome.

NF-1 produces lesions that affect many organ systems. Hypertension resulting from renal artery stenosis or pheochromocytoma and scoliosis caused by tumors or bony abnormalities are among the presenting signs that lead to further evaluation. Because the pathologic lesions often evolve slowly, with the development of neurofibromas occurring predominantly after the onset of puberty, clinicians should screen patients closely who have a lesion suggestive of neurofibromatosis. Other lesions that should heighten the suspicion of NF-1 include tibial pseudarthrosis (often recognized when the child begins to bear weight), sphenoid wing dysplasia, and optic pathway gliomas.

Evaluation

Because NF-1 is a progressive disease, the use of screening techniques at various times during the patient's development may help to detect lesions before they become symptomatic. The American Academy of Pediatrics Committee on Genetics has made recommendations for screening patients who have NF that include the following:

- Evaluation of the patient for the development of plexiform neurofibromas with attention to any abnormal changes in head size, focal neurologic signs, or persistent headache.
- Blood pressure screening, which may suggest the development of pheochromocytoma, renal artery stenosis, and other vascular hypertrophic lesions.
- Evaluation for skeletal changes, focusing on the development of scoliosis and limb asymmetry (for evidence of localized hypertrophy).
- Evaluation of neurodevelopmental progress and attention to signs of learning disabilities.
- Annual ophthalmologic examination for any evidence of Lisch nodules and optic pathway tumors.
- Evaluation of any rapidly changing lesions, particularly of the skin, which may require surgery to improve the patient's appearance.

Because there is no cure for neurofibromatosis, screening of patients for developing tumors may lead to early intervention and symptomatic relief.

Maryann Buetti-Sgouros, MD, Columbia-Presbyterian Medical Center,
New York, NY

"Allergy" to Beer

PRESENTATION

During a routine health evaluation, a previously healthy 15-year-old boy confides to you that he has been experimenting with alcohol. It will not continue, he assures you, because he has discovered that he is "allergic to beer." Asked for details, he describes drinking several cans of beer over the course of an evening on three occasions. Each subsequent morning, he awoke with nausea and abdominal pain that was predominantly on his left side. By mid-day, he noted what appeared to be blood in his urine. The blood, pain, and nausea all resolved gradually over the next 24 hours. He did not tell his parents about these episodes for fear of punishment. He denies other similar episodes of dark-colored urine or abdominal pain and notes no dysuria. He has been taking no medications or illicit drugs and denies trauma.

On physical examination, the boy's pulse rate is 72 beats/min and his blood pressure is 120/80 mm Hg. He has no edema or rashes. His chest is clear and no heart murmurs or rubs are heard. No abdominal masses are palpable, nor is there costovertebral angle or suprapubic tenderness. Complete blood count, prothrombin time, and partial thromboplastin time all are normal. Urinalysis reveals only a trace of blood on dipstick. His serum creatinine is 115.1 mcmol/L (1.3 mg/dL). One further examination leads to the correct diagnosis.

What is your differential diagnosis at this point?
Are there any elements of history or physical examination that would help you?
What additional diagnostic studies would you like performed?

DISCUSSION

Diagnosis

Renal ultrasonography showed minimal hydronephrosis of the left kidney. A MAGA 3-furosemide radionuclide renal scan revealed blocked flow of urine at the ureteropelvic junction (UPJ). The defect was repaired successfully by a urologist.

Although usually diagnosed prenatally by the finding of fetal hydronephrosis on ultrasonography or in early childhood after the palpation of an abdominal mass, UPJ obstruction may present at any age. As in this patient, a partial obstruction may remain silent until the kidneys are challenged with a large fluid load or a medication-induced diuresis. The resultant distention of the renal pelvis leads to abdominal or flank pain, often accompanied by nausea or vomiting. These symptoms may be attributed to gastrointestinal disease.

Gross hematuria, resulting from overdistention of small renal vessels, often is seen, especially after relatively mild trauma. Urinary tract infection may accompany UPJ obstruction as well; the obstruction will be discovered on subsequent imaging.

UPJ obstructions are more common in males than females; most are unilateral, with the left kidney being affected more commonly. Although not seen in this patient, other congenital anomalies are associated with UPJ obstruction in as many as 50% of affected individuals.

The obstructions often are grouped into those of intrinsic and extrinsic origin.

Although true ureteral strictures have been described, the most common intrinsic obstruction is an aperistaltic segment, which causes a functional abnormality of urine transport between the renal pelvis and the bladder. Extrinsic obstruction is caused most commonly by a fibrous band or an aberrant or accessory renal artery that compresses the ureter as it passes anterior to it. These extrinsic obstructions may be associated with an abnormally high insertion of the ureter onto the renal pelvis. It should be noted that a patient who has an extrinsic obstruction also may have a disturbance in peristalsis of the affected ureteral segment. This possibility should be considered when planning therapy. Any of these obstructions may have a dynamic component, with increased resistance to urine flow as urine volume increases.

Evaluation
Evaluation of the older child in whom UPJ obstruction is suspected may be difficult. Levels of serum creatinine may be elevated or normal, depending on the extent of associated renal damage. Because a partial UPJ obstruction may have a dynamic component, the affected renal pelvis and ureter may appear normal or minimally dilated if renal ultrasonography is performed while the child is asymptomatic. Administration of a diuretic, fluid loading, or repeated scanning while the child is symptomatic sometimes is required. Furosemide renal scan and other radiologic tests also have roles in the evaluation of a possible UPJ obstruction, but these test decisions often are best left to a urologic consultant.

Treatment
Surgical relief of UPJ obstruction, both extrinsic and intrinsic, usually is associated with at least partial recovery of renal function. Younger children and those in whom obstructions are less severe are most likely to regain function. Except in the case of a hopelessly damaged kidney, nephrectomy rarely is required.

Gregory P. Conners, MD, University of Rochester School of Medicine and Dentistry, Rochester, NY

Tender Masses Under the Mandible

PRESENTATION

A 4-year-old girl is brought to the office because of a swollen, tender 3.0-cm mass under her left mandible that has been present for 2 weeks. She has had no respiratory symptoms and no fever. There is no history of a cat scratch or other unusual exposure, and she has not traveled recently. She is diagnosed as having bacterial lymphadenitis and treated with amoxicillin/clavulanic acid. When examined 2 days later, the mass is no longer tender and clearly is smaller.

The child returns 3 weeks later because of further swelling and is found to have several firm, fixed, noninflamed masses measuring 2.0 to 3.0 cm in the same area of her neck; there is no overlying erythema. No other adenopathy is found, but the tip of her spleen is palpable. The remainder of her history and physical examination yields no abnormal findings.

She is referred to a surgeon, who does an excision that eventually reveals the cause of her problem. A simple test in the office, however, could have led to the correct diagnosis much more quickly.

What is your differential diagnosis at this point?
Are there any elements of history or physical examination that would help you?
What additional diagnostic studies would you like performed?

DISCUSSION

Diagnosis

The girl was referred to a surgeon, who excised a mass adherent to the left submandibular salivary gland and drained a small lateral lymph node. The pathologist interpreted the mass as necrotizing granulomatous lymphadenitis, suggestive of cat-scratch disease; special stains for acid-fast, fungal, and bacterial microorganisms were negative. Six weeks later, a positive culture for *Mycobacterium avium* from the excised tissue was reported.

Differential Diagnosis

Noninfectious causes of lymphadenopathy of greatest concern to the primary care physician are the lymphoproliferative malignancies, such as Hodgkin and non-Hodgkin lymphoma, leukemia, and histiocytosis. Infectious etiologies are numerous, with bacterial (*Staphylococcus aureus*, streptococcal groups A, B, C, and H), viral (Epstein-Barr virus, cytomegalovirus, mumps), and fungal causative agents. Cat-scratch disease may be the most common cause of chronic lymphadenopathy and probably is caused by either a pleomorphic bacillus, *Afipia felis*, or a rickettsial pathogen, *Rochalimaea henselae*.

Presentation

Another common cause of lymph node infection is *Mycobacterium* sp, which can be detected by a purified protein derivative (PPD) skin test. Because both *M tuber-*

culosis and nontuberculous mycobacteria (NTM) can be causative agents, it is important to distinguish between the two. Usually a PPD reaction of 15 mm or greater is more indicative of *M tuberculosis*; a reaction of 10 mm or smaller typically is seen in patients infected by NTM. In addition, NTM infections generally cause an isolated cervical lymphadenitis without other systemic signs or symptoms in an otherwise healthy child. NTM less commonly can cause osteomyelitis, cutaneous infection, otitis media, and pulmonary disease, depending on the portal of entry of this ubiquitous organism, which is found everywhere in our environment. Severe pulmonary disease or systemic dissemination usually is found only in immunocompromised hosts.

Histopathologic findings in NTM are nonspecific and depend on the stage of the disease. The adenopathy starts as lymphoid hyperplasia, which then advances to scattered granulomas. These granulomas necrose centrally and eventually coalesce to form microabscesses. Tularemia and lymphogranuloma venereum, as well as cat-scratch disease, have been associated with similar histologic changes.

Treatment

The approach to therapy depends on factors such as the species of NTM isolated, site of infection, drug susceptibility of the organism, and the patient's underlying condition. Many strains of NTM are relatively resistant to antituberculosis drugs. Sensitivity testing is not optimal because the method used was designed for *M tuberculosis* and because in vivo results do not always correlate with in vitro findings.

Synergy between drugs, especially rifampin, can be seen and offers a rationale for combination therapy when antimicrobial treatment is appropriate. Other drugs used in treatment of the various strains of NTM include ethambutol, ethionamide, and less frequently, isoniazid, erythromycin, and aminoglycosides. Multiple drug use is indicated for disseminated infection in immunocompromised patients and in other specific instances. The clinician should realize that cervical lymphadenitis caused by NTM in otherwise healthy children frequently is treated most effectively by surgical excision alone.

This patient probably responded to antibiotics initially because there was a pyogenic infection superimposed on an underlying, indolent NTM lymphadenitis, which is not unusual. She has done well since surgery (with no sequelae), and no further complications are anticipated.

Robert J. Tuite, MD, Rochester, NY

Update: *Rochalimaes henselae* now is called *Bartonella henselae.*

Leg Pain and Refusal to Walk

PRESENTATION

A 2½-year-old boy is brought to the emergency department because of right leg pain. He awoke from a nap, complaining of right leg pain and refusing to walk. The child has been healthy, with no history of fever, cough, vomiting, or diarrhea, although he had the "sniffles" 1 week ago. His parents are not aware of any trauma, but he does fall out of bed frequently. His appetite has decreased slightly.

Physical examination reveals a well-developed, friendly young boy in no distress. His vital signs are normal, as are the results of his entire examination, except that he cries when his right leg is examined and he refuses to stand. The leg appears normal without erythema, swelling, or warmth. He cries when any part of the leg is touched. The boy is given a dose of ibuprofen and sent for a radiograph of the affected leg.

Upon returning from radiology, the child is walking normally, and his radiographs are unremarkable. He is sent home with the diagnosis of muscle strain, to be given ibuprofen.

The following day, the child returns to the emergency department, crying in pain and refusing to walk. His history and examination results have not changed except that he now is pointing to his right ankle. Repeat radiographs of his right ankle are normal.

What is your differential diagnosis at this point?
Are there any elements of history or physical examination that would help you?
What additional diagnostic studies would you like performed?

DISCUSSION

Diagnosis

With this child's presentation, the differential diagnosis includes trauma, transient synovitis, juvenile rheumatoid arthritis, septic arthritis, and osteomyelitis. To help narrow the focus further, laboratory data are needed. A complete blood count revealed: white blood cell (WBC) count, 20.3 x 10^9/L (20.3 x 10^3/mcL), with 3% band forms, 70% segmented neutrophils, 13% lymphocytes, and 4% monocytes; hemoglobin, 1.86 mmol/L (12 g/dL); and platelet count, 403 x 10^9/L (403 x 10^3/mcL). The erythrocyte sedimentation rate (ESR) was 81 mm/h. These findings suggested inflammation and prompted performance of a bone scan, which demonstrated increased activity in the area of the right distal tibial epiphysis. An aspirate of bone from the involved area showed Gram-positive cocci in clusters and later grew *Staphylococcus aureus*, as did the child's initial blood culture, confirming the diagnosis of osteomyelitis.

Osteomyelitis is an infection of bone that can occur by three mechanisms: hematogenous seeding, local invasion from contiguous infected areas, and direct inoculation of the bone (trauma).

Acute hematogenous osteomyelitis is the most common pathogenesis of this infection in children and occurs as a result of bloodborne bacteria localizing in the bone (usually in the metaphysis due to relatively slow blood flow through the capillary bed). Once the bacteria enter the metaphysis, an inflammatory exudate develops that results in increased pressure under the periosteum, which leads to vascular compromise, thrombosis, and necrosis. The periosteum may rupture from the pressure of the inflammatory response, allowing purulent material to drain into the soft tissues and subcutaneous area. The exudate also can travel within the marrow cavity into the epiphysis and then into the joint space, causing septic arthritis. This chain of events is most common in children younger than 12 months of age because transphyseal vessels are present up to that age and disappear later.

Etiology

The most common cause of osteomyelitis is *S aureus*, which accounts for 40% to 80% of cases. Other pathogens include *Streptococcus pyogenes* (the second most common organism), *S pneumoniae* (which is not common), *Haemophilus influenzae* type B (significantly less common because of the vaccine), and Gram-negative bacilli such as *Salmonella* sp (especially in patients who have sickle cell disease) and *Kingella kingae*. Group B streptococci and coliform bacteria are common causes of osteomyelitis in neonates. *Pseudomonas aeruginosa* is the typical organism found in cases of osteomyelitis caused by puncture wounds of the foot; anaerobes must be considered after animal or human bites. Mycobacteria and fungi are rare causes of osteomyelitis. *Neisseria gonorrhoeae* can be a cause of septic arthritis in sexually active adolescents, but it rarely, if ever, causes bone infection.

Presentation

The signs and symptoms of acute hematogenous osteomyelitis vary, depending on the age of the patient, duration of the process, and location of the infection. Systemic signs may be minimal, and fever may not be present. Infants and younger children may present only with irritability, poor appetite, limp, or refusal to walk (pseudoparalysis). As in this young child, the intensity of symptoms can vary, especially when analgesics are introduced.

Older children can describe and localize the pain. Pain is the chief complaint in 50% of cases of osteomyelitis. Diffuse localized tenderness from increased pressure within the bone is the earliest finding, but it is not specific to bone infections. Warmth and swelling also may be present. Point tenderness is a specific finding in those who have osteomyelitis, but it is found in only 15% of patients. Joint motion can be limited because of muscle spasm or septic arthritis. Erythema is a late finding that occurs when the periosteum has ruptured or is very inflamed.

Evaluation

The definitive diagnosis of acute osteomyelitis requires isolation of the etiologic agent. Blood cultures are positive in 50% to 60% of cases. Cultures taken from the bone, either surgically or by needle aspiration, result in a positive culture yield of about 60%, although cultures of synovial fluid aspirated from the joints of children who have both joint and bone infection can raise the total yield to 80%. It may take 10 to 14 days of infection before radiographs show changes in the bone, but obliteration of the normal intermuscular fat planes is evident in 3 to 7 days. The three-phase bone scan, performed with technetium 99m, can detect acute osteomyelitis earlier than conventional radiographs, but during the first 24 to 48 hours, the infected area may be infarcted and, therefore, avascular, resulting in a normal or cold scan. The bone scan also can detect multiple sites of involvement.

The gallium-67 citrate bone scan and the indium-111 oxide WBC scan also have been used to diagnose osteomyelitis, but the length of time required for these studies, the excessive radiation dose, and the low yield make them useful only in certain circumstances. Computed tomography (primarily to detect pelvic and vertebral osteomyelitis) and magnetic resonance imaging have been used as diagnostic tools; both have limitations.

Treatment

The treatment of osteomyelitis consists of intravenous antibiotics and sometimes surgical debridement. In uncomplicated cases that are diagnosed and treated promptly and have a good clinical response to treatment (resolution of fever and diminution of local findings), antibiotic therapy can be switched from the intravenous to the oral route after 5 to 7 days. Acute-phase reactants such as the ESR or serum C-reactive protein should be monitored to evaluate the response to therapy.

Lesson for the Clinician

Several aspects of this child's situation had the potential for misleading his physicians. His history of falling out of bed suggested trauma, while the recent nasal congestion could have represented a viral infection associated with a transient synovitis. The absence of fever would decrease the likelihood of infection. (This boy did develop high fever the night after he was admitted to the hospital.) The initial dramatic response to ibuprofen might suggest minor trauma. His clinical picture reminds the clinician to consider osteomyelitis in a young child whose signs and symptoms may be subtle but are persistent.

Scott A. Barron, MD, Lincoln Pediatric Associates, Lincoln, NE

Intermittent, Sudden Palpitations, Lightheadedness, and Difficulty Breathing

PRESENTATION

A 15-year-old girl comes to your office complaining that she has experienced inter-mittent, sudden episodes of chest pain, fatigue, palpitations, and sensations of dif-ficulty breathing and lightheadedness for 2 months. These episodes occur several times daily and are unaccompanied by other symptoms such as syncope, wheez-ing, swelling of the extremities, or fever. She denies being worried, but reports that her parents are very frightened because a 16-year-old male cousin died recently while playing soccer, and two other relatives, a 27-year-old cousin and a 29-year-old uncle, died suddenly during exercise.

The physical examination reveals a somewhat anxious girl complaining of mild precordial chest pain. Her temperature is 36.9°C (98.4°F) orally, respiratory rate is 16 breaths/min, heart rate is 110 beats/min, and blood pressure is 100/60 mm Hg; weight and height are at the 75th percentile. Her examination is completely nor-mal except for a grade 1 to 2 systolic ejection murmur heard best at the left lower sternal border and point tenderness over the third left costochondral junction.

A radiograph of the chest reveals clear lungs and a mild prominence of the left ventricular border. The electrocardiogram (ECG) shows a sinus rhythm with deep Q waves over the left precordium and left ventricular hypertrophy for her age. The complete blood count, antistreptolysin-O titer, and erythrocyte sedimentation rate are normal.

What is your differential diagnosis at this point?
Are there any elements of history or physical examination that would help you?
What additional diagnostic studies would you like performed?

DISCUSSION

Diagnosis

The symptoms described by this adolescent girl clearly are those of chest wall pain followed by anxiety and hyperventilation. The soft ejection murmur at the lower left sternal border together with a family history of relatives dying at an early age induced an alert physician to obtain an ECG. Left ventricular hypertrophy and deep Q waves raised the suspicion of cardiomyopathy, which was confirmed by echocar-diography.

Hypertrophic cardiomyopathy occurs equally in males and females; one third of these patients have a positive family history with autosomal dominant transmission. In 75% of symptomatic patients, the primary complaint is exertional dyspnea or fatigue. Patients also may experience syncope, palpitation, and chest pain.

The chest pain may be typical of ischemia-induced angina or may feel dull. Arrhythmias such as ventricular tachycardia may cause pain through insufficient coronary blood flow. This patient's pain originated in the chest wall and was brief and intermittent, not like the sustained pain of coronary insufficiency, which often is associated with exercise.

Presentation

Physical findings in patients who have hypertrophic cardiomyopathy characteristically include a systolic ejection murmur, most prominent along the left lower sternal border or apex and sometimes associated with a thrill. There may be a sharp upstroke of the arterial pulse.

Evaluation

Findings on the ECG are abnormal in the great majority of patients. Although there is no characteristic pattern, left ventricular hypertrophy and ST-segment changes are seen. Deep Q waves (5 mm) also may be noted and reflect septal hypertrophy. Associated ventricular arrhythmias are common. Echocardiography is diagnostic, demonstrating diffuse or confined areas of hypertrophy of the ventricular wall or septum. The echocardiogram also differentiates this disorder from aortic stenosis, which may have a similar clinical presentation. Specific molecular diagnosis now is possible for many cardiomyopathies.

Treatment

Management of hypertrophic cardiomyopathy consists of beta-adrenergic blockade and use of calcium channel blocking agents, which reduce the degree of outflow tract obstruction. Inotropic agents, such as digoxin, increase the degree of obstruction and may induce arrhythmias. Sudden cardiac death may occur at any age, but is most common in the second and third decades of life. One third of deaths occur during strenuous exercise, which may precipitate more severe outflow obstruction or arrhythmia. A history of ventricular tachycardia and marked left ventricular hypertrophy are significant risk factors for sudden cardiac death in these patients.

Differential Diagnosis

Chest pain has many causes, one of the most common of which is costochondritis, in which the pain is augmented, as in this patient, by palpation during an episode of discomfort. Chest pain also may be associated with anxiety with or without associated hyperventilation. Pericarditis may present with severe retrosternal pain aggravated by coughing and lying supine. Fever is common, and a pericardial rub usually is heard. The ECG classically demonstrates low voltage and initial ST-segment elevation.

A pulmonary embolism may cause the abrupt onset of severe, pleuritic chest pain. The most frequent etiologies of the embolism are a hypercoagulable state, postoperative status, long-term immobilization, and trauma. Severe pulmonary hypertension, either primary or secondary to chronic lung disease, may be associated with chest pain and exertional dyspnea. This condition should produce an exaggerated pulmonary component of the second heart sound and findings of right ventricular hypertrophy on ECG.

In patients who have acute congestive heart failure as well as chest pain, etiologies to suspect include acute myocarditis, disruption of the mitral valve apparatus by infective endocarditis or trauma, myocardial infarction, arrhythmias, or any of these factors in combination. Acute myocarditis usually is associated with fever and elevation of acute phase reactants. The ECG typically reveals low-voltage QRS complexes. Infective endocarditis usually is associated with underlying valvular disease, spiking fevers, new or altered murmurs, and vegetations noted on echocardiography. Myocardial infarction can be diagnosed by characteristic ECG findings and elevations of circulating enzyme levels.

Lesson for the Clinician

This patient had a serious cardiac disorder as well as chest pain caused by costochondritis and aggravated by hyperventilation. Attention to all the details of the history and physical examination allowed a complete and accurate diagnosis.

Sanjiv B. Amin, MD, University of Rochester School of Medicine and Dentistry, Rochester, NY; Jeffrey M. Devries, MD, MPH, Henry Ford Health System, Detroit, MI

Update: In addition to beta-adrenergic blockers, verapamil has proven useful in the treatment of patients who have hypertrophic cardiomyopathy.

Cervical Mass and Fever

PRESENTATION

A 4-month-old girl is seen in the clinic because of fever as high as 38.8°C (102°F) for 4 days and an anterior cervical mass. She appears only mildly ill. The mass measures 4 x 2 cm and is firm and very tender. No erythema or warmth is noted. Lymphadenitis is diagnosed and she is given an oral cephalosporin. Two days later, because she has not improved, she is admitted to the hospital, where a computed tomographic (CT) scan reveals a cluster of large lymph nodes without evidence of abscess. Intravenous nafcillin is administered, and she is discharged 4 days later on oral medication when her temperature is close to normal.

The baby is readmitted less than 1 week later because the mass has enlarged and fever has returned. Her liver edge is palpable 2 cm below the right costal margin. There is an erythematous, scaling rash on her scalp that is thought to be seborrhea. Testing for human immunodeficiency virus is negative, but serology for Epstein-Barr virus is positive. She is sent home on an oral cephalosporin; when seen 2 weeks later, her adenopathy has regressed markedly. She still has low-grade fever, and her mother reports that she has decreased appetite and activity, but she does not look ill.

One week later the baby is brought to the emergency department because of 2 days of fever and 1 day of vomiting. Her temperature is 40.8°C (105.5°F), and her abdomen is strikingly distended. After intravenous rehydration, an abdominal CT scan is performed that leads to an additional procedure, revealing her diagnosis.

What is your differential diagnosis at this point?
Are there any elements of history or physical examination that would help you?
What additional diagnostic studies would you like performed?

DISCUSSION

Diagnosis

The abdominal CT scan showed a massively enlarged liver containing multiple hypodense lesions and a slightly enlarged spleen that had similar lesions. Liver biopsy demonstrated histiocytes, confirming a diagnosis of Langerhans cell histiocytosis. Characteristic tennis racquet-shaped Birbeck granules were seen in the cytoplasm of the histiocytes on electron microscopy. The baby's condition at the time of her third admission was a result of an intercurrent viral gastroenteritis that had caused moderate dehydration. Her white blood cell count was 12.4×10^9/L (12.4×10^3/mcL) with a normal differential count. Chest radiography findings were normal, and all cultures for bacterial infection yielded negative results. She stabilized quickly with intravenous fluids and supportive care.

Histiocytosis is a rare disorder that results from the abnormal or uncontrolled proliferation of normal antigen-presenting cells. Langerhans histiocytosis, which is synonymous with class I histiocytosis, encompasses the group of disorders previously called histiocytosis X and includes Letterer-Siwe disease, Hand-Schüller-Christian disease, and eosinophilic granuloma. Class II consists of infection-associated hemophagocytic syndrome and familial erythrophagocytic lymphohistiocytosis. Class III is the malignant form of the disease and includes acute monocytic leukemia and histiocytic lymphoma. These patients have the cell markers for histiocytosis as well as for the specific malignancy. Their cell counts also meet the criteria for the given malignancy. The lymphoma is specifically histiocytic.

Presentation

Histiocytosis often mimics other diseases. The rash of histiocytosis, which is seen in 30% to 50% of patients, is an erythematous flaky or scaly rash that usually involves the scalp but also may involve the back, palms, and soles. As in this case, it may be mistaken for seborrheic dermatitis. Petechiae and hemorrhage also are found. Bone is the organ affected most frequently (80% to 100% of patients), and the presentation usually is osteolytic lesions of the skull or vertebral body collapse. Free-floating teeth are seen when the mandible or maxilla is involved. Lymph node involvement can cause strikingly enlarged nodes, but tenderness and warmth are not typical. As in this patient, lymphadenopathy is the presenting feature in many cases, particularly in children; lymph node involvement is found in 33% to 42% of patients. Bone pain, rash, and lymphadenopathy, in combination or alone, are the most common clinical characteristics of histiocytosis.

Chronic otitis media is common; persistently draining ears can result from involvement of mastoid bones. Liver disease is present in 20% of older patients and up to 71% of infants and can manifest as hepatomegaly, jaundice, ascites, fibrosis, and liver failure.

Lung involvement is seen in 15% to 25% of patients, but it is the most common cause of mortality in long-term survivors. Central nervous system involvement is much less frequent and includes pituitary dysfunction with diabetes insipidus, growth failure, and exophthalmos due to granulomatous lesions behind the orbit. Some patients may present with constitutional signs and symptoms such as fever, irritability, and malaise.

Treatment and Prognosis

Treatment and prognosis depend on the number of organ systems involved. Single bony lesions may resolve spontaneously or require only curettage. Multiorgan disease may require chemotherapy, as in this case. Current thinking about treating histiocytosis is to do what is necessary to restore the patient's functioning to normal and to prevent disability, aiming at control while allowing the disease to resolve over time.

Children older than 2 years who have only bone involvement have a 5-year survival rate of 95%. Children older than 2 years who have one or more systems involved have a survival rate as high as 90%. Children younger than 2 years as well as those who have hepatosplenomegaly, lymph nodes larger than 5 cm, honeycomb lung disease, or bone marrow involvement have a 5-year survival rate of 60%. This child received chemotherapy and looked very well at 7 months of age. Her prognosis, however, must remain guarded because her liver was involved.

Lesson for the Clinician

This infant's situation is instructive in that she presented with fever and lymphadenopathy and only later developed more features of histiocytosis. It is not unusual for the rash of histiocytosis to mimic that of seborrhea. The liver edge 2 cm below the right costal margin on her second hospitalization is consistent with normal liver size or mild hepatomegaly. A liver span is not recorded in her record and may have indicated more than mild enlargement. At the time, it was believed that any hepatomegaly was caused by Epstein-Barr infection. In retrospect, it is likely that she had significant liver enlargement at the time of the clinic visit 1 week prior to her third admission. Because she looked well and her adenopathy had regressed significantly, it is possible that the hepatomegaly was overlooked.

A number of other disorders can cause lymph node involvement, including the more common forms of bacterial adenitis, mycobacterial adenitis, cat-scratch disease, lymphoma, infectious mononucleosis, and malignant processes. Histiocytosis, although rare, should be considered in a child who has lymphadenopathy that does not fit well into other categories. As always, careful follow-up of any child in whom illness does not resolve completely is necessary if the clinician is to detect the true cause.

Debbie West, MD, Medical Center of Central Georgia, Macon, GA

Painful Swollen Joints and Dyspnea on Exertion

PRESENTATION

A previously healthy 13-year-old Asian girl is seen because of a 4-week history of general malaise, anorexia, intermittent fever to 37.7°C (101°F), and pains in her ankles, knees, and hands. Over the past 3 weeks, her hands and ankles have become swollen. She has developed dyspnea on exertion and is short of breath at night in bed unless she props herself on pillows.

When the fevers began, the girl was diagnosed as having a urinary tract infection because her urine contained 30 white blood cells per high-power field; the culture was negative. Her past medical and family histories are free of serious illnesses.

On physical examination, the girl is afebrile and has a pulse of 125 beats/min, respirations of 32 breaths/min, and a blood pressure of 92/50 mm Hg. Crackles are heard at both lung bases, and muffled heart sounds accompany a friction rub. Her liver is palpable 1 cm below the right costal margin. An effusion is noted in the proximal interphalangeal joints of both index fingers, as is 1+ pitting edema over both tibias. She walks favoring her left leg. Electrocardiography documents sinus tachycardia and normal voltages. A radiograph of the chest reveals moderate pulmonary edema and bilateral effusions.

What is your differential diagnosis at this point?
Are there any elements of history or physical examination that would help you?
What additional diagnostic studies would you like performed?

DISCUSSION

Differential Diagnosis

Findings on the patient's examination were suggestive of a pericardial effusion, the presence of which was confirmed by echocardiography. Approximately 600 mL of serosanguinous fluid was removed by pericardiocentesis.

The differential diagnosis of pericardial disease is extensive. Infectious etiologies include viral infection (coxsackievirus B, Epstein-Barr virus), bacterial infection (*Streptococcus*, pneumococcus, *Staphylococcus*, and *Mycoplasma*), tuberculosis, fungal infection (histoplasmosis), and parasitic infection (toxoplasmosis). Uremia and hypothyroidism can cause pericardial disease, as can primary and metastatic malignancy and trauma. Connective tissue disorders (rheumatoid arthritis, rheumatic fever, systemic lupus erythematosus [SLE], sarcoidosis) also can present as pericarditis.

Presentation

Typical manifestations of pericardial disease include precordial pain, cough, dyspnea, and fever. Physical findings include the presence of a friction rub, which will vary with the position of the patient and the volume of the effusion, muffled heart sounds, narrowed pulses, tachycardia, neck vein distention, and pulsus paradoxus.

Evaluation

Electrocardiography may reveal low voltages, mild ST-segment elevations, and generalized T-wave inversion. Chest radiographs may reveal an enlarged cardiac shadow (the "water bottle" appearance).

Echocardiography is a sensitive technique for evaluating the size of the effusion and following its progress.

Diagnosis

In this adolescent, the fever and joint pains suggested SLE as the cause of her pericardial disease. The diagnosis was confirmed by a positive antinuclear antibody (ANA) level, the presence of anti-double-stranded DNA antibody (anti-dsDNA), decreased levels of C3 and C4 complement, and an elevated erythrocyte sedimentation rate.

Pericarditis occurs in 25% of patients who have SLE and may be asymptomatic. A rub may or may not be associated. Tamponade is a rare complication. Libman-Sacks endocarditis is a noninfectious endocarditis detected on autopsy in 50% of patients. Individuals who have endocarditis require bacterial prophylaxis against subacute bacterial endocarditis. Myocarditis occurs in fewer than 10%.

Although this patient presented primarily with pericarditis and pleural effusion, other organs were involved. She excreted 0.51 g/d (528 mg/24 h) protein in a urine sample, representing 384 mg/M^2 per 24 hours (normal, 200 mg/M^2 per 24 hours), her ANA titer was greater than 1:1,280, and her hematocrit was 0.29 (29%).

A hallmark of SLE is that it can affect many organs and create a variety of clinical pictures. The condition is diagnosed when the patient manifests four of the following 11 signs: immunologic disorder (anti-dsDNA, anti-Smith antigen); renal involvement (cellular casts, proteinuria); arthritis; neurologic dysfunction (psychosis, seizures); malar rash; elevated ANA level; discoid rash; serositis (pleuritis, pericarditis); hematologic abnormalities (anemia, thrombocytopenia, leukopenia); oral or nasopharyngeal ulcers; and photosensitivity. The clinician may find handy the mnemonic I RAN MAD SHOPS, in which the letters stand for the 11 criteria, with the final S representing SLE.

The leading causes of death from SLE are infection and renal failure. Most patients have immunoglobulin deposits in their glomeruli, but only 50% manifest clinical nephritis, defined as proteinuria of 0.48 g/d (500 mg/24 h). Approximately 50% will have cellular casts, 25% will show the edema of nephrotic syndrome, and 10% will demonstrate acute renal failure with elevated blood urea nitrogen and creatinine levels. Most patients who have mesangial or mild focal proliferative nephritis maintain good renal function; those who have diffuse proliferative nephritis will develop renal failure unless aggressive immunosuppression is pursued. A renal biopsy may be necessary to determine the extent of renal involvement because this aspect of the disease will largely determine the treatment course and aggressiveness of therapy.

Almost all patients experience arthralgias, most frequently of the proximal interphalangeal and metacarpophalangeal joints, although any joint may be affected. Joint erosions and deformities are rare. The anemia of chronic disease occurs in 70% of patients at some point. Leukopenia (usually lymphopenia) is common, but rarely is associated with recurrent infections. Mild thrombocytopenia also is common.

Anemia and leukopenia rarely require treatment; severe thrombocytopenia associated with purpura and bleeding responds to high-dose glucocorticoids.

Any region of the central or peripheral nervous system can be involved in SLE; 60% of patients have some involvement during the course of their illness. Although mild cognitive dysfunction is the most frequent finding, seizures of any type may occur. Laboratory findings that indicate neurologic involvement include abnormal findings on electroencephalography and increased protein and mononuclear cells in cerebrospinal fluid. Neurologic problems usually improve with immunosuppressive therapy, but recurrences are common.

Screening
The ANA titer is the most useful screening test for SLE because it is elevated in almost all children who have active disease. Juvenile rheumatoid arthritis, Sjögren syndrome, and scleroderma also may cause the ANA level to rise. Anti-dsDNA is elevated in 50% to 70% of children who have active renal disease, which also is associated with decreased C3 and C4 levels. Antibodies to the Smith antigen complex occur in only 30% of SLE patients, but when present, they are highly specific for the disorder.

Treatment
Treatment of SLE consists of controlling acute flares and suppressing symptoms. Glucocorticoids and anti-inflammatory agents such as cyclophosphamide are the primary therapeutic agents. The aggressiveness of treatment must be titrated to the desired level of effectiveness and the tolerated extent of side effects. Establishing a strong therapeutic alliance between the patient and the treatment team is essential for optimal management of this serious chronic disorder. Survival among patients who have SLE is approximately 70% over 10 years. A less favorable prognosis exists for nonwhite patients, individuals from low socioeconomic groups, and those who have severe involvement of kidneys, brain, or heart. New techniques derived from the rapid expansion of knowledge about the immune system on the molecular level carry the promise of more effective therapy.

Lesson for the Clinician
Although SLE is not common in childhood, pediatricians should be aware of its many manifestations so they can detect the disease early and provide appropriate treatment.

L. Gregory Lawton, MD, Norma Allgood, MD, David Grant Medical Center,
Travis Air Force Base, CA

Abdominal Pain and Vomiting Leading to Diarrhea and Penile Pain

PRESENTATION

A 17-year-old Taiwanese exchange student comes to the emergency department because of abdominal pain and vomiting that began 1 hour after eating pizza. He has normal vital signs, including temperature, but appears ill. He has diffuse abdominal tenderness without distension, guarding, or rebound pain. Bowel sounds are present and normal in quality. His white blood cell (WBC) count is 18 x 10^9/L (18 x 10^3/mcL) with 80% neutrophils and 5% band forms. The boy is admitted to the hospital for observation.

During the first hospital night he develops diarrhea. Stool studies are requested, including culture, examination for ova and parasites, and Clostridium difficile toxin determination. The next morning he develops penile pain, with discharge and urinary retention that requires catheterization. The discharge is cultured, and he receives one dose of ceftriaxone as well as oral doxycycline for a presumed sexually transmitted disease. The following day, he develops chest pain and shortness of breath. A chest radiograph shows a small right lower lobe effusion with a possible infiltrate. Antibiotic coverage for pneumonia is added to the treatment regimen.

Over the next 3 days, his vomiting and diarrhea resolve, and he seems to have less pain. Cultures of penile discharge and stool studies are negative, and he is discharged on the fifth day with a diagnosis of viral gastroenteritis. Several hours after discharge, he returns because of severe abdominal pain and diarrhea and is found to have pronounced abdominal tenderness. Computed tomographic (CT) imaging of his abdomen is performed.

What is your differential diagnosis at this point?
Are there any elements of history or physical examination that would help you?
What additional diagnostic studies would you like performed?

DISCUSSION

Diagnosis

The abdominal CT scan showed multiple fluid collections in the pelvis. The boy was taken to the operating room where a diagnostic laparoscopy revealed a perforated appendix with multiple pelvic abscesses. An open appendectomy with drainage of the abscesses was performed. His postoperative course was uncomplicated, and he was discharged on the sixth postoperative day with plans to return home to Taiwan.

Appendicitis is the most common abdominal emergency requiring surgery in children. Clinicians are familiar with the classic presentation, which can lead directly to the correct diagnosis. However, many patients, especially children, do not present in a classic fashion. Acute appendicitis can mimic a variety of other conditions, and misdiagnosis of appendicitis is one of the most common causes of litigation in pediatrics. This patient's clinical course offers several valuable teaching points.

Presentation

This boy initially presented with abdominal pain and vomiting and was admitted with a diagnosis of possible appendicitis. The next day he developed some urinary tract symptoms, leading to the erroneous diagnosis of a urethritis due to a sexually transmitted disease. Urologic signs and symptoms, such as painful urination, urinary retention, hematuria, and pyuria, all have been reported to be presenting signs of acute appendicitis. There even have been several reports of appendicitis presenting as acute scrotal pain and swelling. The following day, this patient developed chest symptoms, and a radiograph showed a small pleural effusion, leading the clinicians to believe that he had pneumonia. His radiographic findings may have been caused by atelectasis due to splinting from pain or to pleural irritation from peritonitis.

Evaluation

The diagnosis of appendicitis still relies on a detailed history and a careful physical examination; unfortunately, there is no definitive test. Laboratory tests such as WBC and differential cell count, erythrocyte sedimentation rate, and C-reactive protein all have been investigated for their value in predicting the presence of an inflamed appendix. Although somewhat useful if they are positive, normal values do not exclude the diagnosis of appendicitis. Radiologic examinations have been used to aid in the diagnosis, but plain radiographs are helpful only if a fecalith is seen.

Ultrasonography has been used widely in evaluating patients who have abdominal pain. A positive ultrasonographic study is helpful, but a negative study does not exclude appendicitis. CT scan is somewhat more sensitive and specific than ultrasonography, but it is not practical in the initial evaluation of most patients who have abdominal pain.

The goal of the primary care physician should be early recognition of acute appendicitis; delay in diagnosis can lead to perforation and numerous complications. Having the patient examined by an experienced surgeon as soon as appendicitis becomes a viable diagnostic option can speed the process of diagnosis and expedite surgery if it is needed. Unexplained abdominal pain and tenderness of greater than 6 hours duration, even if they vary in intensity, are findings consistent with appendicitis, as is persistent vomiting. A diagnostic clue to rupture of the appendix may be a sudden feeling of relief in a patient who has had abdominal pain and tenderness, followed by a worsening of the symptoms. This so-called "lucent interval" results from the rupture releasing the tension on the wall of the appendix.

Lesson for the Clinician

One cannot overemphasize the value of repeated physical examinations. Over time, valuable insights into the nature of the patient's condition may appear, but they will not be appreciated if the clinician does not keep an open mind and repeatedly evaluate the clinical situation.

Dina B. Morrissey, MD, Teresa Kim, MS, Memorial Health Care, Worcester, MA

Sudden Tachycardia, Hypertension, and Acidosis During Surgery

PRESENTATION

A 7-year-old Hispanic boy in good health is admitted for cosmetic ear surgery. He has no medical or family history of major illness, and his preoperative evaluation is unremarkable. He undergoes general anesthesia with standard inhalational agents (halothane and nitrous oxide). Two hours into the surgery, he suddenly develops tachycardia of 200 beats/min and an elevated blood pressure of 150/90 mm Hg. Arterial blood gas results are: pH, 7.05; Pco_2, 67 torr; Po_2, 435 torr; and base excess, -10. After appropriate management, his vital signs normalize rapidly and the acidosis resolves. The remainder of the surgery is canceled, and he is transferred to the pediatric intensive care unit for postoperative monitoring. The signs and symptoms do not recur. He has a prompt and satisfactory recovery and is discharged home the next morning after follow-up is arranged.

What is your differential diagnosis at this point?
Are there any elements of history or physical examination that would help you?
What additional diagnostic studies would you like performed?

DISCUSSION

Diagnosis

Although pediatricians rarely deal directly with malignant hyperthermia (MH), the condition exhibited by this child, they should be familiar with this disorder because prior knowledge and anticipation may be lifesaving.

MH is an acute hypermetabolic reaction triggered by inhalational anesthetic agents and succinylcholine. The combination of halothane and succinylcholine is strongly associated with MH, but either agent alone can trigger an episode.

The primary biochemical abnormality in MH appears to occur in skeletal muscle, where metabolism is enhanced due to abnormally high concentrations of calcium in the myoplasm of the muscle cells. Myoplasmic calcium regulates adenosine triphosphate (ATP) synthesis by mitochondria. MH-susceptible patients appear to have abnormal calcium release channels that are sensitive to various triggering agents. Exposure to these agents causes calcium to be taken up by mitochondria in excess amounts, resulting in abnormal muscle contraction, accelerated cellular metabolism, and uncoupling of oxidative phosphorylation.

Presentation

MH is a clinical diagnosis usually made intraoperatively by the anesthesiologist. Signs and symptoms are consistent with a hypermetabolic state and include tachycardia, tachypnea (if the patient is breathing spontaneously), unstable blood pressure, hyperthermia, and varying degrees of muscle rigidity. Hyperthermia usually is a late sign. It can be extreme, with reported temperatures exceeding $42\,°C$ ($107.6\,°F$); on the other hand, hyperthermia may not occur at all if treatment is instituted early.

Laboratory evaluation may reveal hyperkalemia, respiratory and metabolic acidosis, hypoxia, and elevated levels of creatine phosphokinase. Renal failure, hepatic failure, disseminated intravascular coagulation, and neurologic injury are potential complications. Conditions that can mimic MH include light anesthesia, thyroid storm, pheochromocytoma, cocaine toxicity, and other drug reactions.

Many patients who have an MH reaction have a strong family history of similar reactions, indicating a genetic basis for the disorder. On further investigation, this patient's family recalled a paternal aunt who experienced hyperpyrexia during surgery. Other muscle disorders, such as congenital myotonia and the muscular dystrophies, have a strong association with and may predispose to the MH syndrome. There is no definitive screening test for MH, although testing of a skeletal muscle biopsy specimen for in vitro contracture response to drugs such as caffeine and halothane may identify susceptible individuals. Careful questioning about prior anesthetic reactions should be part of every preoperative evaluation to identify MH-susceptible patients and allow special planning for their anesthesia. All potential trigger agents should be avoided. Newer anesthetic agents such as propofol will allow for trigger-free general anesthesia.

Treatment
If recognized early and treated promptly, mortality from MH should be low. When the condition is diagnosed, all potential trigger agents should be stopped, as they were in this case. This patient then was treated with dantrolene, the therapy of choice for acute MH reactions. Dantrolene relaxes skeletal muscle directly by inhibiting intracellular calcium release. It is given as an intravenous bolus of 2.5 mg/kg and may be repeated until symptoms are controlled. Supportive therapy is crucial and includes ventilation with 100% oxygen, aggressive cooling, treatment of acidosis and hyperkalemia, and maintenance of urine output.

Lesson for the Clinician
MH is a rare condition, occurring in 1 in 15,000 individuals at most. Because pediatric anesthesiologists tend not to elect to use succinylcholine, the incidence of MH has decreased dramatically in recent years. Pediatricians should be aware, however, that the condition does occur and should alert anesthesiologists of any family history of MH in their patients.

Liliana D. Gutierrez, MD, Jackson Memorial Medical Center, Miami, FL

Chronic Cough

PRESENTATION

A 14-year-old boy comes to the office because he has been coughing for 2 weeks. A mild upper respiratory tract infection was present initially, evolving into a cough that is paroxysmal in nature and described as "wet and mucousy" and occasionally productive of clear mucus. The patient has had no fever, sore throat, or headache, and he has had no contact with anyone having a chronic cough. He already has completed a 10-day course of cephalexin prescribed by another physician for presumed acute sinusitis.

The boy's physical examination yields all normal findings except for a clear posterior pharyngeal discharge and a slight prolongation of his expiratory breathing. Although he has no past history of asthma, reactive airway disease is considered as a possible mechanism for his cough, and he is placed on albuterol and a 5-day course of prednisone.

He returns 3 days later because his cough has persisted and he has developed a cloudy nasal discharge. Palpation over his sinuses causes discomfort, and he is placed on a 10-day course of clarithromycin for sinusitis. He returns 1 week later, and although his nasal discharge is less pronounced, he continues to have paroxysms of coughing. An evaluation results in a normal complete blood count, negative cold agglutinins, a nonreactive tuberculin skin test, negative smear and culture of sputum for mycobacteria, normal radiographs of chest and sinuses, and normal pre- and postbronchodilator pulmonary function tests.

Two weeks later, he is still experiencing episodic coughing. Additional studies reveal the etiology of his chronic cough.

What is your differential diagnosis at this point?
Are there any elements of history or physical examination that would help you?
What additional diagnostic studies would you like performed?

DISCUSSION

Diagnosis

Chronic cough in an adolescent can result from many causes, including asthma, sinusitis, pneumonia, *Mycoplasma pneumoniae* or *Chlamydia pneumoniae* infections, tuberculosis, pertussis, psychogenic cough, smoking, cystic fibrosis, and recurrent viral upper respiratory tract infections. This patient's laboratory evaluation included serologic testing with an enzyme-linked immunosorbent assay (ELISA) for immunoglobulins to pertussis, as well as a nasopharyngeal culture and a fluorescent antibody test for the presence of pertussis antigen in nasopharyngeal secretions. He had significantly elevated immunoglobulin (Ig) M and IgA antibodies. (These studies were done by a reference laboratory.) Although the nasopharyngeal tests were negative, the serologic findings were highly suggestive of pertussis.

Presentation

The catarrhal stage of classic pertussis, which is the most infectious period, generally lasts for about 1 week and is followed by the paroxysmal stage, which is characterized by episodic paroxysms of forceful coughing, typically more frequent at night. This stage lasts for approximately 1 to 4 weeks. The convalescent stage, in which the symptoms of the paroxysmal stage persist in milder form, can last from 1 to 6 months.

It is important to realize that pertussis in older individuals may not follow the classic pattern, but may manifest instead as a prolonged illness limited primarily to a dramatic paroxysmal cough, which may not have the characteristic "whoop." Usually there is no history of previous lower respiratory tract disease, although the onset of the cough is likely to be well defined over several days or a week. The cough can be debilitating, keep the patient out of school for long periods, and fail to respond to symptomatic medications. A similar clinical pattern can result from infections with *Mycoplasma* organisms or some viruses.

Evaluation

Pertussis is not easy to diagnose because growth of the *Bordetella pertussis* organism from nasopharyngeal culture is particularly difficult and usually can be achieved only during the initial 3 to 4 weeks of illness, when the diagnosis often is not entertained. Fluorescent antibody tests from nasopharyngeal specimens can yield both false-positive and false-negative results.

Serologic tests often are used in the diagnosis of pertussis. Serologic confirmation of pertussis is indicated most reliably by the demonstration of at least a fourfold rise in IgG or IgA antibody. However, because acute-phase sera often are not obtained, antibody titer increases are documented only rarely. The ELISA is used widely to detect antibody to specific *B pertussis* antigens. Single measurements of high IgA and IgM titers indicate a recent infection. The demonstration of specific nasopharyngeal IgA *B pertussis* antibody also aids in diagnosis. Pertussis immunization induces serologically detectable IgM and IgG, but not IgA, antibodies. After infection, IgA antibodies may be detectable for up to 2 years. The presence of high IgM and IgA titers has been considered evidence of *B pertussis* infection. Recently, polymerase chain reaction assay has been shown to be more sensitive and more rapid than culture in detecting *B pertussis* in nasopharyngeal aspirates. Physicians who want to employ some of the newer serologic tests might have to look beyond their local laboratory services.

Lesson for the Clinician

The incidence of pertussis has increased recently, particularly among persons 10 years of age and older. Adolescents and young adults play an important role in transmission because vaccination-induced immunity to pertussis wanes with increasing age, beginning at about 4 years after the last dose. In addition, pertussis among adolescents and adults usually is manifested by a persistent cough and often goes undiagnosed. These infected adolescents may serve as a reservoir of infection, exposing susceptible individuals. The attack rate for pertussis infection in family contacts is very high, and one study showed that two thirds of cases in these immunized contacts were subclinical. The clinical picture of pertussis among adolescents and adults typically includes protracted coughing attacks that worsen at night, a sign that should alert the physician to this infection.

In the future, new acellular pertussis vaccines may reduce the disease prevalence among adolescents and young adults as well as among young children. For optimal control of the disease, immunity must be maintained in older children and adults via booster immunization. This practice, coupled with early childhood immunization, will protect infants and toddlers from this serious disease.

James A. Waler, MD, Jacksonville Health Care Group, Jacksonville, FL

Vaginal Bleeding

PRESENTATION

A 7-year-old African-American girl is seen in the emergency department because she has noticed spots of blood on her underwear. She has experienced discomfort with urination, but denies having urinary frequency, hematuria, or vaginal discharge. The child has been well; is receiving no medications; and has not had fever, abdominal pain, other unusual bleeding, trauma, gynecologic disorders, or urinary tract infections. She denies having inserted any foreign bodies into her vagina. She has a history of constipation (her last bowel movement was 5 days ago), and she has sickle cell trait. Her mother experienced menarche at age 15 years and her sister at 14 years.

On physical examination, the girl looks well and has normal vital signs. Serosanguinous discharge is noted on her underwear and at the opening of the vagina. The vulva appears normal except for a dark red mass visible at the introitus. The genital examination is difficult to perform because the child is apprehensive and the lesion is tender. The remainder of her examination, including evaluation of the abdomen, anus, and rectum, is completely normal, and there are no signs of pubertal changes. Urinalysis yields normal results except for 6 to 10 red blood cells per high-power field.

After being moved to a quiet room and left alone with her mother for a while, the girl is re-examined gently, and the examiner can see clearly a dark red, doughnut-shaped mass at the introitus.

What is your differential diagnosis at this point?
Are there any elements of history or physical examination that would help you?
What additional diagnostic studies would you like performed?

DISCUSSION

Diagnosis

The cause of vaginal bleeding in a child who is not sexually precocious most commonly is vulvovaginitis. However, when what appears to be a mass is seen at the introitus, additional diagnoses must be considered, including polyp, hemangioma, condylomata, hematoma of the hymen (trauma from a straddle injury or nonaccidental abuse), mesonephric cyst, foreign body (as benign as toilet paper), cervical or urethral prolapse, and botryoid sarcoma. In this case, proper visualization of the lesion made it clear that the girl had a urethral prolapse.

Urethral prolapse is encountered predominantly in African-American girls between 5 and 8 years of age, manifesting as genital bleeding. The prolapse often is associated with increased abdominal pressure that worsens with straining or coughing. The diagnosis usually can be made by visualizing a characteristic doughnut-shaped annular mass anterior to the vaginal orifice. If the clinician is unsure whether the mass is urethral or vaginal in origin, the vulva can be retracted gently in a downward, lateral direction to visualize the normal hymen and anterior vagina or the child can be placed supine in a knee-chest position to appreciate the anatomy more easily. In rare instances, if circumstances do not allow for clear inspection of a child who is bleeding or the appearance of the lesion does not allow precise identification, the child can be examined under anesthesia.

Treatment
Management of this child's urethral prolapse included sitz baths four times a day and the application of vaginal estrogen cream to the urethral area twice a day. If the prolapse is necrotic or keeps recurring, surgical excision and reapproximation of the mucosal edges are curative. If the mass originates from the vagina, the possibility of botryoid sarcoma, a rare pediatric tumor, should be considered urgently because surgery and postoperative chemotherapy are necessary.

Lesson for the Clinician
Knowing the etiologies of vaginal bleeding, obtaining a careful history, performing a thorough physical examination, and proceeding to appropriate investigations should lead to an accurate diagnosis. This case reminds clinicians of the need to take a sensitive and careful approach to pediatric gynecologic problems.

Janine Flanagan, MD, Jennifer Cram, MD, Hospital for Sick Children,
Toronto, Ontario, Canada

Difficulty in Arousing From a Nap

PRESENTATION

A mother runs into your office with her 2-year-old son, anxiously stating that he is difficult to arouse. He woke up in the morning without difficulty and had an early breakfast; 2 hours later he fell asleep. After the child had been sleeping for 1 hour, his mother became concerned. When she found that she could not arouse him, she rushed him to the office.

There has been no witnessed trauma, and the only medications said to be in the house are aspirin and acetaminophen, both of which are stored in the bathroom medicine cabinet. The child has never had a similar episode, and there is no family history of metabolic disorders.

On physical examination, the boy's pulse is 110 beats/min, blood pressure is 90/60 mm Hg, respiratory rate is 8 breaths/min, and temperature 36°C (96.8°F) rectally. He is obtunded, responding only to painful stimuli by crying and moving purposelessly. His skin is cool; he is slightly diaphoretic. His pupils are midsize, and findings on his neurologic examination are symmetric, with slight hyporeflexia in all extremities. As you complete your examination, the child has a generalized tonic-clonic seizure. A chemical strip measures his blood glucose at 1.11 mmol/L (20 mg/dL).

What is your differential diagnosis at this point?
Are there any elements of history or physical examination that would help you?
What additional diagnostic studies would you like performed?

DISCUSSION

Diagnosis

The differential diagnosis that the clinician must consider in a child who is obtunded and manifests respiratory depression is broad and includes metabolic disturbances such as ketotic hypoglycemia, ingestion of drugs (clonidine, barbiturates, opiates, carbamazepine, isopropyl alcohol), cerebrovascular accident, central nervous system tumor, and head trauma. An additional possibility is ingestion of ethyl alcohol, which was the cause of this boy's illness. A suspicion of ethanol ingestion often is raised by its common early morning occurrence. Adults leave alcoholic beverages, partially consumed the night before, in a place accessible to the child. One result may be "Sunday morning seizures." The diagnosis in this case was facilitated when questioning of the mother revealed that the parents had held a party the night before that extended late into the night.

Ethanol is a potent toxin that has the potential to induce a number of neurologic and metabolic complications in young children. Formerly present in a number of pediatric medications (to improve solubility and palatability), ethanol now is added to few drugs but can be found in mouthwashes, cough suppressants, and culinary products such as vanilla extract. Its primary source, however, remains alcoholic beverages.

Presentation

In adolescents and adults who ingest ethanol, consequences generally are confined to neurobehavioral effects, including dysarthria, ataxia, poor coordination, and emotional disinhibition. In rare circumstances, acute ethanol ingestion can lead to the development of alcoholic ketoacidosis, manifested by metabolic acidosis with occasional hypoglycemia.

Acute ethanol intoxication in toddlers is associated with a broader range of complications. The triad of hypoglycemia, hypothermia, and coma is considered pathognomonic for ethanol intoxication. Metabolic acidosis often accompanies this clinical picture. The origins of hypoglycemia and metabolic acidosis are unclear, although ethanol metabolism is associated with the generation of reduced nicotinamide adenine dinucleotide (NAD), which not only impairs gluconeogenesis but stimulates conversion of pyruvate to lactate. Findings on physical examination typically are unremarkable, with the exception of profound central nervous system depression. Pupils usually are midsized. Seizures may occur after ethanol ingestion, in association with hypoglycemia.

Significant ethanol toxicity in children is associated with a serum concentration of 21.7 mmol/L (100 mg/dL) (0.1%) or greater. As a general rule, this level is achieved by ingestion of 1 g/kg of ethanol. In an infant weighing 10 kg, this amount corresponds to 6 oz of beer, 40 mL of mouthwash (25% ethanol), or ½ jigger (30 mL) of a mixed drink containing 30 proof (60%) ethanol. As little as 3 to 4 g/kg of ethanol can be fatal to a child.

Evaluation

The laboratory evaluation of patients whose consciousness is altered begins with a bedside blood glucose test. If ethanol ingestion is suspected, electrolyte levels, blood glucose concentration, serum osmolality, and a blood or serum alcohol level should be measured. An osmolar gap can be determined first by calculating serum osmolality (2[Na] + glucose/18 + BUN/2.8). A disparity between the calculated osmolality and the actual (measured) serum osmolality identifies an osmolar gap. Causes of an osmolar gap are confined to ingestion of acetone or any alcohol (ethanol, methanol, ethylene glycol, isopropyl alcohol). Intravenous administration of mannitol or medications containing a high concentration of propylene glycol (such as phenytoin or diazepam for injection) also will produce an osmolar gap. Conversion factors based on the alcohol's molecular weight permit estimation of serum alcohol concentrations from the osmolar gap. In the case of ethanol, the product of the osmolar gap multiplied by 4.5 yields an estimated blood alcohol concentration in mg/dL. A urinalysis may be helpful in ruling out ketotic hypoglycemia or isopropyl alcohol ingestion, both of which are associated with ketonuria. A toxic screen also should be obtained to rule out other toxic ingestions, the effects of which may be masked by the ethanol intoxication.

Treatment

Management of the child who has ethanol intoxication includes stabilization of respiratory and circulatory status, as is required initially in any emergently ill child, immediate therapy for hypoglycemia, treatment of seizures, and warming measures. Hypoglycemia may not respond to glucagon; vascular access, therefore, should be established as quickly as possible to administer dextrose. Ethanol is metabolized at a rate of 15 to 30 mg/dL per hour in children; supportive care during the period of clearance generally is the only level of intervention needed. With ethanol levels greater than 65.1 to 108.5 mmol/L (300 to 500 mg/dL) or in patients whose vital signs are unstable, regardless of serum ethanol concentration, hemodialysis, which rapidly removes ethanol, should be instituted.

Activated charcoal does not adsorb ethanol and should not be administered after ethanol ingestion unless the diagnosis is uncertain or coingestants are suspected.

Michael Shannon, MD, Children's Hospital, Boston, MA

Author Index

Cases by Disease Category

Subject Index